PERSPECTIVES IN PEDIATRIC CARDIOLOGY

Series Editor
Robert H. Anderson, M.D.

PERSPECTIVES IN PEDIATRIC CARDIOLOGY
Volume 1

Editors

Robert H. Anderson, M.D.
Visiting Professor of Pediatrics
School of Medicine
University of Pittsburgh
Pittsburgh, Pennsylvania
Joseph P. Levy Professor of
Paediatric Cardiac Morphology
Cardiothoracic Institute
University of London
London, United Kingdom

William H. Neches, M.D.
Professor of Pediatrics
School of Medicine
University of Pittsburgh
Children's Hospital of Pittsburgh
Pittsburgh, Pennsylvania

Sang C. Park, M.D.
Professor of Pediatrics
School of Medicine
University of Pittsburgh
Children's Hospital of Pittsburgh
Pittsburgh, Pennsylvania

James R. Zuberbuhler, M.D.
Professor of Pediatrics
School of Medicine
University of Pittsburgh
Children's Hospital of Pittsburgh
Pittsburgh, Pennsylvania

Futura Publishing Company, Inc.
Mount Kisco, New York
1988

Contributors

Edward J. Baker, M.D.
Senior Lecturer in Pediatric Cardiology, Evalina Children's Department, Guy's Hospital, London, England

Lionel M. Bargeron, Jr., M.D.
Professor of Pediatrics, Department of Surgery and Pediatric Cardiology, School of Medicine, University of Alabama, Birmingham, Alabama

Lee B. Beerman, M.D.
Associate Professor of Pediatrics, Pediatric Cardiology, Children's Hospital of Pittsburgh, Pittsburgh, Pennsylvania

Anton E. Becker, M.D.
Professor of Pathology, Academic Medical Center, Amsterdam, The Netherlands

Einat Birk, M.D.
Postdoctoral Fellow, Department of Pediatrics and Cardiovascular Research Institute, University of California, San Francisco, California

Eugene A. Blackstone, M.D.
Professor of Surgery, Department of Surgery and Pediatric Cardiology, School of Medicine, University of Alabama, Birmingham, Alabama

Patricia E. Burrows, M.D.
Assistant Professor of Radiology, Faculty of Medicine, University of Toronto, Staff Radiologist, The Hospital for Sick Children, Toronto, Ontario, Canada

Tjark J. Ebels, M.D.
Cardiothoracic Surgeon, Department of Thoracic Surgery, University Hospital, Groningen, The Netherlands

Donald R. Fischer, M.D.
Assistant Professor of Pediatrics, Pediatric Cardiology, Children's Hospital of Pittsburgh, Pittsburgh, Pennsylvania

Robert M. Freedom, M.D.
Head, Division of Cardiology, The Hospital for Sick Children, Professor of Pediatrics and Pathology, Faculty of Medicine, University of Toronto, Toronto, Ontario, Canada

Frederick J. Fricker, M.D.
Associate Professor of Pediatrics, Pediatric Cardiology, Department of Pediatrics, Children's Hospital of Pittsburgh, Pittsburgh, Pennsylvania

William M. Gay, M.D.
Assistant Professor of Pediatrics, Section Pediatric Cardiology, Department of Pediatrics, West Virginia University, Morgantown, West Virginia

Bartley P. Griffith, M.D.
Assistant Professor of Surgery, Department of Surgery, School of Medicine, University of Pittsburgh, Pittsburgh, Pennsylvania

Michael A. Heymann, M.D.
Professor of Pediatrics, Cardiovascular Research Institute and Department of Pediatrics, Physiology and Obstetrics, Gynecology and Reproductive Sciences, San Francisco School of Medicine, University of California, San Francisco, California

Siew Yen Ho, Ph.D.
Senior Lecturer in Paediatrics Cardiothoracic Institute, Brompton Hospital, London, England

Julien I. E. Hoffman, M.D.
Professor of Pediatrics, San Francisco
School of Medicine, University of
California, San Francisco, California

James W. Kirklin, M.D.
Associate Professor of Surgery, Department
of Surgery and Pediatric Cardiology,
School of Medicine, University of
Alabama, Birmingham, Alabama

John W. Kirklin, M.D.
Professor of Surgery, School of Medicine,
University of Alabama, Birmingham,
Alabama

Cora C. Lenox, M.D.
Professor Emeritus of Pediatrics, Pediatric
Cardiology, Children's Hospital of
Pittsburgh, Pittsburgh, Pennsylvania

Robert A. Mathews, M.D.
Associate Professor of Pediatrics,
Children's Hospital of Pittsburgh,
Pittsburgh, Pennsylvania

C. A. F. Moes, M.D.
Professor, Department of Radiology,
University of Toronto, Senior Staff
Radiologist, Department of Radiology, The
Hospital for Sick Children, Toronto,
Ontario, Canada

Albert D. Pacifico, M.D.
Professor of Surgery, Department of
Surgery and Pediatric Cardiology, School
of Medicine, University of Alabama,
Birmingham, Alabama

Donald E. Perrin, M.D.
Associate in Pathology, Division of
Cardiology, Departments of Pediatric
Pathology and Radiology, The Hospital for
Sick Children, Toronto, Ontario, Canada

Marlene Rabinovitch, M.D.
Associate Professor of Paediatrics and
Pathology, Faculty of Medicine, University
of Toronto, Toronto, Ontario, Canada

Abraham M. Rudolph, M.D.
Professor of Pediatrics, Cardiovascular
Research Institute and Department of
Pediatrics, Physiology and Obstetrics,
Gynecology and Reproductive Sciences,
San Francisco School of Medicine,
University of California, San Francisco,
California

Klaus G. Schmidt, M.D.
Postdoctoral Fellow, Department of
Pediatrics and Cardiovascular Research
Institute, University of California, San
Francisco, California

Ralph D. Siewers, M.D.
Associate Professor of Surgery, School of
Medicine, University of Pittsburgh,
Cardiothoracic Surgery, Children's Hospital
of Pittsburgh, Pittsburgh, Pennsylvania

Norman H. Silverman, M.D.
Professor of Pediatrics, San Francisco
School of Medicine, University of
California, San Francisco, California

Jeffrey F. Smallhorn, M.D.
Associate Professor of Pediatrics, Faculty of
Medicine, University of Toronto, Toronto,
Ontario, Canada

Jane Somerville, M.D.
Consultant Cardiologist, National Heart
Hospital, London, England

Benigno Soto, M.D.
Professor of Radiology, Department of
Surgery and Pediatric Cardiology, School
of Medicine, University of Alabama,
Birmingham, Alabama

Susan Stone
Research Secretary, Paediatric and
Adolescent Unit, National Heart Hospital,
London, England

Mary Kay Yurchak
Cardiovascular Technician, Pediatric
Cardiology, Department of Pediatrics,
Children's Hospital of Pittsburgh,
Pittsburgh, Pennsylvania

Preface and Acknowledgments

In the face of the present-day explosion in publication, the shell-shocked potential reader can be forgiven for inquiring "Why another series of books devoted to pediatric cardiology?" There are several reasons why, encouraged by the support from Steven Korn and Futura Publishing Company, we have prepared this volume as the first in a series of "Perspectives in Pediatric Cardiology." First, as editors, we firmly believe that the material presented is well-written, timely, and highly relevant to those concerned with the treatment of children with congenital cardiac malformations. It is our hope and intention that future volumes will, also, meet all these criteria. Second, as consumers, we believe that there is a need for material to be presented in a format intermediate between the highly concentrated manuscript found in peer-reviewed journals and the more generalized reviews in textbooks. In our opinion, the material in this volume bridges this divide and gathers together in detail the various aspects of the subject matter presented. This book is in no way intended to compete with textbooks of pediatric cardiology. By design, it is incomplete. However, because of its eclecticism, it can cover its selected topics more completely than can any textbook. Furthermore, the design also permits each aspect of the chosen subject to be addressed by a recognized expert. Thus, we hope that the book provides expert commentaries on the morphology, diagnosis, and treatment of several important lesions that continually confront and, at times, confound pediatric cardiologists.

Future volumes will likely be of a similar format, while others may well take the form of detailed and in-depth coverage of a single malformation, providing information at present lacking in the bibliography of congenital heart disease. We hope, therefore, that our volume will find a place on the bookshelves of interested practitioners, to be followed, in time, by additional volumes that will provide further *Perspectives in Pediatric Cardiology*.

This volume is based broadly on a symposium held in Pittsburgh in September, 1986. However, there was no transcript of the spoken word, so this book is in no way a verbatim report of the proceedings. Each chapter was specially prepared and edited. As editors, we are greatly indebted to Steven Korn and his colleagues at Futura for their enthusiasm in taking up the concept of "Perspectives." We are also indebted to our hardworking secretarial staff, both in Pittsburgh and London, for efforts over and above the call of duty; namely, Christine Anderson, Beverly Davis, Judith Doubt, Rachel Marinos, and Susan Powell.

Robert H. Anderson, M.D.
William H. Neches, M.D.
Sang C. Park, M.D.
J. R. Zuberbuhler, M.D.

Contents

Section V   The Left Valve in Atrioventricular Septal Defect

Section VI   Aortic Coarctation: Morphology and Investigation

Section VII   Diseases of the Coronary Arteries

Section VIII   Miscellaneous Topics

Patterns of Ventricular Septal Defect: Definition or Description?

1.1

Introduction

Anton E. Becker

Although it is now well over 100 years since Roger correlated the physical signs and morphology of interventricular communications, there is still no consensus about how best to differentiate and describe holes between the ventricles. In part, this is not surprising, since different groups are bound to have some differences in their approach. Ideally, such differences should be minimal, since a broad agreement in terms of description is highly desirable. Other differences seen previously in description may well have related to the difficulties during clinical investigation in obtaining the precision afforded the morphologist at either surgical or autopsy examination. These deficiencies are now largely mitigated by the recently developed sophistication of angiocardiographic, echocardiographic, and magnetic resonance imaging techniques. There remains, however, one major reason why different groups may continue to disagree about the definition of various ventricular septal defects. This is that there is no unanimously accepted criterion of what precisely is *the* ventricular septal defect.

What Is the Ventricular Septal Defect?

Consider three discrete situations in which there is a hole between the ventricles. Take first the arrangement in which there is a deficiency within the inlet or apical parts of the muscular septum (Fig. 1). Few would disagree about the nature of the borders of this hole and its description and definition as a muscular defect. They may disagree about its location within the septum, but we will return to that. Compare now this muscular defect with the morphology of the septal defect in the setting of tetralogy of Fallot in which the aortic orifice overrides the ventricular septum (Fig. 2). The arrangement is much more complex. Operationally, the surgeon will close the right ventricular margin of the cone of space bordered by the attachments of the overriding aortic valve and the crest of the ventricular septum. This procedure will "correct" the malformation by connecting the aorta to the left ventricle. But is this locus repaired by the surgeon *the*

From: Anderson, RH, Neches, WH, Park, SC, Zuberbuhler, JR, eds: *Perspectives in Pediatric Cardiology*: Mount Kisco, New York, Futura Publishing Co., © 1988.

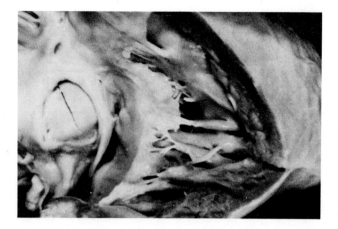

Figure 1. The right ventricular aspect of a hole embedded within the muscular septum and opening to the inlet of the right ventricle. Few, if any, would disagree with the description of this hole as a muscular ventricular septal defect.

ventricular septal defect? Is it better, perhaps, to define the defect as the plane of space roofed by the overriding aortic valve leaflets, this space being the direct basal continuation of the plane of the ventricular septum? This is certainly the space likely to

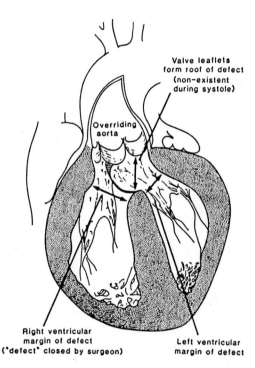

Figure 2. The more complicated situation to be found in tetralogy of Fallot when the aortic orifice overrides the crest of the ventricular septum. This drawing shows the potential candidates for description as the ventricular septal defect.

be nominated by the echocardiographer as the septal defect. In geometric terms, a strong case can be mounted for its being the interventricular communication, even if, during ventricular systole, the "roof" becomes nonexistent with the opening of the valve leaflets. There is a third margin to be considered which may have operational significance. This is the left ventricular margin of the overriding subaortic outflow tract, roofed by the area of the aortic-mitral valvular continuity and the tissues that connect this fibrous area to the crest of the ventricular septum. This tubular space between the body of the left ventricle and the attachments of the overriding aortic valve can become stenotic and may need resection, although few would think of nominating it as the septal defect in the setting of tetralogy of Fallot. Consider finally the arrangement in which both great arteries are connected to the right ventricle and in which there is a hole in the ventricular septum immediately beneath the aortic valve (Fig. 3). It is now well recognized that a spectrum of malformation exists between double outlet right ventricle with subaortic defect and tetralogy of Fallot. What, however, are the borders of the "septal defect" in the setting of double outlet right ventricle? Is the defect still the space that would be closed by the surgeon so as to connect the aorta with the right ventricle? This space is confined by the free edge of the outlet (or infundibular) septum

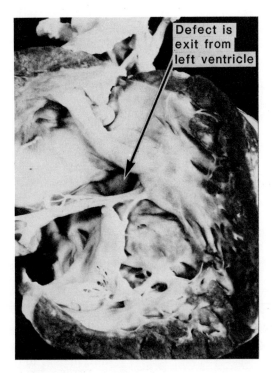

Defect is exit from left ventricle

Figure 3. This is the right ventricular aspect of a case of double outlet right ventricle with a hole opening into the subaortic outflow tract. Although usually described as the "septal defect," the hole is the only exit from the left ventricle. Closing this communication would be disastrous.

(an exclusively right ventricular structure in both double outlet right ventricle and tetralogy), the attachments of the aortic valve leaflets within the right ventricle and the crest of the muscular ventricular septum. This space is, of course, homologous with that closed by the surgeon in tetralogy. Could a case still be made for considering *the* defect to be roofed by the leaflets of the aortic valve itself, since there is often a minimal degree of aortic overriding, even when the aorta is almost exclusively connected to the right ventricle? Or should the defect be defined as the space roofed by the muscular tissue between aortic and mitral valves (in classic double outlet with bilateral infundibulum) and the crest of the ventricular septum? This space would never be closed by the surgeon since it is the only direct exit from the left ventricle to the aorta. Yet most

often it is this hole which is designated as the defect in the setting of double outlet right ventricle (Fig. 3) even though its homolog rarely achieves this accolade in the setting of tetralogy.

Description Rather than Definition

It could be argued that all of this discussion is of pedagogic and pedantic rather than pragmatic significance. We do not consider this to be the case. It makes little sense to have systems of description that recognize one particular hole as *the* defect in one given setting yet another hole in a different setting, particularly since there may be great difficulty in deciding the setting itself when a valve orifice is overriding and is connected almost equally between the two ventricles. The solution to this dilemma is very easy: instead of defining "the defect," it makes more sense to describe the right ventricular borders of the opening to the subarterial outflow tract, the degree of overriding of the arterial valve, and if necessary, the borders and location of the left ventricular exit to the outflow tract. In this way all the information of operational significance will be provided. The concept of right and left ventricular margins to the cone of space beneath the valve (Fig. 4) is also of significance when considering natural history. If the right ventricular margin becomes narrow or closes spontaneously, the lesion will be "corrected." If the left ventricular margin narrows, however, there will be left ventricular outflow tract obstruction.

Previous Approaches to Definition

The process described above will take more time to complete than definition of

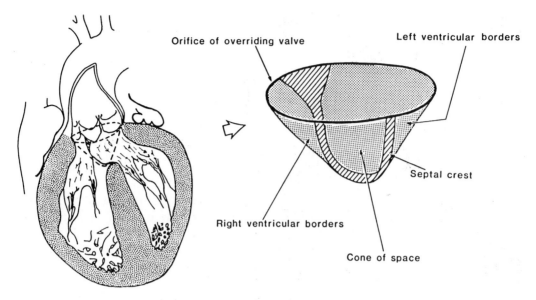

Figure 4. The cone of space found beneath an overriding arterial valve. In these circumstances, it may be necessary to describe both right and left ventricular borders of the cone.

defects as being "high" or "low"; or "supracristal" relative to "infra-" or "intracristal"; or simply being types I through IV. The time taken to provide full description will be well spent, since all the above systems suffer the deficiencies of any procrustean approach in addition to having fundamental deficiencies in terms of science and logic. If we examine such logical deficiencies in the setting of the "cristal" approach, it can be seen that the so-called "supracristal" defect is considered to be above the "crista" because of absence of the outlet (or infundibular) septum (Fig. 5, right panel). The defect is above the branching limbs of the septomarginal trabeculation (septal band) which, presumably, is the crista in this setting. Compare such a defect with a typical "infracristal" defect (Fig. 5, left panel). The infracristal deficiency is roofed by the outlet septum, but is still clasped within the limbs of the septomarginal trabeculation. In this setting, it is the outlet septum that is taken to be the crista and, therefore, it is the change in nature of the crista itself which is recognized by the nomenclature, rather than a clear account being given of the boundaries

of the different defects. This fact, however, seems to have escaped all those who have used the "cristal" approach throughout the years.

Needs of Description

If we strip the argument down to its basics, there are additional features that need description when accounting for the morphology of holes between the ventricles over and above those already discussed. These features are the size of the hole, its position within the ventricular septum, its relationship to the atrioventricular conduction axis, and its relationship to the leaflets and attachments of the atrioventricular and arterial valves. Knowledge of these features should provide the surgeon with all the information he or she needs to repair the septal deficiency successfully. They may also provide the clinician with the information needed to determine which holes will spontaneously close or reduce in size sufficiently to avoid the need for surgical repair. In the

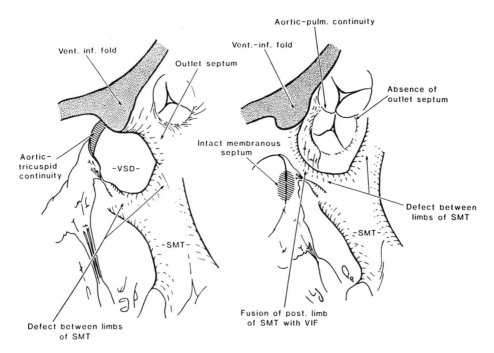

Figure 5. The problems with the convention of describing defects as "infracristal" (left panel) or "supracristal" (right panel). In both examples, the defect is clasped within the limbs of the septomarginal trabeculation. It is the structure nominated as "crista" that has changed, rather than the basic position of the defect.

various chapters of this section, an anatomical description will be given of those different features, and then how well they can be determined using echocardiographic and angiocardiographic investigative techniques will be determined. The natural history of so-called "isolated" defects will then be reviewed, with a concentration on the significance of recognizing different anatomical patterns. The separate role of the pulmonary circulation in determining natural history will be addressed and, finally, all of these different features will be summarized in an overview of treatment.

Ventricular Septal Defect: Anatomical Features as Seen by the Morphologist

Robert H. Anderson

As discussed in the introduction to this section, the major problem in description of a ventricular septal defect is determining precisely what it is. The morphologist has the inestimable advantage of being able to examine all aspects of a heart that has a hole between its ventricles. The anatomy thus described should set the scene for appropriate interpretation of the images seen by the echocardiographer and angiocardiographer and for optimal correction, if necessary, by the surgeon. The discrepancies which still exist in definition of defects by different investigators relate at least in part to the desire to define rather than to describe. Then, if the locus chosen for definition by one group as the defect differs from that chosen by another, there will, of necessity, be disagreement. Such disagreement can be circumvented in the larger part by concentrating upon description and by avoiding definition. Some terms, nonetheless, are so widely used in uniform fashion

that it would be churlish to avoid them. In this chapter, therefore, holes between the ventricular chambers will be described in the simplest fashion we can devise. Unless stated otherwise, they will be described in the setting of the normally constructed heart with concordant atrioventricular and ventriculoarterial connections. The basic descriptions, however, are applicable to all holes between two ventricles irrespective of the nature of the atria and great arteries to which each of those ventricles is or is not connected.

Anatomy of the Normal Septum Relative to Descriptions of Holes Between the Ventricles

The ventricular septum has widely differing appearances when viewed from the

From: Anderson, RH, Neches, WH, Park, SC, Zuberbuhler, JR, eds: *Perspectives in Pediatric Cardiology*: Mount Kisco, New York, Futura Publishing Co., © 1988.

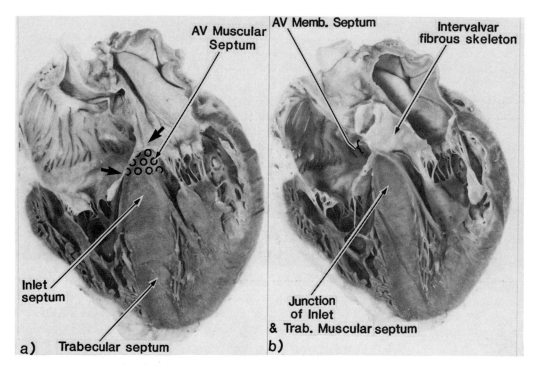

Figure 1. These two simulated "four-chamber" sections through a normal heart show (a) the muscular, and (b) the membranous atrioventricular (AV) septal structures. Note the offsetting of the septal attachments of the atrioventricular valves (arrowed) in (a) giving the muscular atrioventricular septum (stippled).

right and left ventricular aspects. Significantly, the attachments of the mitral and tricuspid valves to the septum are not at the same level. Neither are the attachments of the aortic and pulmonary valves. This is important because, as a consequence of the differential level of attachment, the area between the proximal attachments of the mitral and tricuspid valves separates the right atrium from the left ventricle. It is the atrioventricular muscular septum (Fig. 1a). Deficiencies in this part of the septum are the hallmark of atrioventricular septal defects (Becker and Anderson, 1982; Penkoske et al., 1985). Holes in this region can, rarely, permit only interventricular shunting. Despite this, they are best considered and described as atrioventricular septal defects ("atrioventricular canal malformations" or "endocardial cushion defects"). These defects will not be described in this chapter. The attachment of the leaflets of the aortic

valve to the septum is significantly lower than that of the pulmonary valve, the latter being supported on an extensive sleeve of right ventricular outlet musculature (Fig. 2). This is important because, when seen from the right ventricle, the impression is gained of an extensive area of "outlet septum" supporting the attachments of the pulmonary leaflets (Fig. 3a). This area has been labeled as outlet (or infundibular) septum by several groups of investigators (Soto et al., 1980; Brandt, 1984; Hagler et al., 1985). In reality, most of this area is the external wall of the heart. It can be removed from the heart without entering the cavity of the left ventricle (Fig. 3b).

The morphological features outlined about are pertinent to the way in which we divide the ventricular septum. This, in turn, is significant for description of septal defects. The division into muscular and fibrous components is easy and straightfor-

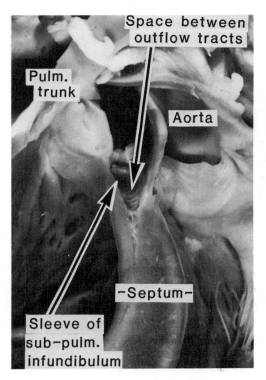

Figure 2. A section through the outlet components of the ventricles showing how the leaflets of the pulmonary (Pulm.) valve are supported by a sleeve of freestanding infundibular musculature.

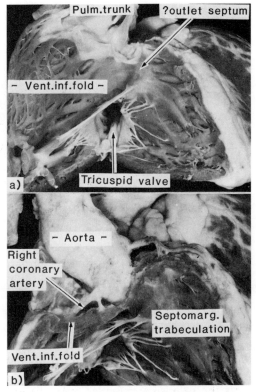

Figure 3. These dissections show (a) the opened outlet component of the right ventricle. At first sight, there is an extensive "outlet septum" beneath the pulmonary valve. As shown in (b), most of this septum is the freestanding sleeve of infundibular musculature which can be removed without damage to the left ventricle. Vent. inf. = ventriculoinfundibular; septomarg. = septomarginal.

ward. The fibrous component of the septum is very small in comparison to the huge bulk of the muscular septum (Fig. 1b). This fibrous component is traditionally termed the membranous septum. It is crossed on its right ventricular aspect by the attachment of the septal leaflet of the tricuspid valve, which further divides the membranous septum into atrioventricular and interventricular parts. The interventricular part tends to be very small at birth. Indeed, in many neonates the entire membranous septum is an atrioventricular structure (Allwork and Anderson, 1979). The membranous septum is an integral part of the fibrous skeleton of the heart. Through its substance, the tricuspid valve achieves fibrous continuity with the aortic valve. Through this area penetrates the atrioventricular conduction bundle (Fig. 1b). Although the membranous septum is small, the muscular septum is huge. Various

attempts have been made conceptually to divide this muscular septum. None of them is perfect because, in its normal state, the septum lacks suitable landmarks for division. When seen from the right side, the attachments of the septal leaflet of the tricuspid valve conveniently demarcate the inlet of the right ventricle. But, because of the "wedged" position of the subaortic outflow tract, this part of the septum separates the inlet of the right ventricle mostly from the outlet of the left (Fig. 4). Therefore, it is not strictly an inlet septum although it has been (and will continue to be) described in that fashion. We have already discussed the deficiencies of the term "outlet septum."

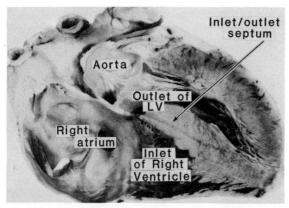

Figure 4. This simulated subcostal oblique cut through the normal heart shows that, because of the wedged position of the subaortic outflow tract, the septum bordering the inlet of the right ventricle is largely an inlet/outlet septal structure.

There is very little septum in the normal heart separating the subaortic from the subpulmonary outlets. Instead, the greater part of the normal muscular ventricular septum separates the apical trabecular components. This part of the septum is coarsely trabeculated on its right and finely trabeculated on its left ventricular aspects. The upper part of the left ventricular side is smooth while the corresponding aspect on the right side supports the extensive muscular trabeculation which we call the septomarginal trabeculation (septal band). This trabeculation branches at the cardiac base and its limbs clasp the extensive supraventricular crest which separates the tricuspid and pulmonary valves. This is the part usually described as an outlet (or infundibular) septum. In reality, it is the ventriculoinfundibular fold of the right ventricle. This is itself significant because defects through or above this crest ("supracristal") would, self-evidently, lead outside the heart were the heart itself normally structured.

Description of Ventricular Septal Defects

To fully describe a hole between the ventricles it is necessary to know its position within the septum, its relationship to the atrioventricular conduction axis, and its relationship to the arterial and atrioventricular

valves. These are not necessarily independent features. Thus, knowledge of the position of a defect within the septum usually permits deduction of its relationship to the atrioventricular conduction axis.

Position Within the Septum

Position within the septum is most readily described when a defect is embedded within and surrounded by the musculature of the septum. Such defects, which are universally called "muscular" defects, can open into the inlet (Fig. 5a), the apical trabecular (Fig. 5b), or the outlet (Fig. 5c) components of the right ventricle. When a defect opens into the inlet of the right ventricle, it is often shielded, in part, by the septal leaflet of the tricuspid valve. However, a muscular bridge always separates the defect from the attachment of the tricuspid valve and, hence, the area of the atrioventricular membranous septum (Fig. 6a). Defects in the extensive apical trabecular components of the right ventricle can empty centrally, apically, or anteriorly. Apical defects are often multiple, and this combination is frequently described as the "swiss cheese septum" (Fig. 6b). Defects opening into the outlet of the right ventricle are usually small. When the superior rim of these defects becomes attenuated, they can be very similar in morphology to the doubly

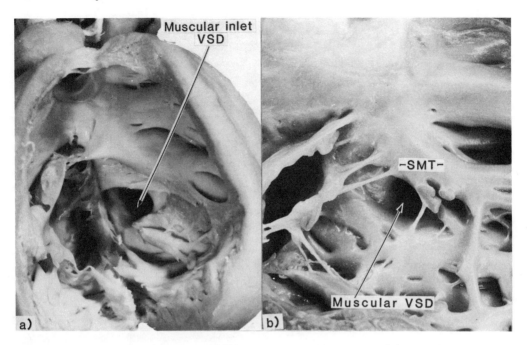

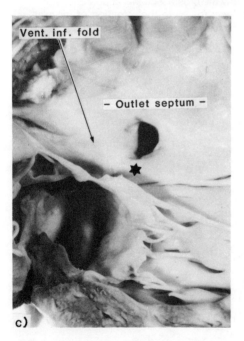

Figure 5. These three hearts show muscular defects (VSD) in the inlet (a), the central trabecular (b) and the outlet (c) components of the septum. Note the muscle bar in (c) between the defect and the tricuspid valve is formed by fusion of the posterior limb of the septomarginal trabeculation with the ventriculoinfundibular (vent. inf.) fold. SMT = septomarginal trabeculation.

committed and subarterial defect (see below). The conduction axis runs anterosuperior to a muscular inlet and posteroinferior to a muscular outlet defect, but is rarely related directly to the margins of these de-

fects (Fig. 7). Apical muscular defects are unrelated to the nonbranching bundle but may be intimately related to fascicles of the bundle branches. As we will see, the septal location of all other defects can also conve-

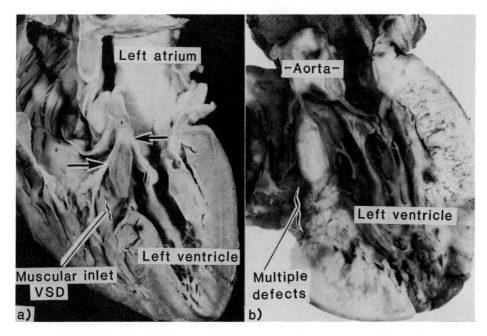

Figure 6. These simulated "four-chamber" cuts show the cross-sectional appearances of a muscular inlet (a) and multiple apical muscular defects (b). Note the retention of valvular offsetting (arrowed) in (a) and how the bulk of the septum is retained in (b).

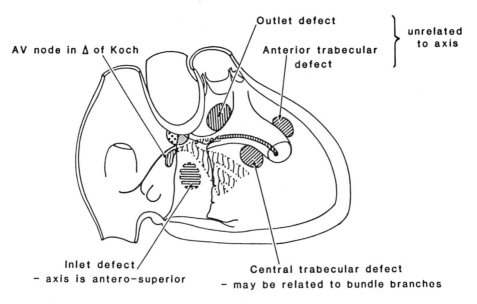

Figure 7. How the relationship of the atrioventricular conduction axis varies with muscular defects according to their position within the septum. AV = atrioventricular; △ = triangle.

niently be described according to whether they open to the inlet, the apical trabecular, or outlet components of the right ventricle.

Relationship to Atrioventricular and Arterial Valves

Holes between the ventricles can be related to the atrioventricular and arterial valves for various reasons. The most common type of ventricular septal defect is usually related to both an arterial and an atrioventricular valve because it has an area of fibrous continuity of the supporting structures of the valves as part of its direct border. These defects are traditionally described as "membranous." They never exist simply because of absence of the interventricular component of the membranous septum. Indeed, as discussed above, in most normal infants there is no interventricular membrane septum at birth (Allwork and Anderson, 1979). The defects exist, as judged morphologically, because of deficiency of the muscular septum in the environs of the cardiac skeleton (Fig. 8). Hence, our preference is to describe them as "perimembranous" defects.

Perimembranous Defects

All perimembranous defects in hearts with concordant atrioventricular and ventriculoarterial connections have the penetrating atrioventricular bundle located on their posteroinferior rim (Fig. 9), although its precise relationship to the edge of the defect varies from case to case (Milo et al., 1979; Ueda and Becker, 1985). Perimembranous defects can vary in precise morphology according to the extent of deficiency of the muscular septum. Some defects are so large that they open into both inlet and outlet components of the right ventricle (Fig. 10a). These defects are de-

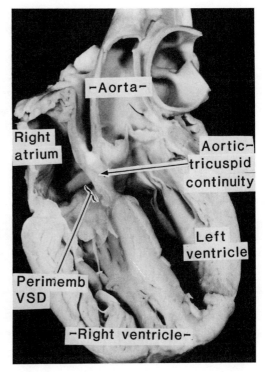

Figure 8. This simulated "four-chamber" section shows how the cardinal feature of a perimembranous defect is that its roof is formed by fibrous continuity between the atrioventricular and an arterial valve. In this heart with concordant ventriculoarterial connection, it is the aortic valve in continuity with the tricuspid and mitral valves.

scribed as being confluent. Usually they are associated with overriding of the aortic valve. Other defects open predominantly into the inlet (Fig. 10b) or outlet (Fig. 10c) components of the right ventricle. The defect opening into the right ventricular inlet, like the muscular inlet defect, is shielded in part by the septal leaflet of the tricuspid valve. It has the medial papillary muscle in an anterosuperior location. It is distinguished from the inlet muscular defect because its roof is formed by fibrous continuity between the mitral and tricuspid valves (Fig. 11). Perimembranous inlet defects have been described as "atrioventricular canal defects" (Neufeld et al., 1961). They differ from atrioventricular septal defects

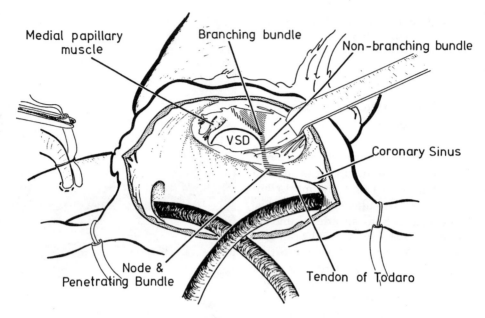

Figure 9. The relationship of the conduction axis as seen by the surgeon in a perimembranous ventricular septal defect. The only exception to this arrangement in hearts with a concordant atrioventricular connection is when there is overriding and straddling of the tricuspid valve (see Fig. 12). VSD = ventricular septal defect.

with exclusively ventricular shunting in that they do not possess the trifoliate left valve which is the hallmark of an atrioventricular septal defect (see Chap. 5.1). The left valve found in hearts with a perimembranous defect that opens into the inlet of the right ventricle is morphologically a mitral valve. Defects opening into the outlet of the right ventricle have the medial papillary muscle in the posteroinferior position. The defect seen in tetralogy of Fallot is usually a perimembranous outlet defect, but one that is associated with overriding of the aortic valve and deviation of the outlet septum. Some small perimembranous defects extend into neither the inlet nor the outlet parts of the right ventricle (Fig. 10d). They certainly border on the inlet and outlet components, but their long axis is orientated toward the ventricular apex and the medial papillary muscle tends to be located at the apex of the defect. These defects can be said to open mostly to the apical trabecular component

or can be described more simply as perimembranous trabecular defects.

Overriding Arterial or Atrioventricular Valves

Ventricular septal defects—whether perimembranous or muscular—can also be directly related to arterial or atrioventricular valves because the valve orifices override the septum. It is in these circumstances that it is most difficult to define the defect. As described in the introduction, problems of definition are circumvented if several features are described. Operationally, the most significant feature is the margin of the cone of space enclosed by the overriding valve orifice that will be patched by the surgeon. In the case of overriding of the tricuspid and pulmonary valves, this will usually be the left ventricular margin. When the aortic or

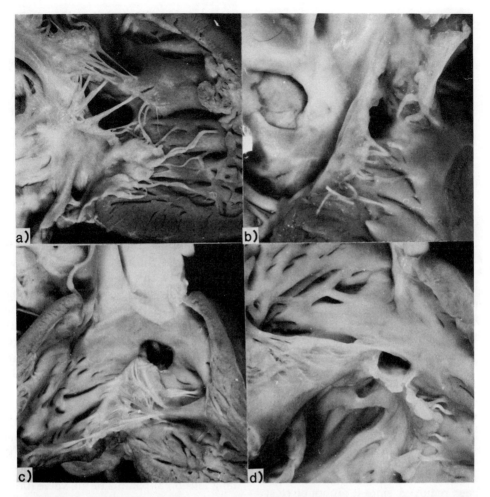

Figure 10. The similarities and differences between perimembranous defects when they are confluent (a), open to the inlet of the right ventricle (b), open to the outlet (c), and are small and confined to the immediate environs of the central fibrous body (d).

mitral valves override, the right ventricular margin is usually closed by the surgeon. In all these circumstances, an account of both right and left ventricular margins may be needed to provide a complete description.

Overriding Tricuspid Valve

The morphologically tricuspid valve overrides in the setting of a defect characterized by malalignment of the atrial and ventricular septal structures (Fig. 12). The ven-

tricular septum reaches the atrioventricular junction at a point well away from the crux; at precisely what point depends on the degree of override. An anomalous atrioventricular conduction axis penetrates from atrial to ventricular musculature at the point where the ventricular septum meets the atrioventricular junction (Milo et al., 1979b). If the tricuspid valve and its tension apparatus were removed surgically, the margins of the defect would be the diverging edges of the atrial and ventricular septal structures. This plane, however, only has opera-

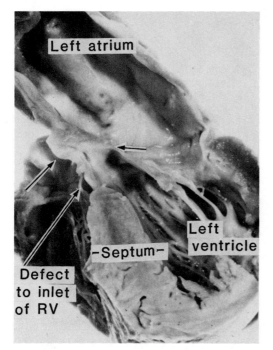

Figure 11. This "four-chamber" section shows how, in a perimembranous defect opening to the inlet of the right ventricle (RV), there is loss of the offsetting of the atrioventricular valves and, hence, loss of most of the muscular atrioventricular septum.

tional significance when the tricuspid valve has been removed, since it cannot be closed surgically while the tension apparatus continues to straddle. When the tricuspid valve is still in place, the left ventricular border of the defect, which Kirklin suggests can be described as a juxtacrux or pericrux defect (personal communication, April 1986), is the area of fibrous continuity of tricuspid and mitral valves on the underside of the atrial septum. The extent of this border within the left ventricle depends upon the degree of straddling of tricuspid valve apparatus, but must surround all the malpositioned chordal support. This plane must be closed to reconnect the straddling valve to the right ventricle. Because much of the left ventricular margin is part of the fibrous skeleton, the defect is perimembranous. The right ventricular border of the defect is

roofed by the attachment of the antero-superior leaflet of the tricuspid valve to the ventriculoinfundibular fold. Its distal extent is the attachment of tricuspid tension apparatus within the right ventricle.

The defect straddled and overriden by the morphologically tricuspid valve, therefore, is an inlet perimembranous defect characterized by atrial and ventricular malalignment.

Overriding Mitral Valve

In contrast, the mitral valve straddles and overrides through a defect opening to the outlet of the right ventricle, almost always in the setting of either a discordant ventriculoarterial connection or double outlet right ventricle. The right ventricular border is the one of operational significance. The defect is almost always also associated with overriding of the pulmonary valve. The roof of the defect therefore may be the right or left ventricular attachments of the pulmonary valve, depending upon whether there is a discordant or double outlet ventriculoarterial connection. The floor of the defect must extend to include the straddling tension apparatus of the valve (unless the valve is removed, when the floor will be the crest of the ventricular septum). The variable border is found posteroinferiorly. This may be a muscular structure when the posterior limb of the septomarginal trabeculation fuses with the ventriculoinfundibular fold. Alternatively, the defect may be bordered directly by fibrous continuity between the atrioventricular and arterial valve (in other words, may become perimembranous).

Overriding Aortic Valve

Most frequently it is the aortic valve that overrides the ventricular septum. Almost all "isolated" perimembranous defects

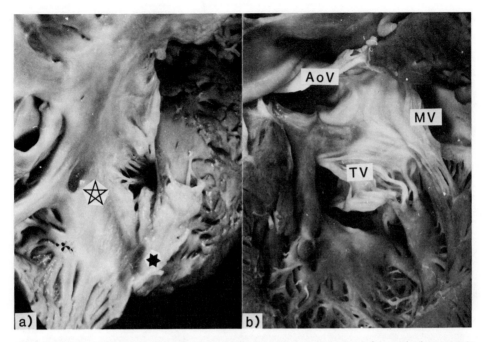

Figure 12. These illustrations show a) the right ventricular and b) the left ventricular aspects of a heart in which the tricuspid valve straddles and overrides the muscular ventricular septum (shown by the solid star in a). This is malaligned relative to the atrial septum (open star). The left ventricular aspect reveals fibrous continuity between aortic (AoV), mitral (MV), and tricuspid (TV) valves.

have a small degree of aortic override, but it is not obvious morphologically when the valve is connected largely to the left ventricle. The override becomes more noticeable with more commitment of the aortic valve to the right ventricle. This is seen typically in the so-called "Eisenmenger" defect and in the setting of tetralogy of Fallot (Fig. 13). Detailed measurements have shown that these entities are morphologically distinct (Oppenheimer-Dekker et al., 1985). With all these defects, it is easy to see how the overriding leaflets of the aortic valve can be considered as the roof of the defect. The margin of operational significance, however, is that seen by the surgeon from the right ventricle across which a patch will be placed to reconnect the aorta to the left ventricle. This margin may be formed in part by fibrous continuity between the aortic and tricuspid valves (i.e., a perimembranous defect, Fig. 13a). Alternatively, the borders may be ex-

clusively muscular, composed in turn of the limbs of the septomarginal trabeculation, the ventriculoinfundibular fold, the parietal wall of the right ventricle and the outlet septum (Fig. 13b). There is also a third possibility; namely, that the outlet septum is lacking and part of the border is fibrous continuity between the leaflets of the aortic and pulmonary valves. This is the defect we describe as being doubly-committed and subarterial: it can extend to become perimembranous (see below). When an overriding aortic valve is connected mostly to the right ventricle, then the left ventricular margins of its border can also be significant should the defect be restrictive, since this margin may require surgical enlargement. Variability is seen in the roof of this margin, which may be made up of aortic-mitral fibrous continuity (even when there is aortic-tricuspid discontinuity and the defect has a muscular margin as seen from the ventricle) or

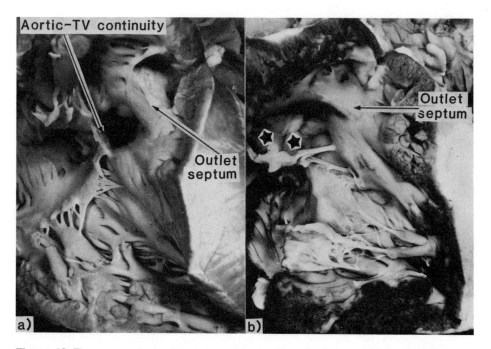

Figure 13. These two photographs show the view from the right ventricular apex of hearts with tetralogy of Fallot and (a) a perimembranous defect (note the continuity between aortic and tricuspid valves [TV]) and (b) a defect with a muscular posteroinferior rim (starred) between the aortic and tricuspid valves.

can be formed by a muscular ventriculoin-fundibular fold (subaortic muscular infundibulum). If this margin needs enlargement, it is the part of the septal crest overlain by the anterior limb of the septomarginal trabeculation which can safely be resected.

Overriding Pulmonary Valve

The pulmonary valve overrides the septum most frequently in the setting of the Taussig-Bing malformation. This is also the arrangement in which there may be straddling and overriding of the mitral valve. The description of the defect in this setting is comparable for that of the overriding aortic valve. Overriding by the pulmonary valve is also seen with deviation of the outlet septum into the left ventricle and concomitant narrowing of the subaortic outflow tract (Fig. 14). It is the left ventricular border of this defect that is of operational signifi-

cance. This may be muscular when the outlet septum, septomarginal trabeculation, and ventriculoinfundibular fold are fused together. Alternatively, the defect may be perimembranous when there is fibrous continuity between the mitral and tricuspid and/or the pulmonary or aortic valves. These are the defects associated with coarctation or interruption of the aortic arch. It may well be necessary to resect the outlet septum so as to provide adequate left ventricular flow into the aorta if an attempt is to be made to close the defect.

Defects with Fibrous Continuity Between the Aortic and Pulmonary Valves

The final situation in which the arterial valves can be related directly to the margin of a ventricular septal defect is when the

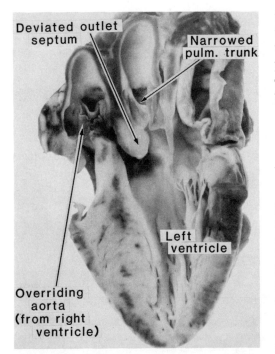

Deviated outlet septum

Narrowed pulm. trunk

Left ventricle

Overriding aorta (from right ventricle)

Figure 14. This illustration shows how malalignment of the outlet septum into the left ventricle produces overriding of the aorta and subpulmonary obstruction in this heart with a discordant ventriculoarterial connection (complete transposition).

outlet septum is lacking and the facing leaflets of the aortic and pulmonary valves are directly continuous with one another. If a surgical attempt is made to close such a defect, the patch will be placed along the area of aortic-pulmonary continuity (unless the patch is placed around both arterial valves and a conduit used to provide right ventricular-pulmonary circulation). Absence of the outlet septum with aortic-pulmonary fibrous continuity can be found in the setting of concordant, discordant or double outlet ventriculoarterial connections (Fig. 15). An analogous situation exists when there is a common arterial trunk and the roof of the defect is the overriding leaflets of the truncal valve (Fig. 16). Our preference is to describe these defects as being doubly committed and juxtaarterial (or simply juxtatruncal in the setting of a common

trunk). The right ventricular margin of all these defects can be muscular when the ventriculoinfundibular fold fuses with the posterior limb of the septomarginal trabeculation. This structure, when present, protects the atrioventricular conduction axis.

Summary of Relationship to Conduction Axis

Possibly the single most important piece of information for the surgeon who is closing a ventricular septal defect is the precise location of the atrioventricular conduction axis. As we have indicated above, this information can be deduced with considerable precision if the nature of the borders of the defect is known, along with its position within the septum. In all hearts with concordant atrioventricular and ventriculoarterial connections (with one exception; see below), the conduction axis runs posteroinferiorly relative to perimembranous defects. The guide to the location of the atrioventricular node is the apex of the triangle of Koch (Anderson et al., 1983). From this situation in the atrial septum, the conduction axis penetrates through the atrioventricular membranous septum (tricuspid-aortic-mitral continuity) and reaches the left ventricular aspect of the septal crest. The precise relationship of the bundle to the crest varies from heart to heart. Generally speaking, it is farther from the crest when the defect opens to the outlet of the right ventricle and closer when there is an inlet defect. These are, however, only guidelines. The bundle may branch directly astride the septum (Titus et al., 1974) and, in rare circumstances, may be encased within tension apparatus to the tricuspid valve on the right side of the defect (Ueda and Becker, 1985). Considered overall, the crest of the septum (seen from the right ventricle) is best avoided between the posteroinferior margin of the defect and the origin of the medial papillary muscle. The only exception to the above description for perimembranous defects in the concor-

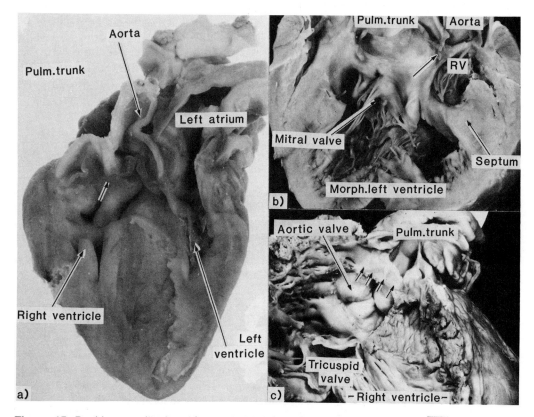

Figure 15. Doubly committed and juxtaarterial defects in the setting of concordant (a), discordant ventriculoarterial connections (b), and double outlet right ventricle (c). In both hearts there is no evidence of muscular outlet septum so that there is fibrous continuity between the leaflets of the aortic and pulmonary valves (arrowed). The heart shown in b also has a discordant atrioventricular connection (congenitally corrected transposition). RV = right ventricle.

dantly connected heart is when there is straddling and overriding of the morphologically tricuspid valve, in which case the penetrating atrioventricular bundle is located at the fusion point of the ventricular septum with the atrioventricular junction rather than at the apex of the triangle of Koch.

The relationship of the conduction axis to muscular defects depends on their position. The axis always runs anterosuperiorly to defects opening within the inlet of the right ventricle. The proximity of the axis to the edge of the defect depends upon how closely the defect approximates the central fibrous body. Muscular defects within the extensive apical trabecular components are never related directly to the nonbranching or branching components of the axis. Ramifications from the axis, however, may course over the edges of the defects and extensive trauma to these areas could result in hemorrhage and exudate tracking retrogradely through the sheaths that enclose the conduction fibers (Latham and Anderson, 1972). In any defect opening between the ventricular outlets, the significant feature of the conduction axis is whether a muscular strand separates the edge of the defect from the central fibrous body (membranous septum). The muscle strand is produced by fusion of the ventriculoinfundibular fold with the posterior limb of the septomarginal trabeculation, and it overlies the conduction axis. The degree of protection provided is proportional to its size. When the strand is

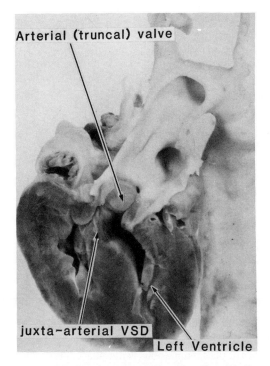

Arterial (truncal) valve

juxta-arterial VSD

Left Ventricle

Figure 16. This paracoronal section through the outlet of a heart with a common arterial trunk shows the juxtaarterial defect which is roofed during ventricular diastole by the coapted leaflets of the truncal valve.

lacking, there is tricuspid-aortic fibrous continuity and the defect is perimembranous. The most significant feature in all respects, therefore, is whether or not the defect is perimembranous.

Summary of Anatomical Differences

Operationally, the most significant border of a defect is that seen by the surgeon from the right ventricle. Three distinct patterns stand out. The first includes all those defects embedded within the substance of the ventricular septum. These defects are universally described as "muscular." The most common pattern, however, is the second one, in which part of the margin of the defect is formed directly by the car-

diac skeleton (central fibrous body). Our preference is to describe these defects as "perimembranous." The third, and most rare, pattern is that in which an area of fibrous continuity between the aortic and pulmonary valves forms an edge. We describe this third type of defect as "doubly committed and juxtaarterial." Also of operational significance is the location of the defect within the septum. This can be described in various ways. One approach is to account for location relative to the valves, describing subaortic or subtricuspid defects, and so on (Capelli et al., 1983). Our preference is to state the part of the right ventricle into which the defect opens, in other words to account for those opening into the inlet, apical trabecular, or outlet components (or else describing a defect as confluent). A further feature of major surgical importance is the presence of overriding leaflets of the arterial or atrioventricular valves. This can also be described in terms of subaortic or subtricuspid defects, and so on. Our preference in this situation is simply to describe the presence of the overriding valve together with the atrioventricular or ventriculoarterial connection we judge to be present. It is in this setting that it is most difficult to judge the precise defect. We would account for the margins of both right ventricular and left ventricular entrances to the overriding outflow tract if there were any possibility for ambiguity in our description, since situations of potential ambiguity have the greatest potential for disagreement. In this setting we would urge most strongly that description is preferable to definition. Brevity has little value. Understanding and communication must be the primary considerations.

References

Allwork SP, Anderson RH. Developmental anatomy of the membranous part of the ventricular septum in the human heart. *Br Heart J* 1979;41:275–280.

Anderson RH, Ho SY, Becker AE. The surgical

anatomy of the conduction tissues. *Thorax* 1983;38:408–420.

Becker AE, Anderson RH. Atrioventricular septal defects. What's in a name. *J Thorac Cardiovasc Surg* 1982;83:461–469.

Brandt PWT. Axial angled angiocardiography. *Cardiovasc Intervent Radiol* 1984;7:166–169.

Capelli H, Andrade JL, Somerville J. Classification of the site of ventricular septal defect by 2-dimensional echocardiography. *Am J Cardiol* 1983;51:1474–1480.

Hagler DJ, Edwards WD, Seward JB, Tajik AJ. Standardized nomenclature of the ventricular septum and ventricular septal defects, with applications for two-dimensional echocardiography. *Mayo Clin Proc* 1985;60:741–752.

Latham RA, Anderson RH. Anatomical variations in atrioventricular conduction system with reference to ventricular septal defects. *Br Heart J* 1972;34:185–190.

Milo S, Ho SY, Wilkinson JL, Anderson RH. The surgical anatomy and atrioventricular conduction tissues of hearts with isolated ventricular septal defects. *J Thorac Cardiovasc Surg* 1980;79:244–255.

Milo S, Ho SY, Macartney FJ, et al. Straddling and overriding atrioventricular valves: morphol-ogy and classification. *Am J Cardiol* 1979; 44:1122–1134.

Neufeld HN, Titus JL, DuShane JW, et al. Isolated ventricular septal defect of the persistent common atrioventricular canal type. *Circulation* 1961;23:685–696.

Oppenheimer-Dekker A, Gittenberger-de-Groot AC, Bartelings MM, et al. Abnormal architecture of the ventricles in hearts with an overriding aortic valve and a perimembranous ventricular septal defect ("Eisenmenger VSD"). *Int J Cardiol* 1985;9:341–355.

Penkoske PA, Neches WH, Anderson RH, Zuberbuhler JR. Further observations on the morphology of atrioventricular septal defects. *J Thorac Cardiovasc Surg* 1985;90:611–622.

Soto B, Becker AE, Moulaert AJ, et al. Classification of ventricular septal defects. *Br Heart J* 1980;43:332–343.

Titus JL, Daugherty GW, Edwards JE. Anatomy of the atrioventricular conduction system in ventricular septal defect. *Circulation* 1963;28:72–81.

Ueda M, Becker AE. Morphological characteristics of perimembranous ventricular septal defects and their surgical significance. *Int J Cardiol* 1985;8:149–157.

1.3

Echocardiographic Manifestations of Ventricular Septal Defects

Donald R. Fischer, Edward J. Baker, and Robert H. Anderson

Our understanding of the morphological characteristics of ventricular septal defects has been greatly aided by the segmental approach and descriptive terminology advocated by Becker and Anderson (1983). It is quite a different exercise, however, to define the extent and location of a ventricular septal defect when holding the heart in one's hand as a morphologist or surgeon, than determining the same information by echocardiography. With careful scanning and thorough analysis, it is indeed possible to determine the type of a ventricular septal defect accurately by echocardiography, although one must be aware of pitfalls involved in this procedure that might lead to confusion and erroneous diagnoses (Sutherland et al., 1982).

Our mission as echocardiographers is to distinguish the three types of defects discussed in the preceding chapter: the peri-membranous defect, the doubly committed subarterial defect, and muscular defects. The perimembranous defect is defined as one having the central fibrous body as a border, that is, the area of the heart where there is fibrous continuity between the atrioventricular valves or between these valves and an arterial valve. These defects may range in size from small holes with virtually no extension into the remainder of the septum, or large defects that may extend into the various components of the extensive muscular septum. The doubly committed subarterial defect has as its superior margin fibrous continuity between both arterial valves. Muscular defects have an entirely muscular border and may be located within the inlet, trabecular, or outlet portions of the septum. Muscular defects may themselves be multiple or can coexist with the other morphological types.

From: Anderson, RH, Neches, WH, Park, SC, Zuberbuhler, JR, eds: *Perspectives in Pediatric Cardiology*: Mount Kisco, New York, Futura Publishing Co., © 1988.

Location of the defect by echocardiography depends on obtaining multiple cross-sectional planes through the heart from the standard positions, including the parasternal long and short axis, apical, and subxiphoid views. One must scan slowly from a given projection through multiple planes in order to visualize the relationships among the cardiac valves, their support apparatus, and the ventricular septum. A single still frame is inadequate to define a defect completely. Mistakes in definition of a defect are most easily made if the diagnosis is based on limited information. The advantage of echocardiography over angiography is the ability to scan through multiple planes and consolidate this information to give a three-dimensional image enabling more precise definition of type and extension of a ventricular septal defect. The crucial information needed is the relationship of the defect to the central fibrous body and to the arterial and atrioventricular valves, and the presence or absence of exclusively muscular borders. This review will serve to demonstrate the correlation between the morphological and echocardiographic characteristics of the major types of ventricular septal defects.

Perimembranous Defects

Perimembranous defects are the most common type of ventricular septal defect. In order to identify a defect as perimembranous, the echocardiographer must demonstrate that the superior margin of the defect is formed by fibrous continuity between either the atrioventricular valves or between an atrioventricular valve and one of the arterial valves. Figure 1 demonstrates a large perimembranous defect with the superior margin formed by fibrous continuity between the tricuspid and aortic valves. This can usually be best demonstrated echocardiographically from an apical projection an-

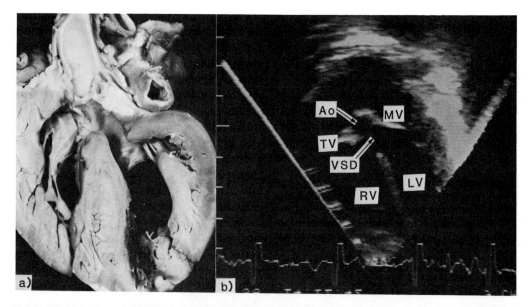

Figure 1. These anatomical (a) and echocardiographic (b) sections (not from the same patient) in apical four-chamber projection show the salient features of large perimembranous defect, namely that the superior margin is formed by fibrous continuity between tricuspid and aortic valve. Ao = aorta; LV = left ventricle; MV = mitral valve; RV = right ventricle; TV = tricuspid valve; VSD = ventricular septal defect.

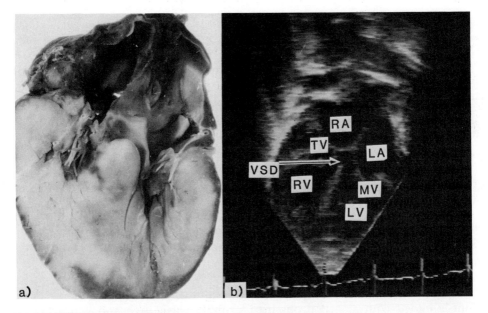

Figure 2. These sections in apical four-chamber projection (not from the same patient) show the features of a perimembranous defect extending to open between the ventricular inlets. LA = left atrium; RA = right atrium.

gling gradually from posterior to anterior so as to demonstrate the inlet and outlet components of the right ventricle.

If they are large, perimembranous defects may extend into adjacent portions of the muscular septum. Those that extend to open into the inlet of the right ventricle (Fig. 2) can be best demonstrated echocardiographically angling posteriorly to the level

of the atrioventricular valves. A defect in this region has as its superior border fibrous continuity between the tricuspid and mitral valves. The anticipated offsetting of the two atrioventricular valves is lost. A perimembranous defect may be present and yet the inlet septum may be intact. Figure 3 shows anatomical sections obtained from the same heart demonstrating a section at the level of

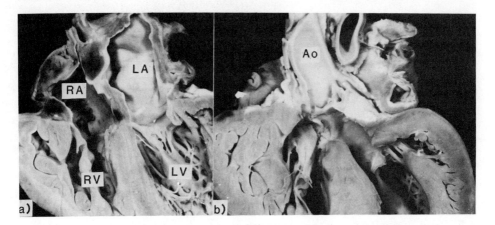

Figure 3. These sections through a heart with a perimembranous defect opening to the outlet of the right ventricle (b) show how the inlet part of the septum (a) can be intact.

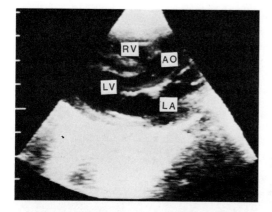

Figure 4. This parasternal long-axis echocardiogram demonstrates a large ventricular septal defect with override of the aortic root.

the atrioventricular valves in which the septum is intact, with a section obtained more anteriorly clearly demonstrating a perimembranous defect extending to open into the outlet of the right ventricle. This type of hole reinforces the concept that a single cross-sectional cut is inadequate to define a ventricular defect.

Echocardiography is quite capable of identifying perimembranous defects and their extension. Other complicating features of perimembranous defects may also be present and should be specifically sought at the time of the study. Overriding of an arterial valve is relatively common and can be seen in a variety of views. Controversy still exists as to the method for determining degree of override, but this can probably best be visualized from either the long axis or apical projections. Figure 4, a long-axis projection, shows the posterior great artery overriding a ventricular defect that was determined to be perimembranous by scanning in other planes. The anterior great artery may also override if there is posterior deviation of the outlet septum, as can be seen in patients with the complex of interrupted aortic arch and ventricular septal defect.

Overriding and straddling of an atrioventricular valve is less common, but has important surgical implications and must be sought by identifying support structures of the atrioventricular valves and noting relative sizes of the ventricles (Fig. 5).

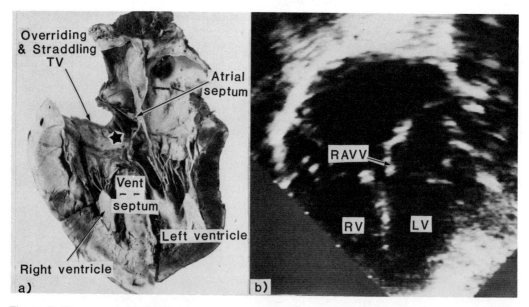

Figure 5. These anatomical and echocardiographic sections in apical four-chamber projection during diastole illustrate how the right-sided atrioventricular valve (RAVV) overrides and straddles an inlet perimembranous ventricular defect. The central fibrous body and the ventricular septum are grossly malaligned.

Another feature commonly associated with perimembranous defects is the presence of tissue tags derived from the tricuspid valve which partially close the defect and create the so-called "aneurysm" of the membranous septum (Fig. 6). This tissue may make it difficult to gauge the functional size of the defect accurately and is known to play a role in spontaneous closure.

Muscular Defects

Muscular ventricular septal defects are distinctive by their separation from the fibrous tissue supporting the leaflets of the valves by echo-dense muscular tissue. The defect may be far removed, as with an apical trabecular defect, or near to the valves with minimal muscle separating the valve plane from the defect. The major significance of this differentiation is that one can assure the surgeon that the defect with exclusively muscular borders will be free of conduction tissue around its immediate pe-

rimeter, but that a particular border may be adjacent to the conduction axis. The distinction among muscular defects in the inlet, trabecular, and outlet portions may be somewhat arbitrary and controversial, but it should suffice if the echocardiographer can simply describe the relative position of the muscular defect in relation to the atrioventricular valves in order for the surgeon to plan an appropriate approach to closure.

Figure 7 demonstrates a pathological specimen and echocardiographic cross-section of a heart with a muscular inlet defect. Note that the usual offsetting of the atrioventricular valves is present and a discrete bar of dense septal tissue is seen superior to the defect, separating it from the central fibrous body. These defects are particularly significant since the conduction axis is related to their anterosuperior quadrant (Milo et al., 1980). Muscular defects may also be found more distal in the trabecular septum, in which case they may be quite hard to identify echocardiographically. The anatomical specimen in Figure 8 shows multiple defects near the apex. These defects might

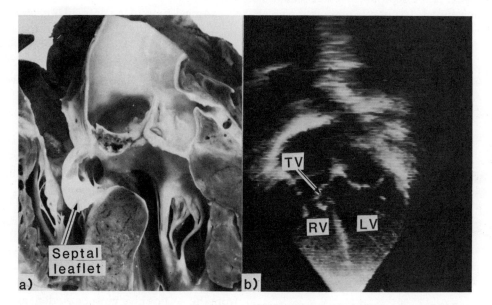

Figure 6. Anatomical and echocardiographic sections (not from the same patient) in apical four-chamber projection showing the septal leaflet of the tricuspid valve closing a perimembranous ventricular septal defect opening into the right ventricular inlet and creating a so-called "aneurysm" of the membranous septum.

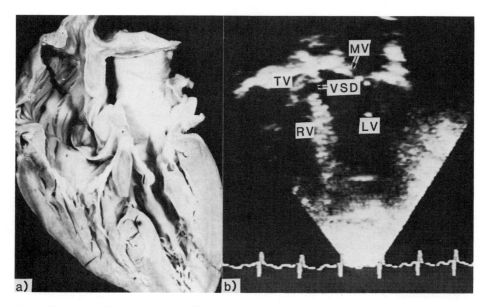

Figure 7. Anatomical and echocardiographic sections (not from the same patient) in apical four-chamber view demonstrating a muscular ventricular septal defect opening to the right ventricular inlet. A small area of echo-dense tissues separates the superior margin of this defect from the plane of the atrioventricular valves.

be quite difficult to visualize in cross-section, especially if small. Similarly, a trabecular muscular defect can be difficult for the surgeon to visualize from the right ventricular aspect of the septum since trabeculations in the ventricle frequently obscure the holes. The corresponding long-axis echocardiographic projection in Figure 8 is an example of a similar case of multiple muscular defects that are quite large and are seen to be clearly separated from the aortic valve by muscular tissue.

Apical muscular ventricular septal defects are probably the easiest to miss by echocardiography (Fig. 9). In this situation, Doppler sampling on the right ventricular side of the defect is able to show turbulent systolic flow confirming left-to-right interventricular shunting in this location. The addition of Doppler information with very small ventricular septal defects can be very helpful in confirming the clinical impression that a ventricular septal defect is present.

The short-axis projection may also yield a good view of muscular defects as one angles inferiorly from the apex of the heart superiorly to the plane of the aortic valve. Short-axis cross-sections from hearts with muscular trabecular defects are illustrated in Figure 10. Distinct muscular separation from the aortic valve must be evident as one scans in order to make this diagnosis.

Muscular outlet defects are more rare

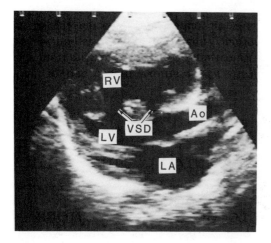

Figure 8. This echocardiogram in parasternal long-axis projection shows multiple large muscular defects in the apical trabecular septum.

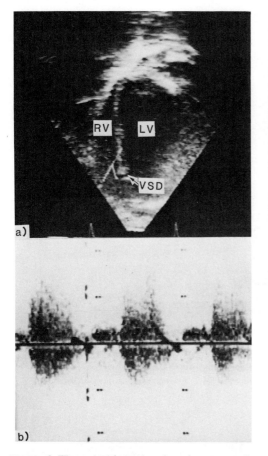

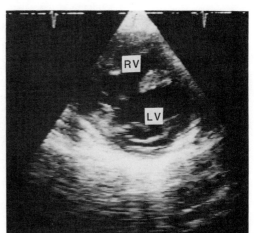

Figure 10. This echocardiogram in short-axis projection demonstrates a muscular defect in the apical trabecular septum.

Figure 9. The apical four-chamber view suggests a tiny defect in the apical muscular septum (a). Doppler sampling on the right ventricular side of this defect (b) demonstrates turbulent systolic flow, confirming the presence of interventricular shunting.

and can be confused with doubly committed subarterial defects. The distinction lies in identifying tissue that is echo-dense beneath the plane of the arterial valves. If the tissue is minimal, it may be virtually impossible to distinguish these defects without visualizing the defect directly at surgery. The anatomical specimen in Figure 11 is oriented in a long-axis view and shows a defect beneath the plane of the arterial valves with minimal muscular tissue as a superior margin. The distinction might be impossible to make by echocardiography, but the crucial information to be relayed is that this defect

is nearly adjacent to the arterial valves and might require a pulmonary arterial approach at the time of surgical repair.

Doubly Committed Subarterial Defects

Doubly committed subarterial defects have as their hallmark continuity between the pulmonary and aortic valves, with no tissue present immediately inferior to the plane formed by the conjoined leaflets of the arterial valves. These defects are best demonstrated as one angles from a parasternal view from a long axis toward a short-axis projection (Fig. 12). Often associated with these defects is dilation of the right coronary sinus of Valsalva with prolapse of the right coronary leaflet of the aortic valve inferiorly and with occasional bulging of this leaflet into the defect itself. This is correlated clinically with the development of aortic insufficiency and may limit the magnitude of the left-to-right interventricular shunt. These doubly committed defects can extend to become perimembranous or may have a muscular posteroinferior rim, the

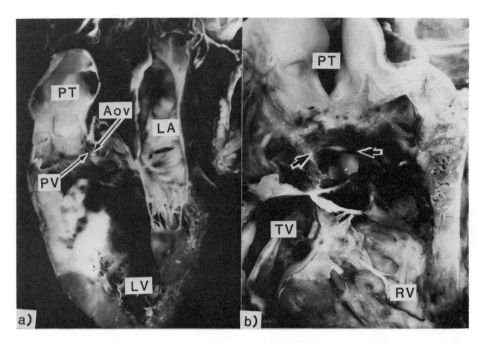

Figure 11. This anatomical specimen shows the difficulties in distinguishing muscular outlet from doubly committed and subarterial defects. In this case, a small muscle bar (between arrows) produces offsetting of the aortic (AoV) and pulmonary (PV) valves. It may not be possible to visualize such a bar echocardiographically. (a) is a long-axis section of the heart viewed from the right ventricle in (b).

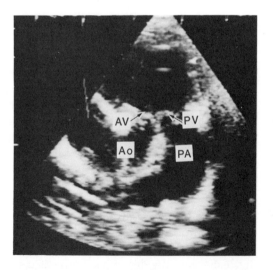

Figure 12. This diastolic frame obtained by angling from a parasternal long-axis to short-axis projection shows fibrous continuity between the aortic and pulmonary valves, identifying the defect as being committed and subarterial. AV = aortic valve; PV = pulmonary valve.

latter structure, if present, protecting the atrioventricular conduction axis (Milo et al., 1980).

Summary

Careful echocardiographic imaging can indeed allow identification of the type and extent of a ventricular septal defect. Difficulties may arise with positive identification of small muscular trabecular ventricular septal defects or multiple muscular ventricular septal defects of the "swiss cheese" variety. In addition, differentiation between doubly committed subarterial and muscular outlet defects may be difficult if the muscular rim inferior to the arterial valves is minimal. Similarly, muscular inlet defects may be difficult to differentiate from perimembranous inlet defects if there is little muscular tissue inferior to the atrioventricular valves. This is not merely an academic exercise, but has important clinical significance. Knowledge of the borders of the defect correlates with location of the conduction tissue, guiding suture placement to avoid atrioventricular block. One can assure the surgeon that if there is a muscular inlet defect, the conduction axis will be anterosuperior as opposed to the posteroinferior location found with all perimembranous defects (Milo et al., 1980). The surgical approach to closure of a ventricular septal defect depends on its location. Those opening to the inlet of the right ventricle may be closed from a right atrial approach, while it may be impossible to close those opening between the outlets from this incision. Doubly committed subarterial defects, on the other hand, are in most instances best approached from the pulmonary trunk.

Finally, location has significance with regard to spontaneous closure. Perimembranous defects opening toward the inlet of the right ventricle with tricuspid valve tissue tags surrounding them are much more likely to become smaller than are perimembranous outlet defects and large trabecular muscular defects. This information can be useful in planning follow-up and providing prognostic information for children when the indications for surgical intervention are borderline.

References

Becker AE, Anderson RH. Anomalies of the Ventricles. In: *Cardiac Pathology: An Integrated Text and Colour Atlas.* New York, Churchill Livingston, 1983.

Milo S, Ho SY, Wilkinson JL, Anderson RH. Surgical anatomy and atrioventricular conduction tissues of hearts with isolated ventricular septal defects. *J Thorac Cardiovas Surg* 1980;79:244–255.

Sutherland GR, Godman MJ, Smallhorn JF, et al. Ventricular septal defects: Two-dimensional echocardiographic and morphological correlations. *Br Heart J* 1982;47:316–328.

The Angiocardiographic Recognition of Types of Ventricular Septal Defects

Robert M. Freedom, C. A. F. Moes, Patricia E. Burrows, Donald E. Perrin, and Jeffrey F. Smallhorn

The Nature of the Ventricular Septum in Humans

In the preceding chapter, the curvilinear nature of the human ventricular septum and its components have been demonstrated. Indeed, because the perimembranous and infundibular components of the septum are relatively anterior when compared to the posterior muscular inlet septum, such portions of the ventricular septum can be imaged separately using the technique of axial angiography (Bargeron et al., 1977; Ceballos et al., 1981; Fellows et al., 1977; Green et al., 1981; Puyau and Burko, 1966; Santamaria et al., 1983; Soto et al., 1985). Standard approaches to axial projections have to be modified when considering hearts whose atrioventricular and/or ventriculoarterial connections depart from the normal. Thus, the ventricular septum, especially the outlet portion, is not curved in individuals with complete transposition whose arterial outlets are relatively parallel, and not spiralled. Similarly, the ventricular septum assumes a saggital configuration among patients with a discordant atrioventricular connection, and it assumes a more or less horizontal disposition in hearts exhibiting superoinferior ventricles or in many of those exhibiting crossed atrioventricular connections (Fig. 1).

Much anatomical information about the type of atrioventricular connection, and indeed about the disposition of the interventricular septum, can be gleaned noninvasively from cross-sectional echocardio-

From: Anderson, RH, Neches, WH, Park, SC, Zuberbuhler, JR, eds: *Perspectives in Pediatric Cardiology*: Mount Kisco, New York, Futura Publishing Co., © 1988.

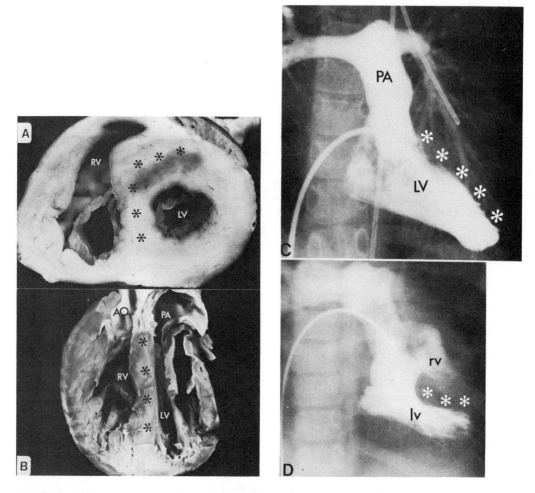

Figure 1. (A) The normal heart. A cross-sectional view of the interventricular septum (asterisks) somewhat inferior to the arterial outlets. (B) The relatively straight interventricular septum (asterisk) in the patient with complete transposition. (C) Frontal left ventricular (LV) angiocardiogram in a patient with discordant atrioventricular and ventriculoarterial connections. (D) Horizontal interventricular septum in a patient with superoinferior ventricles. MPA-main pulmonary artery; LV and RV-left and right ventricle; Ao-aorta.

graphic examination. Such echo scanning can provide considerable aid when planning the specific angiocardiographic projection (Capelli et al., 1983; Smallhorn et al., 1983; Sutherland et al., 1982).

Nomenclature

There is no unanimity in the nomenclature of the integral components of the ventricular septum, or in the designation of the various types of ventricular septal defects (Anderson et al., 1984; Capelli et al., 1983; Freedom, 1979; Santamaria et al., 1983; Soto et al., 1985; Wenink et al., 1979). Ventricular septal defects can be classified as perimembranous, muscular, or doubly committed and subarterial. Defects that involve the membranous septum and the immediately contiguous perimembranous areas and surrounding muscular structures are designated perimembranous. Muscular

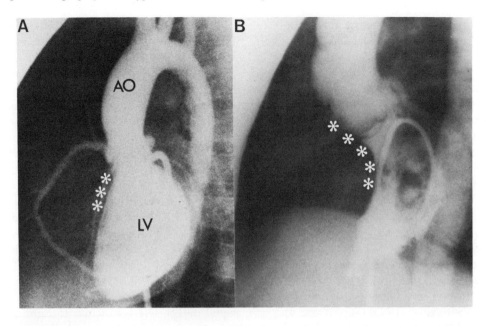

Figure 2. The so-called sigmoid interventricular septum. (A) Normal left ventricular outflow; a relatively straight path between left ventricle (LV) and aorta (Ao); the plane of the interventricular septum is noted (asterisk). (B) A sigmoid (white asterisk) septum: relative angulation between the infundibular and trabecular septum.

defects are located in the inlet, trabecular, or outlet portions of the ventricular septum. Such defects may coexist with perimembranous ones. The third type of ventricular defect involves that portion of the ventricular myocardium that separates the arterial outflow tracts. These defects are termed subarterial and infundibular. In addition to the integral components of the ventricular septum, there may be normal variations in the contour of the left ventricular outlet that may influence angiographic projections. When the left ventricular septal wall lacks a special prominence, it provides for a straight channel between the left ventricle and aorta. In other individuals, the base or infundibular portion of the ventricular septum seemingly protrudes toward the cavity of the left ventricle, producing the so-called sigmoid configuration (Goor et al., 1969) (Fig. 2). The implications of such an angled interventricular septum on echocardiographic interpretation have been discussed elsewhere (Bernstein et al., 1983).

The Perimembranous Ventricular Septal Defect

There is a convincing body of evidence that some perimembranous ventricular septal defects, especially those whose original size is small to moderate, tend to become smaller or even to close (Anderson et al., 1983A; Beerman et al., 1985; Freedom, 1979; Freedom et al., 1974; Ramaciotti et al., 1986). While we and others suggested that the mechanism of closure might be related to a so-called aneurysm of the membranous ventricular septum, we are aware that the designation "aneurysm of the membranous ventricular septum" embraces a host of morphological-pathological mechanisms, only one of which is truly derived from membranous septum (Anderson et al., 1983A; Freedom, 1979; Chesler et al., 1968). Anderson and his colleagues (1983A) have addressed this conundrum, providing the following observations: those anatomical structures most frequently responsible for reduction in size of a perimembranous ventricular septal defect were reduplication of the tricuspid valve, adhesion of the tricuspid valve leaflets to the ventricular defect, prolapse of an aortic valve leaflet, or subaortic tissue tags possibly derived from the remnant of the membranous septum. These authors conclude that partial closure is only rarely related to the so-called aneurysm of the membranous septum.

Selective biplane left ventriculography filmed in the long-axial oblique projection and its reciprocal projection should nicely profile the perimembranous ventricular septal defect and contiguous tricuspid valve tissue (when present) (Bargeron et al., 1977; Ceballos et al., 1981; Santamaria et al., 1983; Soto et al., 1985) (Figs. 3 and 4).

Ventricular Septal Defect with Left Ventricular–Right Atrial Shunting

An isolated deficiency of the atrioventricular membranous septum (with none of the anatomical stigmata of an atrioventricular septal defect) which permits left ventricular to right atrial shunting must be extremely uncommon (Anderson et al., 1984; Elliott et al., 1965). Most individuals considered to have the so-called Gerbode defect (Gerbode et al., 1958) have a perimembranous defect with left-to-right shunting from the left ventricle through the ventricular defect which is shrouded by tricuspid tissue. Indeed, of the nine patients studied by Burrows and her colleagues (1983), all had so-called aneurysm of the membranous ventricular septum and some had obvious adherence of deformed leaflets of the tricuspid valve to the perimembranous defect. Burrows et al. (1983) concluded that, in the presence of a perimembranous ventricular septal defect, left ventricular to right atrial shunting is often the result of tricuspid valve deformities, including isolated clefts, perforations or duplicate orifices, adherence of tricuspid valve tissue to the margins of the ventricular septal defect, and to commissural defects. Biplane left ventriculography filmed in the long axial oblique and

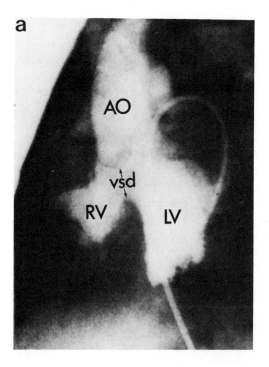

Figure 3. Perimembranous ventricular septal defect. (a) Large defect profiled by long axial oblique left ventriculogram; (b and c) Smaller perimembranous defect shrouded by tricuspid tissue, producing a small so-called aneurysm of membranous ventricular septum (black asterisk) shown nicely in this long axial oblique left ventriculogram; the trabecular muscular septum appears intact; the tricuspid orifice (white asterisk) is clearly profiled in (c); (d and e) A larger so-called aneurysm of the membranous septum; (d) Right long axial oblique left ventriculogram shows shunting (curved arrow) of contrast into outflow tract of right ventricle. The diaphragmatic surface of the left ventricle (multiple white asterisks) does not show any posterior small marginal defects; the infundibular septum (IS) (solitary white asterisk) is shown; (e) The "aneurysm" is clearly evident.

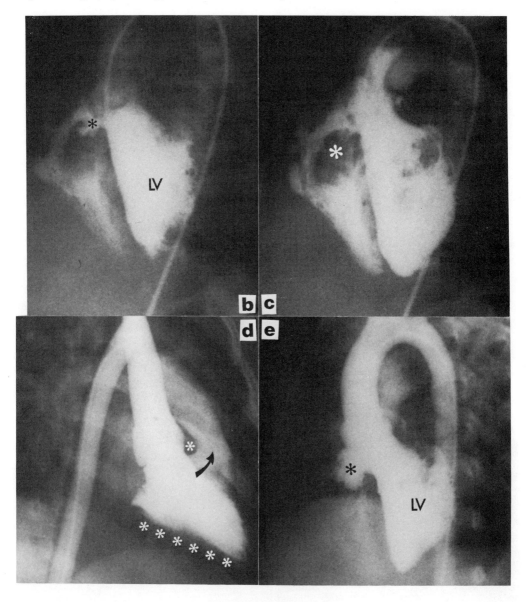

Figure 3. *Continued.*

reciprocal right anterior oblique projections probably best demonstrates the anatomy of such a perimembranous defect with a deformity of the tricuspid valve which permits left ventricular–right atrial shunting (Burrows et al., 1983; Santamaria et al., 1983) (Figs. 5 and 6). It is important in this assessment to exclude a true atrioventricular septal defect (Soto et al., 1981).

Acquired Right Ventricular Outflow Tract Obstruction and the Perimembranous Ventricular Septal Defect

It is well established that progressive right ventricular outflow tract obstruction can complicate the natural history of the patient with a ventricular septal defect. A re-

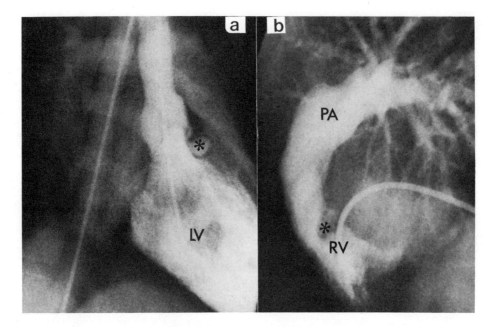

Figure 4. Perimembranous defect with a "windsock" protruding into the right ventricular outflow tract. (a) left ventricular angiogram in right axial oblique showing the windsock (asterisk) protruding into the outflow tract of the right ventricle; (b) lateral right ventriculogram (RV) showing the narrowing of the subpulmonary outflow tract by the aneurysmal windsock (asterisk).

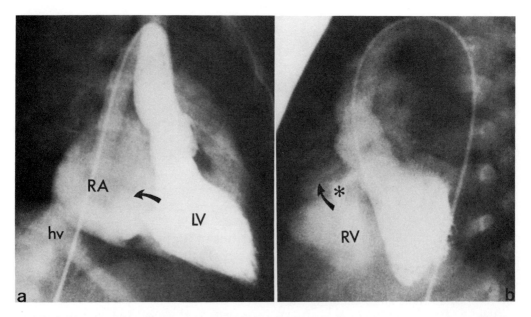

Figure 5. Perimembranous defect with left ventricular-to-right atrial shunt. (a and b) Right and left long axial oblique left ventriculogram. (a) Contrast passes (arrow) from LV to the right atrium (RA) and refluxes into the hepatic veins (hv); (b) the adherent tricuspid tissue (asterisk) and the intact trabecular septum are clearly shown in the long axial oblique left ventriculogram.

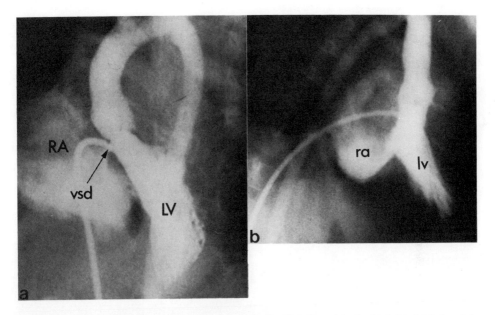

Figure 6. A relatively small perimembranous defect with left ventricular to right atrial shunt. (a and b) Right and left long axial oblique projections from selective left ventriculography.

view previously published from this institution (Freedom, 1979) has summarized those diverse morphological expressions poten-tially responsible for acquired right ventricular outflow tract obstruction. Data subsequently published by Pongiglione and his

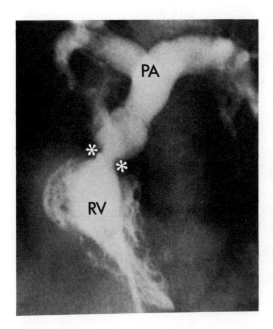

Figure 7. Anomalous muscle bundles of the right ventricle (white asterisk) demonstrated by this right ventriculogram (RV) filmed with caudocranial tilt.

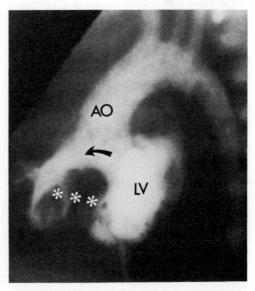

Figure 8. Hypertrophic obstructive cardiomyopathy with perimembranous ventricular septal defect. This left ventricular angiogram in the left long axial oblique projection clearly demonstrates the disproportionately enlarged (white asterisk) interventricular septum.

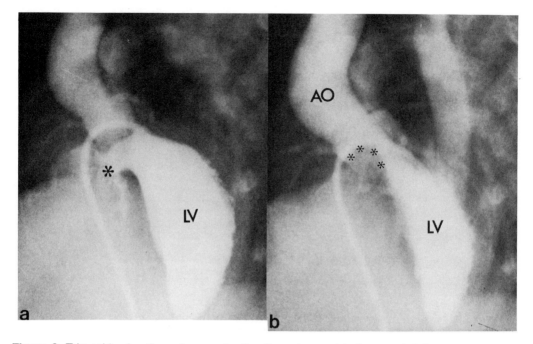

Figure 9. Tricuspid valve tissue tags protruding through a ventricular septal defect, producing left ventricular outflow tract obstruction. Two frames of long axial oblique left ventriculogram (LV) showing herniation of tricuspid valve tissue (asterisk) through the defect, resulting in subaortic stenosis.

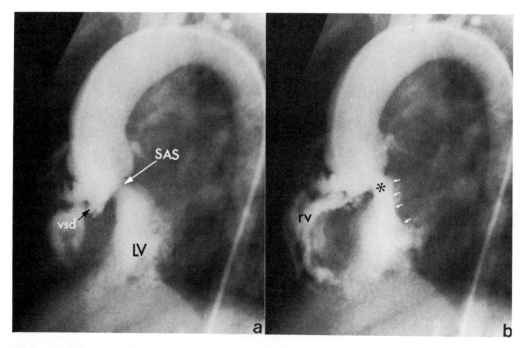

Figure 10. Fibromuscular left ventricular outflow tract obstruction (SAS) in a child with a small perimembranous defect and aneurysmal tissue. Long axial oblique left ventriculogram. Note the very narrow LV outflow tract (asterisk) in b. The mitral valve is noted by white arrows.

colleagues from Toronto (1982) clearly demonstrated that, among most patients with a perimembranous ventricular septal defect, hypertrophy of so-called right ventricular muscle bundles (producing a two-chambered right ventricle) and not hypertrophy of a malaligned outlet septum is responsible for right ventricular outflow tract obstruction (Fig. 7). Both mechanisms, however, have been recognized as responsible for the so-called Gasul transformation.

The Perimembranous Ventricular Septal Defect and Left Ventricular Outflow Tract Obstruction

Among patients with usual atrial arrangement, concordant atrioventricular and ventriculoarterial connections and ventricular septal defect, a variety of mechanisms have been identified that can obstruct the left ventricular outflow tract (Anderson et al., 1983B; Baumstark et al., 1978; Chung et al., 1984; Dirksen et al., 1978; Feigl et al., 1986; Fisher et al., 1982; Freedom et al., 1977A, 1977B, 1985; Moene et al., 1981, 1982, 1986; Moulaert and Oppenheimer-Dekker, 1976; Moulaert et al., 1976; Nanton et al., 1979; Sellers et al., 1964; Sennari, 1985; Shore et al., 1982; Smallhorn et al., 1983; Vogel et al., 1983). Such mechanisms include fibromuscular obstruction with aortic mitral discontinuity; caudal displacement of the outlet septum with the left ventricular outflow tract wedged between the displaced septum and the left-sided ventriculoinfundibular fold; muscular abnormalities of the left ventricle; tissue tags derived from membranous septum, tricuspid or mitral valves; tensor apparatus of the aortic leaflet of the mitral valve attached to the left ventricular septal surface; hypertrophic cardiomyopathy; or some combination of the above.

It has become increasingly evident that subaortic stenosis of the fibrous-fibromuscular type may complicate the course of the

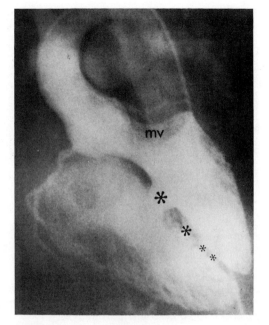

Figure 11. Left ventriculogram in four-chamber projection showing multiple posterior muscular inlet ventricular septal defects (asterisk). Note the normal mitral valve (MV). Toward the apex of the left ventricle, the ventricular septal defects are probably more in the midtrabecular zone.

patient with an isolated perimembranous ventricular septal defect. While once considered an uncommon concurrence, we recently analyzed the occurrence of subaortic stenosis in 41 patients with ventricular septal defect (Vogel et al., 1983). Thirty-one of the 41 patients had fibrous or fibromuscular obstruction of the left ventricular outlet. Thirty-eight of the 41 patients had a perimembranous ventricular septal defect, and fully half of these patients had a so-called aneurysm of the membranous ventricular septum. The subaortic stenosis was inferior to the ventricular septal defects in 30 patients. Eleven of the 41 patients had some form of right ventricular outflow tract obstruction, often due to anomalous muscle bundles.

Demonstration of such a perimembranous ventricular septal defect and its associated subaortic stenosis is usually best

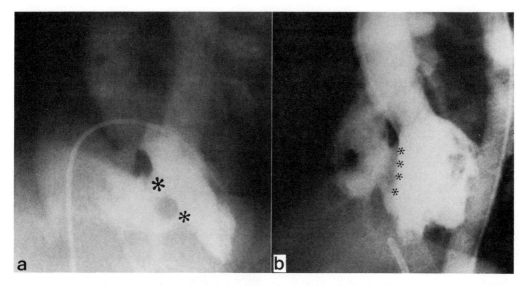

Figure 12. Two large posterior inlet muscular ventricular septal defects shown by a left ventricular angiogram filmed in four-chambered projection. (a) Four-chamber projection showing two defects (asterisk). (b) In the same patient, a long axial oblique angiogram erroneously suggests one large defect, but the plane of ventricular septum (asterisk) is clearly seen, suggesting the defects are not clearly profiled.

achieved from selective biplane left ventricular angiography filmed in the long axial oblique and its reciprocal projection. When obstruction to the left ventricular outlet is relatively posterior, then the four-chamber projection left ventriculogram may be required (Figs. 8–10).

Muscular Ventricular Septal Defects

In this section, we will discuss those ventricular septal defects occupying the muscular portion of the ventricular septum (excluding outlet defects) (Anderson et al., 1984; Capelli et al., 1983; Green et al., 1981; Moene et al., 1981; Santamaria et al., 1983). Axial angiography is the ideal method of profiling the various portions of the interventricular septum. Because the posterior muscular inlet ventricular septal defect has a predilection for straddling and overriding of the tricuspid valve, anomalies of the right atrioventricular junction must be anticipated when one recognizes a ventricular

septal defect occupying the posterior portion of the interventricular septum. Peculiar muscular anomalies of the left ventricle predisposing to left ventricular outflow tract obstruction and/or obstructive anomalies of

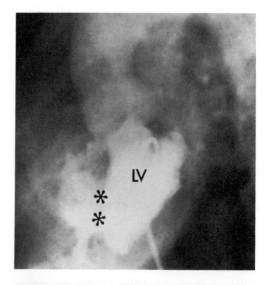

Figure 13. Large posterior inlet muscular defect (asterisk) shown by four-chamber left ventricular angiocardiography.

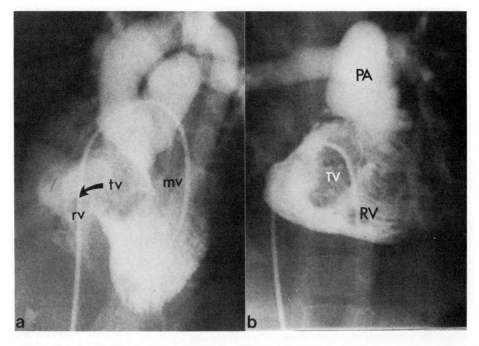

Figure 14. Straddling tricuspid valve in a patient with a posterior inlet ventricular septal defect. (a) This LV angiogram filmed in four-chamber projection shows the straddling tricuspid valve (TV) connecting with the LV; the smaller RV is seen. (b) This frontal RV angiogram demonstrates a slightly small right ventricle and a medially displaced tricuspid orifice (TV).

the aortic arch have been associated with so-called central muscular trabecular defects (Anderson et al., 1983B, 1984; Dirksen et al., 1978; Freedom et al., 1977B; Moene et al., 1981, 1982, 1986; Moulaert et al., 1976; Vogel et al., 1983; Wenink et al., 1979). Because the hemodynamic sequels of such left ventricular myocardial abnormalities may be masked in a grieviously ill infant with a large pulmonary blood flow together with systemic levels of pulmonary arterial hypertension and severe congestive heart failure, the mere recognition of a central or midtrabecular defect should alert one to the potential of left ventricular muscular abnormalities.

The Posterior Muscular Inlet Ventricular Septal Defect

The posterior or inlet muscular ventricular septal defect may occur in isolation or

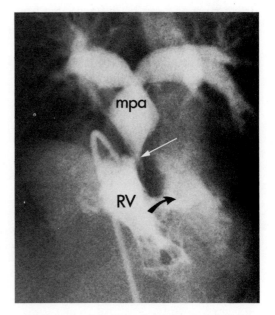

Figure 15. A central muscular defect (black arrow) shown by this right ventricular angiogram in a patient with a previously banded pulmonary trunk and dynamic (white arrow) subpulmonary obstruction.

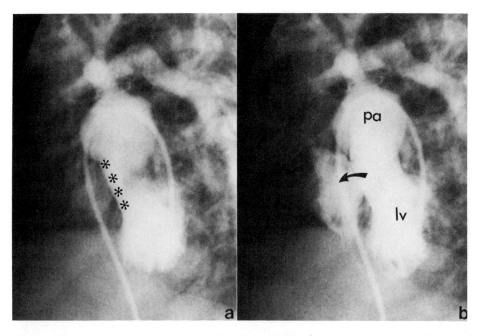

Figure 16. Large trabecular muscular defect in a patient with complete transposition and previously banded pulmonary trunk. (a) The intact perimembranous septum (black asterisk); (b) the large trabecular defect (arrow).

in combination with other defects. Such a defect must and can be differentiated from the ventricular septal defect component of an atrioventricular septal defect (Anderson et al., 1984; Green et al., 1981; Santamaria et al., 1983; Soto et al., 1985; Wenink et al., 1979).

As illustrated in the elegant angiocardiographic study of Green and his colleagues (1981), axial angiography is mandatory in the assessment of this defect. The posterior defect is best visualized in the four-chambered projection (Figs. 11–13). Such a posterior defect may coexist with other defects, and occasionally two or more posterior ventricular septal defects may be present. Furthermore, once an inlet ventricular septal defect is identified, careful scrutiny must be focused on the tricuspid valve. Override of the atrioventricular junction and/or minor or major degrees of straddling of the tricuspid valve demand the presence of an inlet ventricular septal defect (Fig. 14),

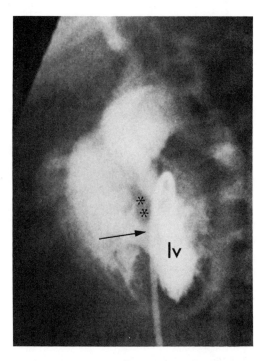

Figure 17. Central muscular trabecular defect and small subaortic area demonstrated by long axial oblique left ventriculogram.

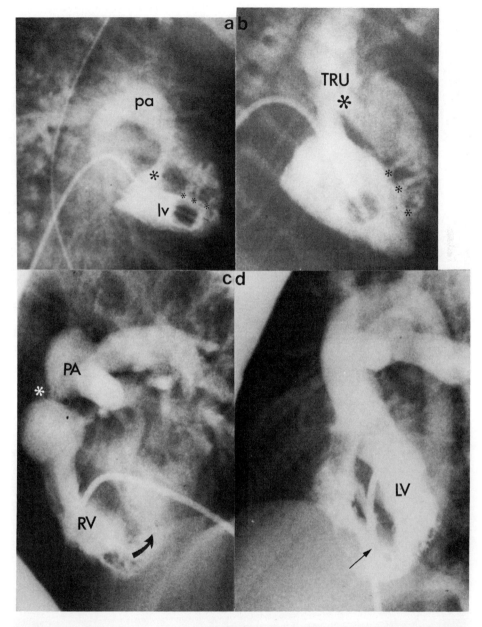

Figure 18. Multiple anterior trabecular ventricular defects shown by right long axial oblique left ventriculogram. (a) A patient with Taussig-Bing double-outlet right ventricle and coarctation. The large asterisk notes the subpulmonary defect. (b) Common arterial trunk with multiple anterior trabecular ventricular septal defects. (c and d) Apical trabecular muscular defects (arrow) shown by right ventricular and left ventricular angiography. The left ventricular injection is performed in a four-chamber projection.

but not one with exclusively muscular rims. While selective right atriography filmed in the four-chambered projection should demonstrate tricuspid override and/or straddle, one would hope that cross-sectional echocardiographic interrogation of the atrio–ventricular junction would provide this diagnosis.

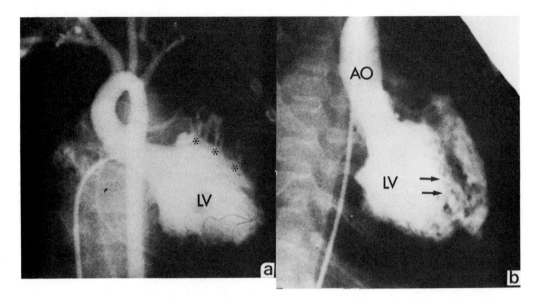

Figure 19. Multiple small and large anterior trabecular muscular defects in two different patients. (a) Shallow right axial oblique. (b) A steeper projection.

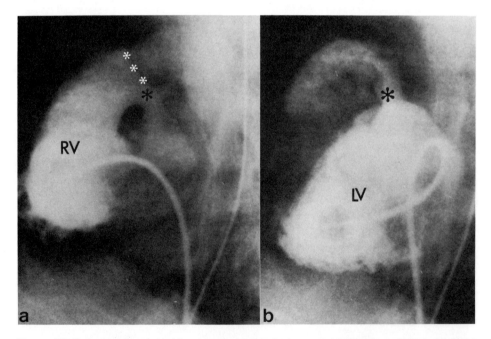

Figure 20. Subarterial and doubly committed ventricular septal defect in an infant. (a) Right ventriculogram (RV) in lateral projection shows the subarterial defect (black asterisk) is roofed by the pulmonary valve (white asterisk); (b) the lateral left ventriculogram shows the direction of the defect (asterisk) entering the right ventricular outflow tract.

Muscular Central Trabecular Ventricular Septal Defects and Left Ventricular Muscular Abnormalities (Figs. 15–17)

Moene and his colleagues (1981, 1982, 1986) have defined a spectrum of left ventricular muscular abnormalities that may coexist with central muscular (trabecular) ventricular septal defects. The three basic types of abnormal left ventricular muscular structures include prominent anterolateral muscle bundles, a posteromedial muscle, and the so-called anteroseptal twist. Patients with such central muscular ventricular septal defects and associated left ventricular muscular abnormalities may exhibit aortic arch hypoplasia of variable severity. These muscular abnormalities of the left ventricle and the central muscular trabecular ventricular septal defects can be profiled by a combination of selective left ventricular angiograms filmed in the four-chambered and long axial oblique projections (Bargeron et al., 1977; Elliott et al., 1984; Freedom, 1984; Green et al., 1981; Santamaria et al., 1983; Soto et al., 1985).

The Muscular Anterior Trabecular Defect

Wenink and his colleagues (1979) have reviewed the anatomy of muscular ventricular septal defects, classifying such muscular defects into three types: posterior defects, central defects, and marginal. Often such marginal defects are multiple, and may be found anterior to the septomarginal trabeculation at the apex of the heart. Because these defects are often relatively anterior to the trabecular septum, they are often best profiled in the right axial oblique projection (Bargeron et al., 1977; Ceballos et al., 1981; Fellows et al., 1982; Santamaria et al., 1983; Soto et al., 1985) (Figs. 18 and 19).

Subarterial and Doubly Committed Ventricular Septal Defect

Ventricular septal defects in this area of the ventricular septum result from maldevelopment of the outlet components of both ventricles such that there is no outlet septum (Anderson et al., 1984; Capelli et al., 1983; Freedom, 1979; Momma et al., 1985). When the defect is large, with a major deficiency of the outlet septum, both arterial valves in fibrous continuity may form the roof of the ventricular septal defect. Such a defect may be confluent with perimembranous ventricular deficiencies. The importance of the subarterial ventricular septal defect to the etiology of aortic valve prolapse and aortic regurgitation is clearly established. One must be reminded, however,

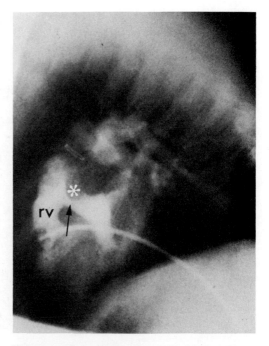

Figure 21. Subarterial and doubly committed defect with mild prolapse of pulmonary valve shown by lateral right ventricular angiography. The prolapsed pulmonary leaflet (white asterisk) forms the roof of the defect.

that deformation of the aortic root can also occur with perimembranous ventricular septal defects.

Doubly committed and subarterial defects can probably best be recognized from a left ventriculogram performed in the long axial oblique projection, and specifically the elongated right anterior oblique view (Ceballos et al., 1981; Santamaria et al., 1983; Soto et al., 1985). Early opacification of the right ventricular outflow tract is also supportive evidence of the subarterial position of the ventricular septal defect (Figs. 20–22).

When one suspects and/or confirms the presence of a subarterial type of ventricular septal defect, retrograde aortography is mandatory. The prolapsing and deformed right or noncoronary leaflet is usually nicely demonstrated by a thoracic aortogram performed in the biplane mode. The inferior border of the prolapsing and regurgitant leaflet is deformed with lobulations, the involved leaflet is usually larger than the noninvolved leaflet(s) (Fig. 22).

Malalignment Type of Outlet Ventricular Septal Defect

Posterior displacement of the outlet septum will encroach on the left ventricular outflow tract (Anderson et al., 1983B, 1984; Freedom et al., 1977A, 1977B; Moulaert et al., 1976; Smallhorn et al., 1983; Vogel et al., 1983). When the ventriculoarterial connections are concordant, such posterior displacement of the outlet septum will result in subaortic stenosis. In the most severely affected patients, aortic valve stenosis with annular hypoplasia may contribute to diffuse stenosis of the left ventricular outflow tract. The ventricular septal defect resulting

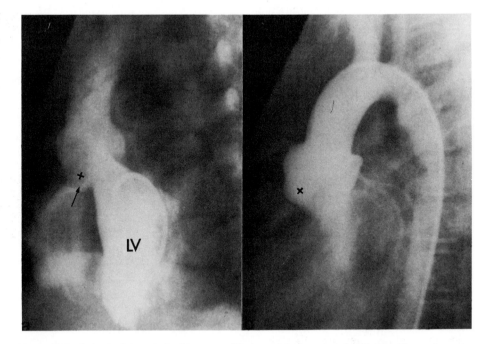

Figure 22. Subarterial and doubly committed ventricular septal defect with aortic valve prolapse. Deformed right aortic leaflet prolapses into the defect, effectively reducing its size. (a) Long axial oblique left ventricular angiogram shows the prolapsed aortic valve (×), seemingly roofing the defect (arrow). (b) Retrograde aortogram demonstrates the prolapsed and deformed right aortic leaflet (×).

from caudal displacement of the outlet septum is inferior to the muscular subaortic obstruction, and this particular type of defect is commonly found in patients with interruption of the aortic arch (Freedom et al., 1977C). It may also be observed in patients with less severe forms of obstructive anomalies of the aortic arch.

Aortic atresia can be found with a normal-sized left ventricle. With rare exception, patients with aortic atresia and a normal-sized left ventricle have an associated ventricular septal defect. We have previously shown that in some of these patients the ventricular septal defect results from caudal displacement of the outlet septum which, when it fuses with the left-sided ventriculoinfundibular fold, will result in subaortic atresia (Freedom et al., 1977D).

When the atrioventricular connections are concordant but the ventriculoarterial connections are discordant, caudal displacement of the outlet septum will result in subpulmonary obstruction of varying severity. Abnormal prominence of the left-sided ventriculoinfundibular fold in such patients may further contribute to a tunnel form of left ventricular outflow tract obstruction in complete transposition (Moene et al., 1983; Vogel et al., 1984; Waldman et al., 1984) (Fig. 23).

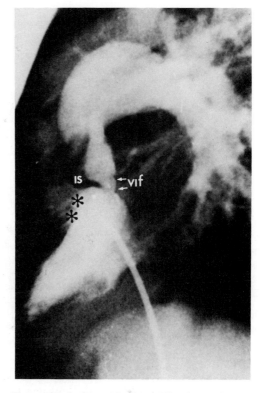

Figure 23. Left ventricular outflow tract obstruction in complete transposition. The caudally displaced outlet septum (IS) and the left-sided ventriculoinfundibular fold (VIF) wedge the outflow tract, producing a tunnel deformity. The defect (asterisk) is inferior to the displaced infundibular septum.

The Ventricular Septum and the Left Ventricular Outflow Tract in the Patient with Complete Transposition

While a defect in any portion of the ventricular septum can occur in the patient with complete transposition, such patients have a predilection toward the outlet type of ventricular septal defect (Oppenheimer-Dekker, 1978). Posterior or caudal displacement of the outlet septum in these patients can obstruct the left ventricular outflow tract, with the malalignment type of defect

inferior to the displaced outlet septum. Anterior displacement of the outlet septum will encroach on the right ventricular outflow tract, producing subaortic stenosis in the setting of complete transposition (Fig. 24). Isolated defects of the outlet septum with neither caudal nor anterior displacement can also occur. When there is no muscular rim beneath the arterial valves, then the defect is doubly committed and subarterial.

Fibrous or fibromuscular obstruction of the left ventricular outflow tract, diffuse hypoplasia of the left ventricular outflow tract, accessory tissue tags, cordal attachments from the mitral valve, or pulmonary valvular stenosis can all compromise the left

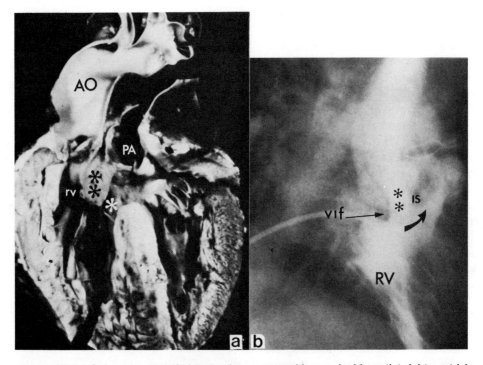

Figure 24. (a) Subaortic stenosis in complete transposition or double outlet right ventricle. Anterior displacement of the infundibular septum (asterisk) clearly narrows the right ventricular outflow tract in complete transposition. (b) This shallow right anterior oblique right ventriculogram shows the narrowed subaortic area (asterisk) wedged between the ventriculoinfundibular fold (vif) and the malaligned infundibular septum. Note the defect resulting from the displacement (asterisk).

ventricular outflow tract in complete transposition independent of the site(s) of the ventricular septal defect (Shrivastava et al., 1976; Tonkin et al., 1980). Guidelines to profile the ventricular septal defect have been discussed elsewhere in this chapter. Frequently, the long axial oblique and its reciprocal projection clearly demonstrate the nature of the subpulmonary obstruction (Freedom et al., 1984).

Multiple Ventricular Septal Defects (Figs. 25 and 26)

Multiple ventricular defects can involve any portion of the interventricular septum (Anderson et al., 1984; Fellows et al., 1982;

Santamaria et al., 1983; Soto et al., 1985; Wenink et al., 1979). Thus, no single angiographic projection can obviously fully define the potential for multiple ventricular septal defects. The long axial oblique and its reciprocal projection together with the hepatoclavicular four-chamber projection should adequately profile the posterior, perimembranous, outlet, and mid- and anterior trabecular septal structures. The use of low-ionic contrast media will allow two or more ventriculograms performed with 1.5 ml to 2.0 ml/kg body weight without jeopardizing the patient. Such multiple ventricular septal defects have been likened colloquially to a "swiss cheese" ventricular septum. But just as there are many types of swiss cheese, so too, the specific sites of the many ventricular defects require anatomical specification.

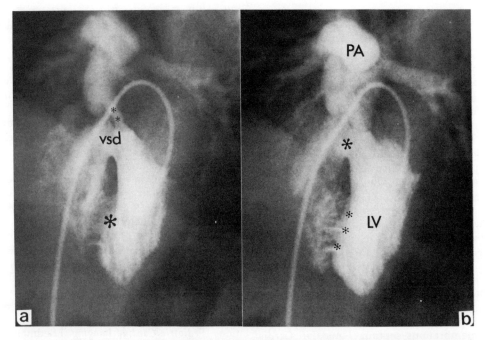

Figure 25. Multiple ventricular septal defects. (a and b) An infant with complete transposition. Left long axial oblique left ventricular angiograms. (a) A substantial perimembranous defect, and seemingly muscular defects as well. (b) The multiple defects (asterisk) are clearly seen.

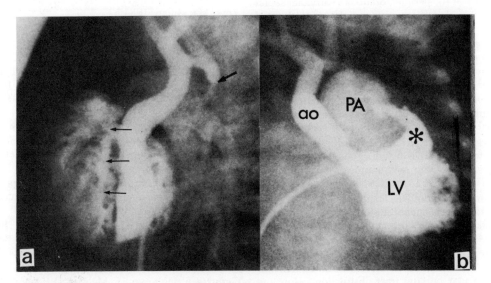

Figure 26. "Swiss cheese" ventricular septum in a neonate with coarctation (broad arrow). (a) Long axial oblique left ventriculogram shows the multiple defects (arrows). (b) Shallow right anterior oblique left ventricular angiogram demonstrates a large anterior trabecular and a low infundibular defect (asterisk) jetting into the pulmonary trunk.

References

Anderson RH, Lenox CC, Zuberbuhler JR. Mechanisms of closure of perimembranous ventricular septal defect. *Am J Cardiol* 1983A;52:341–345.

Anderson RH, Lenox CC, Zuberbuhler JR. Morphology of ventricular septal defect associated with coarctation of aorta. *Br Heart J* 1983B; 50:176–181.

Anderson RH, Lenox CC, Zuberbuhler JR. The morphology of ventricular septal defects. *Persp Pediatr Pathol* 1984;8:235–268.

Baumstark A, Fellows KE, Rosenthal A. Combined double chambered right ventricle and discrete subaortic stenosis. *Circulation* 1978;57: 299–302.

Bargeron LM Jr, Elliott LP, Soto B, et al. Axial cine-angiography in congenital heart disease. Section I. Concept, technical and anatomic considerations. *Circulation* 1977;56:1075–1083.

Beerman LB, Park SC, Fischer DR, et al. Ventricular septal defect associated with aneurysm of the membranous septum. *J Am Coll Cardiol* 1985;5:118–123.

Bernstein RF, Tei C, Child JS, Shah PM. Angled interventricular septum on echocardiography: Anatomic anomaly or technical artifact? *J Am Coll Cardiol* 1983;2:297–304.

Burrows PE, Fellows KE, Keane JF. Cineangiography of the perimembranous ventricular septal defect with left ventricular-right atrial shunt. *J Am Coll Cardiol* 1983;1:1129–1134.

Capelli H, Andrade JL, Somerville J. Classification of the site of ventricular septal defect of 2-dimensional echocardiography. *Am J Cardiol* 1983;51:1474–1480.

Ceballos R, Soto B, Bargeron LM Jr. Angiographic anatomy of the normal heart through axial angiography. *Circulation* 1981;64:351–359.

Chesler E, Korns ME, Edwards JE. Anomalies of the tricuspid valve including pouches resembling aneurysm of the membranous ventricular septum in childhood. *Am J Cardiol* 1968;21:661–668.

Chung KJ, Fulton DR, Friedberg MB, et al. Combined discrete subaortic stenosis and ventricular septal defect in infants and children. *Am J Cardiol* 1984;53:1429–1432.

Dirkson TG, Moulaert AJ, Buis-Liem TN, Brom AG. Ventricular septal defect associated with left ventricular outflow tract obstruction below the defect. *J Thorac Cardiovasc Surg* 1978;75:688–694.

Elliott LP, Bargeron LM Jr, Green CE. Angled angiography. General approach and findings. In Friedman W, Higgins CB (Eds): *Pediatric Cardiac Imaging*. Philadelphia: Saunders, 1984:1–25.

Elliott LP, Gedgaudas E, Levy M, Edwards JE. The roentgenologic findings in left ventricular-right atrial communication. *Am J Roentgenol* 1965;93:304–314.

Feigl D, Sweetman KM, Lobo KV, et al. Accessory tissue of the tricuspid valve protruding into the left ventricle through a septal defect. *Arch Pathol Lab Med* 1986;110:144–147.

Fellows KE, Keane JF, Freed MD. Angled views in cineangiocardiography of congenital heart disease. *Circulation* 1977;56:485–490.

Fellows KE, Westerman GR, Keane JF. Angiocardiography of multiple ventricular septal defects in infancy. *Circulation* 1982;66:1094–1099.

Fisher DJ, Snider AR, Silverman NH, Stanger P. Ventricular septal defect with silent discrete subaortic stenosis. *Pediatr Cardiol* 1982;2:265–269.

Freedom RM. The natural history of ventricular septal defect with morphologic considerations. In Moss AJ (Ed): *Pediatrics Update*. New York: Elsevier, 1979:251–272.

Freedom RM. Axial angiocardiography in the critically ill infant. Indications and contraindications. *Pediatric Cardiac Imaging*. Friedman W, Higgins CB (Eds): Philadelphia: WB Saunders, 1984:26–50.

Freedom RM, Bain HH, Esplugas E, et al. Ventricular septal defect in interruption of aortic arch. *Am J Cardiol* 1977C;39:572–582.

Freedom RM, Culham JAG, Moes CAF. *Angiocardiography of Congenital Heart Disease*. New York: MacMillan, 1984:525–530.

Freedom RM, Culham JAG, Rowe RD. Angiocardiography of subaortic obstruction in infancy. *Am J Roentgenol* 1977A;128:813–824.

Freedom RM, Dische MR, Rowe RD. Pathologic anatomy of subaortic stenosis and atresia in the first year of life. *Am J Cardiol* 1977B;39:1035–1044.

Freedom RM, Dische MR, Rowe RD. Conal anatomy in aortic atresia, ventricular septal defect and normally developed left ventricle. *Am Heart J* 1977D;94:689–698.

Freedom RM, Pelech A, Brand A, et al. The progressive nature of subaortic stenosis in congenital heart disease. *Int J Cardiol* 1985;8:137–143.

Freedom RM, White RD, Pieroni DR, et al. The natural history of the so-called aneurysm of the membranous ventricular septum in childhood. *Circulation* 1974;49:375–384.

Gerbode F, Hultgren H, Melrose D, Osborn J. Syndrome of left ventricular-right atrial shunt. Successful surgical repair of defect in five cases with observation of bradycardia on closure. *Ann Surg* 1958;148:433–446.

Goor D, Lillehei CW, Edwards JE. The "Sigmoid Septum". Variation in the contour of the left ventricular outlet. *Am J Roentgenol* 1969;107:366–376.

Green CE, Elliott LP, Bargeron LM Jr. Axial cineangiocardiographic evaluation of the posterior ventricular septal defect. *Am J Cardiol* 1981;48:331–335.

Moene RJ, Oppenheimer-Dekker A, Bartelings MM. Anatomic obstruction of the right ventricular outflow tract in transposition of the great arteries. *Am J Cardiol* 1983;51:1701–1704.

Moene RJ, Oppenheimer-Dekker A, Gittenberger-DeGroot A. Morphology of ventricular septal defects (VSD) occurring with coarctation of the aorta (COA). In: *Abstracts for the Annual Meeting of the Association of European Paediatric Cardiologists.* Dubrovnik, 1986, p. 15.

Moene RJ, Oppenheimer-Dekker A, Wenink ACG. Relation between aortic arch hypoplasia of variable severity and central muscular ventricular septal defects: Emphasis on associated left ventricular abnormalities. *Am J Cardiol* 1981;48:111–116.

Moene RJ, Oppenheimer-Dekker A, Moulaert AJ. The concurrence of dimensional aortic arch anomalies and abnormal left ventricular muscle bundles. *Ped Cardiol* 1982;2:107–114.

Momma K, Toyama K, Takao A. Natural history of subarterial infundibular ventricular septal defect. *Am Heart J* 1985;108:1312–1317.

Moulaert AJ, Oppenheimer-Dekker A. Anterolateral muscle bundle of the left ventricle. Bulboventricular flange and subaortic stenosis. *Am J Cardiol* 1976;37:78–81.

Moulaert AJ, Bruins CC, Oppenheimer-Dekker A. Anomalies of the aortic arch and ventricular septal defects. *Circulation* 1976;53:1011–1015.

Nanton MA, Belcourt CL, Gillis DA, et al. Left ventricular outflow tract obstruction owing to accessory endocardial cushion tissue. *J Thorac Cardiovasc Surg* 1979;78:537–541.

Oppenheimer-Dekker A. Interventricular communications in transposition of the great arteries. In Van Mierop LHS, Oppenheimer-Dekker A, Bruins C (Eds): *Embryology and Teratology of the Heart and Great Arteries.* The Hague: Leyden University Press, 1978:139–159.

Pongiglione G, Freedom RM, Cook D, Rowe RD. Mechanisms of acquired right ventricular outflow tract obstruction in patients with ventricular septal defects. An angiocardiographic study. *Am J Cardiol* 1982;50:776–780.

Puyau FA, Burko H. The tilted left anterior oblique position in the study of congenital cardiac anomalies. *Radiology* 1966;87:1069–1073.

Ramaciotti C, Keren A, Silverman NH. Importance of (perimembranous) ventricular septal an-

eurysm in the natural history of isolated perimembranous ventricular septal defect. *Am J Cardiol* 1986;57:268–272.

Santamaria H, Soto B, Ceballos R, et al. Angiographic differentiation of types of ventricular septal defects. *Am J Roentgenol* 1983;141:273–281.

Sellers RD, Lillehei CW, Edwards JE. Subaortic stenosis caused by anomalies of the atrioventricular valves. *J Thorac Cardiovasc Surg* 1964;48:289–302.

Sennari E. Morphological study of ventricular septal defect associated with obstruction of aortic arch among Japanese. *Jap Circ J* 1985;49:61–67.

Shore DR, Smallhorn J, Stark J, et al. Left ventricular outflow tract obstruction coexisting with ventricular septal defect. *Br Heart J* 1982;48:421–427.

Shrivastava S, Tadivarthy SM, Fukuda T, Edwards JE. Anatomic causes of pulmonary stenosis in complete transposition. *Circulation* 1976;54:154–159.

Smallhorn JF, Anderson RH, Macartney FJ. Morphological characterization of ventricular septal defects associated with coarctation of the aorta by cross sectional echocardiography. *Br Heart J* 1983;49:485–494.

Soto B, Bargeron LM Jr, Diethelm E. Ventricular septal defect. *Semin Roentgenology* 1985;20:200–213.

Soto B, Bargeron LM Jr, Pacifico AD, et al. Angiography of atrioventricular canal defects. *Am J Cardiol* 1981;48:492–499.

Sutherland GR, Godman MJ, Smallhorn JF, et al. Ventricular septal defects: Two dimensional echocardiographic and morphologic correlations. *Br Heart J* 1982;47:316–328.

Tonkin IL, Sansa M, Elliott LP, Bargeron LM Jr. Recognition of developing left ventricular outflow tract obstruction in complete transposition of the great arteries. *Radiology* 1980;134:53–59.

Vogel M, Freedom RM, Brand A, et al. Ventricular septal defect and subaortic stenosis: An analysis of 41 patients. *Am J Cardiol* 1983;52:1258–1263.

Vogel M, Freedom RM, Smallhorn JF, et al. Complete transposition of the great arteries and coarctation of the aorta. *Am J Cardiol* 1984;53:1627–1632.

Waldman JD, Schneeweiss A, Edwards WD, et al. The obstructive subaortic conus. *Circulation* 1984;70:339–344.

Wenink ACG, Oppenheimer-Dekker A, Moulaert AJ. Muscular ventricular septal defects. Reappraisal of the anatomy. *Am J Cardiol* 1979;43:259–264.

Ventricular Septal Defect: Anatomy in Relation to Clinical Outcome

Jane Somerville

Even in 1987 it is essential to initiate my essay with a mention of terminology. So mutable, complex, and even emotional, has become "naming the rose" in pediatric cardiology that the reader may not follow what is being discussed unless it is clearly defined. Most gardeners (specialists) are able to recognize their own roses, but terms used do not always convey similar information to the interested bystander. In order, therefore, that my thoughts and findings will be understood, the nomenclature used by myself and colleagues (Capelli et al., 1983) will be described and amplified. This is done in the interests of classification rather than as a proselytizing effort for conversion to a new faith.

An acceptable terminology for ventricular septal defects must be usable by all disciplines who encouter these lesions: clinicians, pediatricians, surgeons, radiologists, anatomists, and echocardiographers. Of equal importance is that the same terminology can, and should, be used in those malformations where a ventricular septal defect is associated with other anomalies such as complete or corrected transposition, double outlet left or right ventricle, double inlet ventricles, tricuspid atresia, and so on. I appreciate that each specialist has a different view of the ventricular septum and, as in life, that what is "up" to one may be "down" to another. It is my belief that terminology derived from embryological concepts, so frequently myths, has no place in clinical use. "What does a structure do?" is more relevant to understanding and management than "where does it come from?" For these reasons, ventricular septal defects are classified here according to whether they are subvalvular, or muscular, the site being determined as viewed from the right ventricle (Fig. 1). It is possible for a ventricular septal defect to be beneath, and bordered

From: Anderson, RH, Neches, WH, Park, SC, Zuberbuhler, JR, eds: *Perspectives in Pediatric Cardiology*: Mount Kisco, New York, Futura Publishing Co., © 1988.

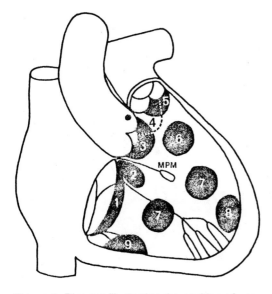

Figure 1. Diagram illustrating the position of ventricular septal defects. 1–5, subvalvular; 6–9, muscular. 1 = inlet; 2 = subtricuspid; 3 = subaortic; 4 = subarterial doubly committed; 5 = subpulmonary; 6 = outlet; 7 = central; 8 = apical; 9 = posterior. MPM = medial papillary muscle (muscle of Lancisi).

by one or more of the four valves in the heart, and it is designated accordingly; when beneath all four, as in some complex anomalies, it is locally referred to as a subcommittee!

Subvalvular defects may be as follows:

1. Subtricuspid: beneath the septal cusp of tricuspid valve.
2. Submitral: this occurs only when it is beneath both atrioventricular valves (see no. 5).
3. Subaortic: as in Fallot.
4. Subpulmonary: outflow or supracristal.
5. Subtricuspid and submitral: when both valves are at the same level (inlet defects or so-called canal-type).
6. Subaortic and subpulmonary: doubly committed subarterial.

Muscular defects are simply designated according to their site in muscular septum: apical, central, outflow, or posterior. Valve leaflets do not form their border, although they may be close, and muscle surrounds the defect.

The weakness in this simple but effective approach is in the description of the defects immediately beneath both arterial valves. The subpulmonary defect (outlet or "supracristal") appears from the right ventricular side to be related to the pulmonary valve leaflets but, when small, it is not obvious that it is also contiguous to the aortic valve lying on the other side. This becomes evident when the aortic leaflet prolapses, which is an important part of the natural history of such defects. This subpulmonary defect is sometimes large, extending beneath much of the pulmonary valve. When there is no pulmonary valve stenosis, there is inevitable pulmonary hypertension and prolapse of the pulmonary leaflets may partially close the hole. When subpulmonary defects, as viewed from the right ventricle, extend more posteriorly to be placed beneath the aortic valve (because of absence or deficiency of infundibular septum), they are called doubly committed and subarterial. Similarly, the different and readily recognized subaortic defect (found with Fallot), which is separated from the pulmonary valve by the subpulmonary infundibulum, is easily recognized from the right ventricular aspect.

In studies on changing form and function of congenital cardiac anomalies, it was clear to me that the most important determinant of natural history of large ventricular septal defects was their site (Somerville, 1979). When we looked at a group of infants presenting with failure in infancy with documented large ventricular septal defects, cardiomegaly, and elevated pulmonary arterial pressure and flow, but who did not have surgery for various reasons, it was revealed that the defect became smaller or closed spontaneously in about half over an observation period of 4 to 12 years (Table 1). In contrast, 15% of defects remained large. These patients died, developed the Eisenmenger reaction, remained in chronic failure, or developed the signs of hyperkinetic pulmonary hypertension and cardiomegaly such that they needed to have surgery later.

Table 1
Natural History 92 Pts. Large VSD
Causing Failure Infancy

Age 6/52–8 mths.—1964–1970
(Selected Series)

Stay Same (Death 1st yr.–3)	8%
↑ PVR (Eisenmenger)	7%
→ Fallot	6%
Severe Inf. St. ± Small VSD	2%
→ Small VSD	64%
Close completely	13%

85% have change in form

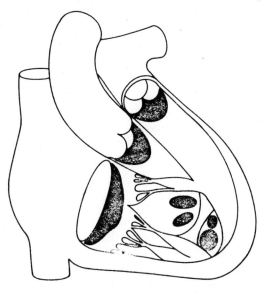

Figure 2. This diagram illustrates those defects that do not close. They are the subvalvular ones that are roofed by large expanses of valve leaflet (submitral and subtricuspid; subaortic; and doubly committed and subarterial) along with multiple muscular defects.

The anatomy of those defects that stay open and remain large is shown in Figure 2. The reason that closure of subaortic and doubly committed defects cannot take place is because, in every systole, the cephalad borders (formed by the leaflets of the arterial valves) are open. Similarly, the inlet defect that is both submitral and subtricuspid is too long to be sealed off completely by extensive and separated cusp tissue derived from the septal leaflet of the tricuspid valve. Sometimes the anterior portion may be closed off by this leaflet, but not the rest, since the leaflet is mobile, billows backwards in systole, and increases the size of the functioning defect. Large and multiple muscular ventricular septal defects with strands of tissue between them have no way of becoming smaller in systole. This is in contrast to smaller muscular defects, adequately surrounded by muscle, which can close off.

It is noteworthy that the type of ventricular septal defect found in older patients with the Eisenmenger reaction is the same as in the infants whose ventricular septal defects remain large (Table 2). Thus, it is clear that such defects are associated with a bad clinical outcome and, when identified in infancy, they should be closed without delay.

The anatomy of those ventricular septal defects that become smaller or close is different. Fewer close completely than become spontaneously smaller in the first three to eight years. The process of closure, however, can go on into adult life. This fact probably accounts for the rarity of the small ventricular septal defect in middle age or the elderly. There are three types of ventricular septal defect that close or become smaller (Fig. 3). The most common, in this series, was the subtricuspid defect. Solitary muscular defects, particularly when centrally placed, often closed, as did outflow or apical muscular defects (Fig. 4). Closure was a slower process with these than with subtricuspid defects. The small subpulmonary defect can be sealed by a prolapsing leaflet of the aortic valve. Such patients have a history of a murmur or the diagnosis of ventricular septal defect early in life. Later they present with aortic regurgitation, sometimes without clinical evidence of a ventricular septal defect which may be larger than expected at operation.

There are several different ways in which nature closes subtricuspid ventricular

Table 2
Type of VSD *in Eisenmenger Reaction*

21 Pts. Aged 11–42 yrs. Large–20 (95%)	
Subaortic (like Fallot)	9 (43%)
Subarterial (Doubly Com.)	3
Sub. Tric./Mitral (Inlet)	3
Sub. Pulm. Outflow	2
Multiple Musc. or Mixed	4

septal defects. Either fibrosis starts at the edges and spreads inwards, the septal leaflet of the valve adheres to the edges, or tissue tags are derived from the underside of the leaflets forming an "aneurysm of the membranous septum" in the inflow of the right ventricle (Anderson et al., 1983). If there is added pulmonary stenosis, the "aneurysm" will prolapse into the left outflow, causing subaortic stenosis. This is what happens in classic complete transposition. Exceptionally, the prolapsed leaflet tissue or aneurysm in the right ventricle can be large enough to cause tricuspid stenosis or long

enough to cause right ventricular outflow obstruction. Sometimes the tags derived from the valve leaflet are not enough to close over the whole defect, so that a hole remains surrounded by bulges of tethered valve tissue (Fig. 5). In this setting, the residual shunt may be directed from left ventricle to right atrium. These are the ventricular septal defects that are most likely to be the site of future endocarditis.

As can be seen from Table 1, 6% of patients with large ventricular septal defect and an initial left-to-right shunt changed to present later as mild Fallot's tetralogy with cyanotic attacks and a decrease in heart size. These patients may have had enough left-to-right shunt during early infancy to precipitate failure, but are predestined to develop infundibular stenosis because they were born with an abnormally positioned and structured outlet septum together with muscle bands which encircle the subpulmonary outflow tract. Even when the infant is in failure, the presence of displaced muscle on the right ventricular angiograms can

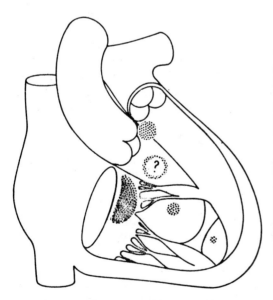

Figure 3. This diagram shows the sites of defects that will close. They are the subtricuspid defect along with small subpulmonary and small muscular defects.

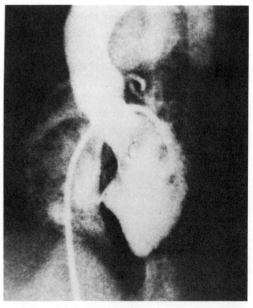

Figure 4. This left ventricular angiogram shows a midmuscular defect that has virtually closed. The "funnel" effect illustrates its initial large size.

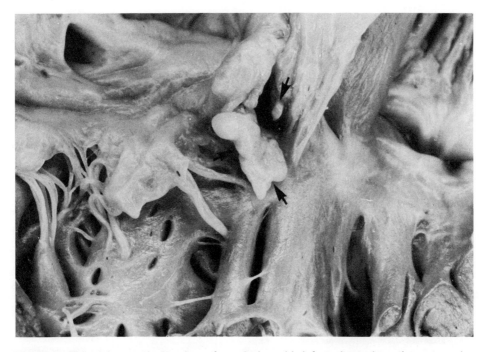

Figure 5. This right ventricular view of a subtricuspid defect shows how tissue tags (arrowed) have almost but not quite closed the hole, leaving a small residual defect.

be recognized even when, at first, they offer no obstruction (Fig. 6). A mild abnormality of the pulmonary valve often coexists. With stimulus of right ventricular work and hypertension, the muscle bands hypertrophy and become obstructive. At first the obstruction is labile but subsequently a fixed narrowing due to fibroelastic tissue is deposited over the muscle as the result of turbulence. It is neither urgent nor mandatory to close these ventricular septal defects during infancy, although doing so might prevent the progression of infundibular stenosis. It is important, however, to recognize the potential for forming infundibular obstruction so that there is warning about cyanotic attacks. As this happens, the chest radiograph shows the heart becoming smaller with reduction in pulmonary flow. Right ventricular hypertrophy increases, as seen on the electrocardiogram, with the electrical axis shifting to the right. Delay in pulmonary valve closure with ultimate loss of the pulmonary sound is usual. The murmur be-

comes obviously ejection and remains loud. The pulmonary arteries are large as the result of carrying a large flow.

Despite spontaneous closure of a ventricular septal defect, some unwanted problems may remain or even develop. Pulmonary vascular disease may already be established by the time the defect closes or becomes smaller. This may not manifest until after puberty or in adult life when the pulmonary arterial pressure rises to cause symptoms. Such patients may appear to have "primary" pulmonary hypertension because the early history is ignored or unknown. This can also occur in patients with acquired infundibular stenosis and large ventricular septal defect. It accounts for the development of progressive pulmonary hypertension after good repair in older children, adolescents, and adults who have had "mild" or "acyanotic" Fallot's tetralogy. In such patients, the significance of a pulmonary arterial pressure of 30 to 50 mmHg distal to the stenosis should not be ignored.

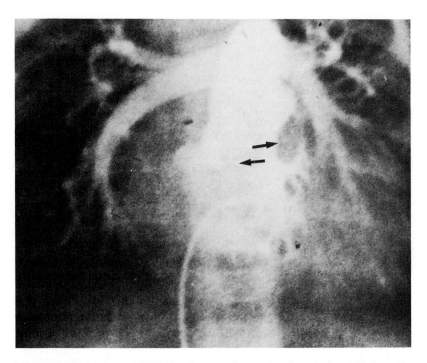

Figure 6. This right ventricular angiogram shows the abnormal muscle bundles in the outflow tract of a patient who, at this stage, has a wide subpulmonary outflow tract but who subsequently developed the appearance of tetralogy of Fallot.

Late heart block can also develop after spontaneous closure of a subtricuspid ventricular septal defect. Initially, left axis deviation may appear and, if block occurs later, presumably the same fibrotic reaction that has been involved in closing the defect affects the conduction tissue (which is adjacent to its posteroinferior margin). In the usual subtricuspid ventricular septal defects, the conduction axis is well separated from the edge of the defect. Hence, the rarity of conduction tissue involvement with such defects. Perhaps the rare development of block after spontaneous closure of this defect is a coincidental late development. The frequent progression to left axis deviation from a normal axis during closure, however, supports the view that it is not.

Another problem that may show after closure of a ventricular septal defect is progressive infundibular stenosis. This requires the combination of the congenital deformity of the right outflow tract which predisposes to the formation of fixed infundibular obstruction together with the type of ventricular septal defect that can close spontaneously. Usually when infundibular obstruction has developed, the associated ventricular septal defect is of the subaortic type, which remains large (Fallot's tetralogy). "Lone" infundibular stenosis with closed ventricular septal defect may take the form of a muscular/fibrous ring obstruction beneath the valve or else a muscular obstruction close to the apex which divides the inflow and outflow portions of the right ventricle, giving rise to so-called "two-chamber" right ventricle. The scar of the closed defect can be found at operation (if looked for), and preoperative left ventricular angiography can disclose an unusual pit or pouch.

There are other morphological correlations that are important in the management of ventricular septal defects. The association of ventricular septal defect with subaortic stenosis and with aortic regurgitation is important. There are two variants found with coexistent subaortic stenosis. The uncommon type is when a subpulmonary ventricular septal defect is proximal to the subaortic obstruction produced by displacement of the muscular outlet septum into the left ventricle. This arrangement (the Becu complex) is present in fetal development and deflects blood flow away from the aorta and results in the commonly associated aortic arch anomalies and early established pulmonary vascular disease (Becu et al., 1955). The subaortic obstruction may progress rapidly. In the other, more frequent, type, the ventricular septal defect is distal to, or beside, the obstruction. The obstructive lesion is acquired and, as in other types of fixed aortic stenosis, manifests later in childhood. Indeed, it may form as the ventricular septal defect is spontaneously closing or closed. This is another reason for careful follow-up of patients with small and closing ventricular septal defects in whom the left ventricular outflow tract should be routinely screened by echocardiography. This type of ventricular septal defect with subaortic stenosis may be found with classic coarctation. More frequently, it is not associated with such anomalies. The anatomical abnormality of the left ventricular outflow which predisposes to formation of such obstructive lesions is difficult to document. In some, the obstructing remnant protrudes from the area of fibrous continuity between the aortic and mitral valves. In most, the obstructive shelf is formed on the septal subaortic surface as in "fixed" subaortic stenosis with an intact ventricular septum. As with the latter (and more common) lesion, the shelf is not membranous and is not congenital (Somerville, 1985). The ventricular septal defect may be subtricuspid or more anterior but separated from the aortic valve.

Aortic regurgitation with ventricular septal defect arises with three forms of defects. These have to be distinguished from one another since their natural history and management are different. In the group most common in the Far East, the defect is subpulmonary (outflow), usually but not always small, and is associated with deformity of the right aortic sinus which is evident before the prolapse of the leaflet. It is likely that the whole outflow portion of the heart is abnormal since the right aortic sinus, irrespective of the presence or degree of aortic valve regurgitation, is unusually anterior and rotated to the left (anticlockwise as viewed by the surgeon; Somerville et al., 1970). It is thus possible, indeed likely, that there is a "weakness" or basic abnormality that may predispose to prolapse, generally of the right, and less often of the noncoronary leaflet, or both. Aortic regurgitation may develop at any age but is rare before the age of three years. It may lead to closure of the defect and is progressive, sometimes with unexpected rapidity. It can cause a windsock-like obstruction of the right outflow tract. In some patients, the defect is obviously doubly committed and large.

When aortic regurgitation complicates ventricular septal defect in our series (U.K. and Northern Europe), the defect is more frequently subaortic, separated from the outflow, and less anterior. This is found in more than half of those patients who present with ventricular septal defect and aortic regurgitation. Because of aortic root dilation, which is usual in large subaortic ventricular septal defect, there may be prolapse of an aortic leaflet, right or noncoronary, into the right ventricle, or all three may fail to coapt centrally. The resulting aortic regurgitation may be directed to the right or left ventricular cavities. This is an age-related and acquired problem and is to be expected in adolescent and adult patients with tetralogy of Fallot, particularly if shunted, and in those with "complex" pulmonary atresia (see Chapter 3.2). It also occurs as a result of endocarditis in these lesions where the aortic valve is the major target. Often the aortic regurgitation is missed because attention is not focused on this possibility (Capelli et al., 1982).

A small group of patients, about 15%, have ventricular septal defects of any type with congenitally abnormal aortic valves which are bicuspid, floppy, stenosed, or regurgitant. The management of these patients depends on the severity of the aortic regurgitation and the size of the ventricular septal defect. These features have to be judged separately.

The principles governing the behavior of the ventricular septal defect work irrespective of the associated lesions, although the effects may be different and even disastrous. Closure of a ventricular septal defect with "aneurysm" formation with complete transposition may cause subpulmonary stenosis and obstruct the outflow of the left ventricle. This may occur after pulmonary vascular disease has become established and even advanced, so that results of surgery may be unexpectedly disastrous. Reduction in the size of a ventricular septal defect with double outlet right ventricle leads to subaortic stenosis when the defect opens beneath the aorta.

The naming of these different roses, with their varying thorns, forms, and habits, is vital for communication and comparison to increase our knowledge. Whatever the size of the ventricular septal defect or its associated lesions, its site and anatomical neighbor remain the most important determination of its effect on the patient's life.

References

Anderson RH, Lenox CC, Zuberbuhler JR. Mechanisms of closure of perimembranous ventricular septal defect. *Am J Cardiol* 1983;52:341–345.

Becu LM, Tauxe WN, DuShane JW, Edwards JE. A complex of congenital cardiac anomalies: Ventricular septal defect, biventricular origin of the pulmonary trunk and subaortic stenosis. *Am Heart J* 1955;50:901–911.

Capelli H, Ross D, Somerville J. Aortic regurgitation in tetrad of Fallot and pulmonary atresia. *Am J Cardiol* 1982;42:1979–1983.

Capelli H, Andrade JL, Somerville J. Classification of the site of ventricular septal defect by 2-dimensional echocardiography. *Am J Cardiol* 1983;51:1474–1480.

Somerville J. Congenital heart disease: Changes in form and function. *Br Heart J* 1979;41:1–22.

Somerville J. Fixed subaortic stenosis—a frequently misunderstood lesion. *Int J Cardiol* 1985;8:145–148.

Somerville J, Brandao A, Ross D. Aortic regurgitation with ventricular septal defect. *Circulation* 1970;41:317–330.

Sommerville J, Stone S, Ross D. Fate of patients with fixed subaortic stenosis after surgical removal. *Br Heart J* 1980;43:629–647

Pulmonary Circulation in Ventricular Septal Defect

Marlene Rabinovitch

The functional and structural responses of the pulmonary circulation to the altered hemodynamics caused by a ventricular septal defect can be major determinants of the timing and the outcome of surgical intervention. Infants with large unrestrictive ventricular septal defects may have severe congestive heart failure if the pulmonary vascular resistance falls rapidly. Alternatively, there may be no congestive heart failure if the response is one of intense vasoconstriction from birth. In both groups, surgical repair may result in normal pulmonary artery pressure in the early postoperative period. Alternatively, severe labile pulmonary hypertension may occur if the vascular bed is hyperreactive. Early surgical intervention is usually associated with regression of even advanced pulmonary vascular structural changes but, rarely, there may be rapid progression despite relatively mild abnormalities at the time of repair.

The patients with intense pulmonary vasoconstriction from birth are less likely to be identified as having a severe cardiac le-

sion prior to the development of advanced pulmonary vascular changes. Those who are "hyperreactive" may succumb in the early postoperative period from low cardiac output secondary to a pulmonary hypertensive crisis. Those who develop rapid progression of pulmonary vascular disease are inevitably ill-fated. It is therefore important to identify the cellular mechanisms responsible for both pulmonary vasoconstriction and for the initiation and propagation of structural changes in the pulmonary arteries. The following, then, describes the nature and time course of pulmonary vascular changes in the setting of an infant with a large ventricular septal defect and the correlation of these abnormalities with the pre- and postoperative hemodynamics of the pulmonary circulation. The discussion which follows addresses the changes in structure, function, and interaction of endothelial and smooth-muscle cells that may govern heightened pulmonary vascular reactivity. New information is presented concerning the potential significance of degra-

From: Anderson, RH, Neches, WH, Park, SC, Zuberbuhler, JR, eds: *Perspectives in Pediatric Cardiology*: Mount Kisco, New York, Futura Publishing Co., © 1988.

dation and synthesis of connective-tissue proteins (collagen, elastin, glycoproteins) in the development of fixed pulmonary hypertension and progressive vascular obstruction.

Nature and Time Course of Pulmonary Vascular Changes

The mechanism that determines the normal fall in pulmonary vascular resistance at birth is not known. But, when this occurs in the presence of a large unrestrictive ventricular septal defect, the hemodynamics of the pulmonary circulation are altered dramatically. The pulmonary vascular bed is exposed to torrential flow, to persistent elevation in systolic and diastolic pressure with a wide pulse pressure, and to a high oxygen saturation. Congestive heart failure usually follows, so there is also elevated venous pressure and pulmonary edema. More rarely, the pulmonary vascular bed may respond by intense vasoconstriction. How each of these pulmonary circulatory changes influences the development of structural changes in the arteries is not understood (DuShane et al., 1976, Hoffman and Rudolph, 1965).

We have, however, shown that there are progressive abnormalities in the normal pattern of growth and remodeling of pulmonary arteries (Fig. 1A,B) (Hislop et al., 1975). These correlate with the general hemodynamic response of the pulmonary circulation to a ventricular septal defect. These structural changes have come to be known as the A,B,C's of pulmonary vascular disease (Rabinovitch et al., 1978).

GRADE A: There is abnormal extension of muscle into small peripheral arteries; in other words, those accompanying alveolar ducts and those within the alveolar walls that are normally nonmuscular. There may, in addition, be a minimal increase in the wall thickness of the normally muscular arteries (less than 1.5 times normal). Patients

Peripheral Pulmonary Arterial Development

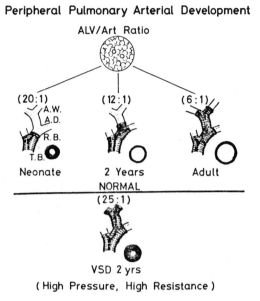

Figure 1A. Schema of normal peripheral pulmonary arterial development and abnormal development in a child with a ventricular septal defect and high pulmonary artery pressure and resistance at two years. Normally, muscle extends with age into arteries more peripheral within the acinus; the wall thickness of the normally muscular arteries decreases and there is a decreasing ratio of alveoli to arteries, indicating an increase in the number of arteries. In a child with a ventricular septal defect, abnormalities in all three features of normal growth and remodeling may be seen, i.e., "precocious" extension of muscle into peripheral arteries, medial hypertrophy of muscular arteries, and a reduced concentration of arteries, i.e., increased alveolar arterial ratio. T.B. = artery accompanying a terminal bronchiolus; R.B. = artery accompanying a respiratory bronchiolus; A.D. = artery accompanying an alveolar duct; A.W. = artery accompanying an alveolar wall; ALV-Art = alveolar-arterial ratio. (Reproduced with permission from Rabinovitch et al., *Circulation* 1978.)

with a ventricular septal defect and these structural features will have increased pulmonary blood flow and widened pulse pressure but normal mean pulmonary arterial pressure. From ultrastructural studies (Meyrick and Reid, 1980), it has been shown that extension of muscle into normally nonmuscular peripheral arteries is due to abnormal differentiation of precursor cells to

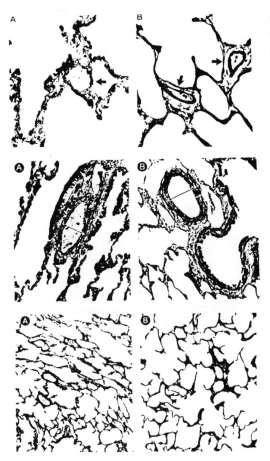

Figure 1B. Morphometric features on lung biopsy tissue. Left: A two-year-old patient with ventricular septal defect and normal pulmonary artery pressure. Right: A two-year-old with a defect of the atrioventicular septum and increased pulmonary artery pressure and resistance. Top: Alveolar wall arteries (arrows) nonmuscularized on left and surrounded by a complete nonmuscularized coat on right ×175. Middle: Artery accompanying respiratory bronchiolus (RB) on left with wall thickness only slightly increased, and on right with wall thickness greatly increased ×70. Arrows denote external diameter and medial width. Bottom: An abundance of small arteries (arrows) relative to alveoli on left and only one small artery in a similar microscopic field on right. (Elastin von Gieson stain.) (Reproduced with permission from Rabinovitch et al., *Circulation* 1978.)

the partially muscular region (Fig. 2). Since peripheral arteries normally become more muscular during childhood as they grow to a certain size, it is tempting to speculate that the stimulus for the precocious change is "stretching" of the cells due to the widened pulse pressure produced by a left-to-right shunt. The intimate relationship between the endothelial cells and the underlying pericytes and intermediate cells begs further speculation that the endothelial cells might "sense" the "stretch" and send a metabolic message to induce differentiation of the precursor cells.

GRADE B: As in so-called Grade A, there is increased extension of muscle but, in addition, there is more severe medial hypertrophy of normally muscular arteries. When medial wall thickness is greater than 1.5 but less than 2 times normal (Grade B mild), mild pulmonary hypertension is usually present. When medial wall thickness is more than twice normal (Grade B severe), pulmonary hypertension is always present, often with pressure values greater than half systemic level. The medial thickness is due to hypertrophy as well as hyperplasia of preexisting smooth-muscle cells and also to an increase in the intercellular ground substance (Meyrick and Reid, 1980). What induces medial hypertrophy is unknown, but our own recent observations in lung biopsy tissue have provided some clues. As medial hypertrophy occurs, there is breakdown of the internal elastic lamina resulting in close interdigitation between endothelial and smooth-muscle cells (Rabinovitch et al., 1986) (Fig. 3). This process may facilitate transfer of endothelial-derived growth factors which stimulate smooth-muscle proliferation. Breakdown of the elastic lamina may occur via direct release of elastase from altered endothelial cells, or indirectly as a result of abnormal endothelial interaction with neutrophils.

GRADE C: In addition to the findings in the so-called severe Grade B variant, arterial concentration is reduced together with arte-

smooth muscle. The precursor cells are the pericyte in the nonmuscular region of the arterial pathway and the intermediate cell in

MUSCULAR   PARTIALLY   NON-MUSCULAR
              MUSCULAR   & CAPILLARY

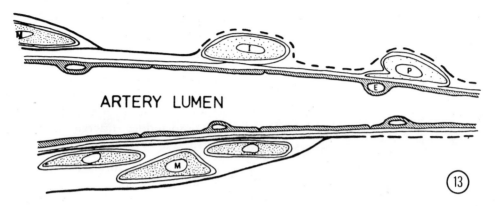

Figure 2. Diagram of the cells in the wall of the distal part of a pulmonary artery. The smooth-muscle cells (M) of the medial muscular coat are surrounded by a discrete basement membrane and are situated between both an internal and external elastic lamina (thick black lines). In the nonmuscular region of the partially muscular artery, the "intermediate" cell (I) is seen. This cell is surrounded by a basement membrane that fuses, in regions, with that of the endothelial cell (E) and is situated internal to the single fragmented internal elastic lamina (broken dashed lines). In the wall of the nonmuscular artery and alveolar capillary, the pericyte (P) is found. This cell is ensheathed by a basement membrane which is continuous with and thereby shares the basement membrane of the associated artery, and like the "intermediate" cell, it is situated internal to the single elastic lamina. (Reproduced with permission from Meyrick and Reid, *Lab Invest* 1978.)

rial size. Patients with these changes usually have an elevation in pulmonary vascular resistance. When arterial number is more than half normal (Grade C mild), pulmonary vascular resistance is usually 3.5–6 U/m². When arterial number is less than half normal (Grade C severe), pulmonary vascular resistance values are often in excess of 6 U/m². The basis of this pattern of grading (Grade C) is likely the failure of new vessels to grow normally, although loss of small arteries through resorption may also occur as has been described in idiopathic pulmonary hypertension (Meyrick et al., 1974).

Whether and to what extent abnormal growth and structural remodeling of the pulmonary vascular bed is associated with heightened pulmonary vascular reactivity or else results in permanent functional impair-

ment has been determined by correlating the morphological features with postoperative hemodynamic studies. We correlated both the quantitative "morphometric" features (A,B,C), and the qualitative changes described by Heath and Edwards (1958) (Fig. 4) with the hemodynamic behavior of the pulmonary circulation. We did this both in the immediate postoperative period in the Intensive Care Unit (Fig. 5A) and one year later at the time of routine cardiac catheter study (Rabinovitch et al., 1984) (Fig. 5B). Morphometric Grades A and B are quantitative refinements of the Grade I of Heath and Edwards (medial hypertrophy), whereas Grade C is a feature not previously considered. In our experience, cellular intimal hyperplasia (Heath-Edwards Grade II) is often associated with Grade C (a reduced number of arteries), whereas occlusive inti-

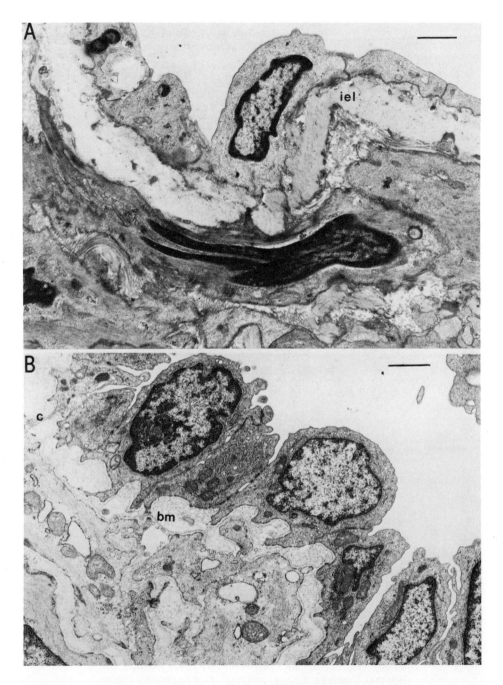

Figure 3. (A) an electron photomicrograph of a respiratory bronchiolus pulmonary artery 92 μm external diameter shows an intact internal elastic lamina (iel). (B) photomicrograph from a terminal bronchiolus pulmonary artery 108 μm external diameter shows only microfibrillar material in the subendothelium but no internal elastic lamina. Endothelial and smooth-muscle cells are separated by only a thick basement membrane (bm). A myoendothelial contact (c) is seen. Bar = 1 μm in both. (Reproduced with permission from Rabinovitch et al., *Lab Invest* 1986.)

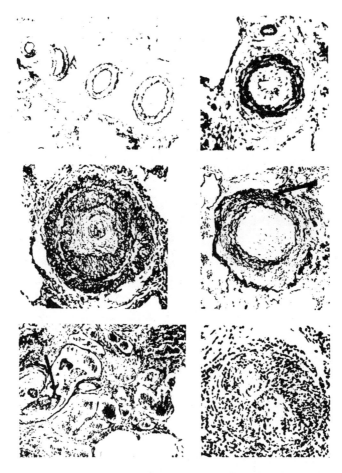

Figure 4. Heath-Edwards classification of pulmonary vascular changes. (A) Grade I: medial hypertrophy. (Elastin van Gieson ×150) (B) Grade II: cellular intimal proliferation in an abnormally muscular artery. (EVG, ×250) (C) Grade III: occlusive changes. Media is thickened due to fasciculi of longitudinal muscle, and vessel is all but occluded by fibroelastic tissue. (EVG, ×150) (D) Grade IV: dilation. Vessel is dilated, and media is abnormally thin (arrow). Lumen is occluded by fibrous tissue. (EVG, ×150) (E) Grade V: plexiform lesion. There is cellular intimal proliferation (arrow); clustered around are numerous thin walled vessels which terminate as capillaries in the alveolar wall. (EVG, ×95) (F) Grade VI: acute necrotizing arteritis. A severe reactive acute inflammatory exudate is seen through all layers of the vessel. (hematoxylineosin, ×250) (Reproduced with permission from Wagenvoort CA, Heath D, Edwards JE: *The Pathology of the Pulmonary Vasculature*. Charles C. Thomas, Springfield, IL, 1964.)

mal hyperplasia with fibroelastosis of the media (Heath-Edwards Grade III) almost always is. Dilation complexes and plexiform lesions (Heath-Edwards, Grade IV), angiomata in the adventitia (Heath-Edwards

Grade V), and fibrinoid necrosis (Heath-Edwards Grade VI) are lesions seen only in very advanced disease. These latter changes exclude corrective surgery.

We observed that patients with Grade

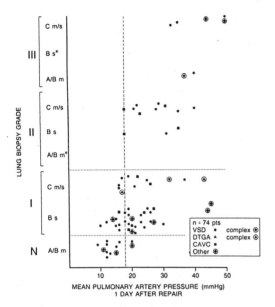

Figure 5A. Lung biopsy grade is correlated with mean pulmonary arterial pressure recorded the day after surgical repair. The dashed vertical lines separate the normal from the abnormally elevated pressure values and the dotted horizontal lines separate the biopsy grades. Note that with the more severe Heath-Edwards changes on lung biopsy tissue, there is a trend toward a greater proportion of patients with elevated pulmonary arterial pressures and higher values. A, B, C, are morphometric grades; m = mild, s = severe; N, I, II, III are Heath-Edwards grades, N = normal, * = no patients in this group; VSD = ventricular septal defect; DTGA = complete transposition; CAVC = complete atrioventricular septal defect; complex = associated abnormality.

A changes have a normal level of pulmonary arterial pressure in the early postoperative period. If the value is increased, it is a minimal change. Patients with more severe medial hypertrophy (Grade B severe, Heath-Edwards I) often have elevated pulmonary arterial pressure and frequently suffer one or more pulmonary hypertensive crises (Jones et al., 1981). Both the presence and the severity of pulmonary hypertension in the early postoperative period are more predictable when there are more advanced changes such as a reduced number of arteries (Grade C) and intimal hyperplasia (Heath-Edwards II-III). The severity of early postoperative pulmonary hypertension is better predicted from the lung biopsy findings than from preoperative pulmonary arterial pressure or resistance values (Fig. 5C).

One year after repair, patients operated within the first eight months of life tend to have normal pulmonary hemodynamics regardless of the severity of vascular changes in the lung biopsy section. So do all patients with vascular abnormalities of only B severity (Heath-Edwards I), regardless of their age at repair. Patients with more advanced vascular changes may have persistent elevation in pulmonary vascular resistance, particularly if they are between nine months and two years of age at the time of repair. This will be even more likely if they are older than two years of age.

This information has encouraged us successfully to apply both quantitative and qualitative methods of analysis to lung biopsy tissue prepared by frozen section to help the surgeon decide between a palliative and a corrective procedure when preoperative hemodynamic data are borderline or difficult to obtain or interpret (Rabinovitch et al., 1981). It must be ensured, however, that the section is adequate. Specifically, several pre-acinar arteries must be included (Haworth and Reid, 1978; Haworth, 1984).

Techniques of quantitative wedge angiography have also been developed to assess the severity of structural abnormalities in the pulmonary vascular bed preoperatively (Rabinovitch et al., 1981) (Fig. 6). The abruptness of tapering of the subsegmental arteries correlates with the severity of vascular disease in the intra-acinar arteries assessed both morphometrically and by the Heath-Edwards classification. Decreased background filling and increased pulmonary circulation time are predictive of patients with advanced changes. There are, however, some pitfalls in the interpretation of the wedge angiogram. An incomplete injection will give the impression of decreased background filling. Incomplete occlusion of the vessel by the balloon will make the circulation time falsely rapid. Previous placement of a pulmonary arterial band will, because of poststenotic dilation, give the false

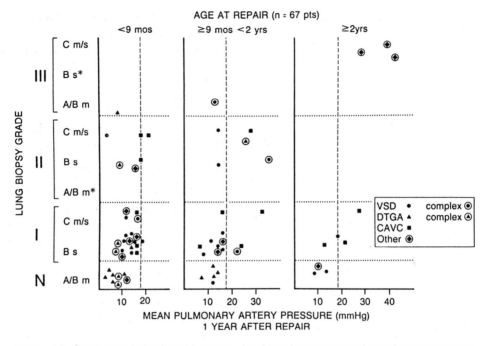

Figure 5B. Graph correlating lung biopsy grade with pulmonary vascular resistance one year after cardiac repair. Patients who underwent repair within the first eight months of life, but not those operated on later, had normal pulmonary vascular resistance regardless of the severity of their structural changes.

impression of "abrupt tapering." Also, some patients with advanced pulmonary vascular disease will not have abrupt tapering because intimal hyperplasia has extended even into larger pre-acinar arteries, narrowing the lumen uniformly. The same will be true of patients who have had severe vasoconstriction from birth and never had much of a left-to-right shunt. Both the latter groups will, however, have a decrease in background filling and a prolongation of the pulmonary circulation time. These features are not seen in patients with mild vascular changes.

The Reactive Pulmonary Circulation

A major challenge in managing the patient with a ventricular septal defect is to understand and control the reactive pulmo-

nary circulation, specifically to prevent or reverse the postoperative pulmonary hypertensive crisis. It has been difficult to establish which factors might be triggering these crises. They are thought to result from the interaction of vascular endothelium with platelets and leukocytes released in the postcardiopulmonary bypass period which, in turn, may more easily release vasoactive agents, thromboxanes, and leukotrienes (Addonizio et al., 1980; Jones et al., 1981). It has been our experience that pulmonary hypertensive crises are most common on the second postoperative day during attempts to wean the patient from assisted ventilation. We have documented that the rapid rise in pulmonary arterial pressure is associated with a subsequent sudden increase in left atrial pressure and an abrupt fall in cardiac output. Various methods of managing these crises have been proposed, including prolonged postoperative anesthesia with fentanyl and the use of pulmonary vasodi-

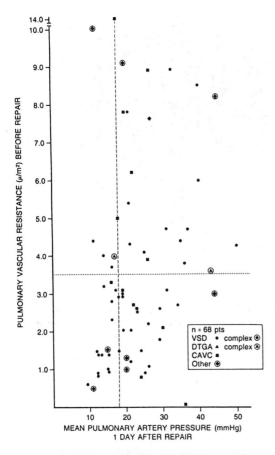

Figure 5C. Graph shows correlation between pulmonary vascular resistance before repair and mean pulmonary artery pressure the day after repair. While a trend is apparent, data points are quite scattered. (Reproduced with permission from Rabinovitch et al., *Circulation*, 1984.)

lators such as tolazoline (Jones et al., 1981). In our own Intensive Care Unit, we have benefited from continuous monitoring of pulmonary arterial and left atrial pressures. We maintain the pulmonary arterial pressure at less than half systemic level by instituting hyperventilation (pCO_2 25–30 torr). If necessary, we continue for several postoperative days. Thereafter, weaning from the ventilator can usually be accomplished slowly and with the help of intravenous vasodilators. Specifically, we give nitroglycerin followed by phenoxybenzamine, particularly if there is evidence of left

ventricular dysfunction. Beta-agonists, salbutamol, or isoproterenol are helpful if there is a component of pulmonary congestion. Almost all patients can be weaned from this therapy after one week.

There will, however, be rare patients who maintain a high level of pulmonary vascular resistance and appear to be refractory to vasodilator therapy despite relatively mild vascular changes on light microscopy (medial hypertrophy). Yet others may develop rapidly progressive pulmonary vascular disease despite early diagnosis and timely intervention. In our most recent lung biopsy studies from patients with congenital heart defects and pulmonary hypertension, we have been trying to learn more about the nature of altered endothelial-platelet-leukocyte, and endothelial-smooth-muscle interactions which may be relevant to the mechanism of heightened pulmonary vascular reactivity and to the development of progressive pulmonary vascular disease.

The Role of Pulmonary Vascular Endothelial Cells

We have identified structural and functional changes in the pulmonary vascular endothelial cells in patients with a ventricular septal defect. On scanning electron microscopy, the endothelial surface of normal pulmonary arteries has a "crinkled" or, when constricted, a "corduroy-like" appearance in that the cells form narrow and even ridges. The endothelial surface of thick-walled pulmonary arteries seen in patients with a large ventricular septal defect has a "cable-like" appearance in that the cells form deep twisted ridges (Rabinovitch et al., 1986) (Fig. 7). This endothelium might be predisposed to interact "roughly" with marginating blood elements such as platelets and leukocytes, facilitating release of vasoactive substances. In patients with advanced vascular changes, the endothelial surface is more uneven and "chenille" in

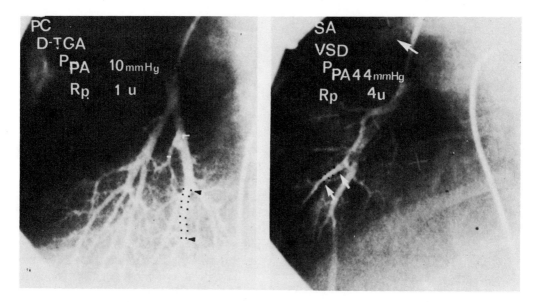

Figure 6. Left: a wedge angiogram shows normal tapering of the pulmonary arteries in an infant with normal pulmonary artery pressure; Right: a wedge angiogram shows abrupt tapering of arteries in an infant with pulmonary hypertension and a ventricular septal defect. Arrows designate length of axial artery segment between 2.5 mm and 1.5 mm lumen diameter. (Reproduced with permission from Rabinovitch et al., *Circulation*, 1981.)

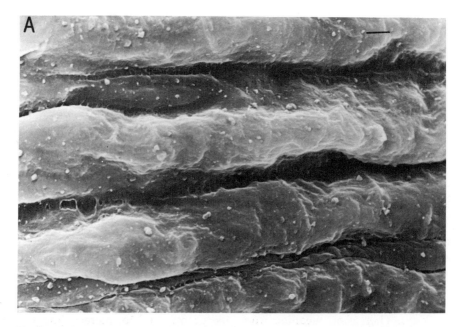

Figure 7. Scanning electron photomicrographs of pulmonary artery endothelial surfaces. (A) Normal pulmonary artery shows "corduroy pattern," neat closely aligned ridges. (B) Hypertensive pulmonary artery shows "cable" pattern, deep knotted ridges, and numerous microvilli (MV). (C) Hypertensive pulmonary artery shows chenille pattern, i.e., high ridges and uneven flattened cells. Bar = 2μm. (Reproduced with permission from Rabinovitch et al., *Lab Invest,* 1986.)

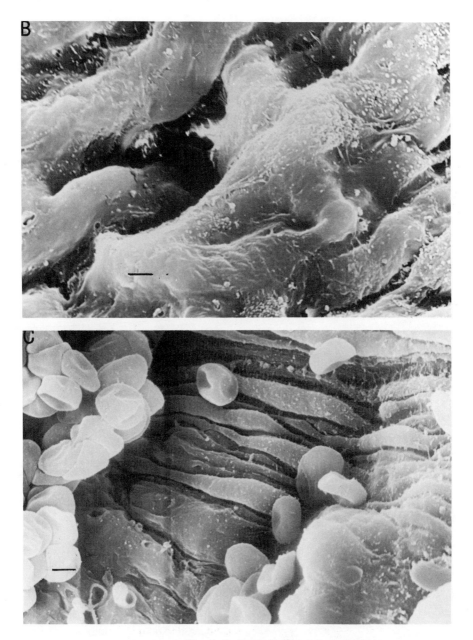

Figure 7. *Continued.*

texture, reflecting areas of obstruction, "high ridges," dilation and "low irregular valleys."

On transmission electron microscopy, endothelial cells from thick-walled pulmonary arteries have an increased volume proportion of microfilament bundles and rough endoplasmic reticulum suggesting a "fortified" cytoskeleton, heightened metabolic activity and protein synthesis. In patients with advanced vascular disease there is no longer an increase in these elements. Moreover, the rough endoplasmic reticulum is sometimes replaced by concentric mem-

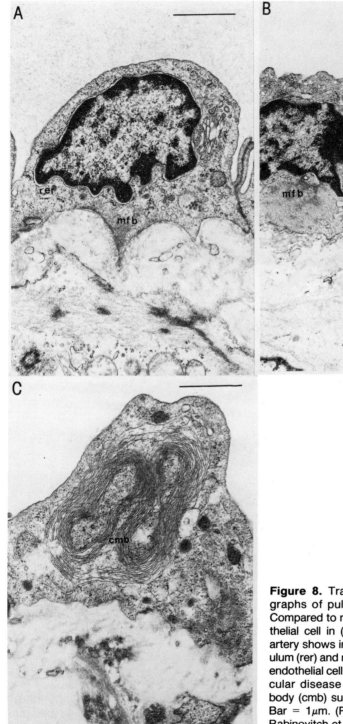

Figure 8. Transmission electron photomicrographs of pulmonary artery endothelial cells. Compared to normal endothelial cell in (A), endothelial cell in (B), from hypertensive pulmonary artery shows increased rough endoplasmic reticulum (rer) and microfilament bundles (mfb). (C) an endothelial cell from a patient with advanced vascular disease with a concentric membranous body (cmb) suggesting a degenerative process. Bar = 1μm. (Reproduced with permission from Rabinovitch et al., *Lab Invest,* 1986.)

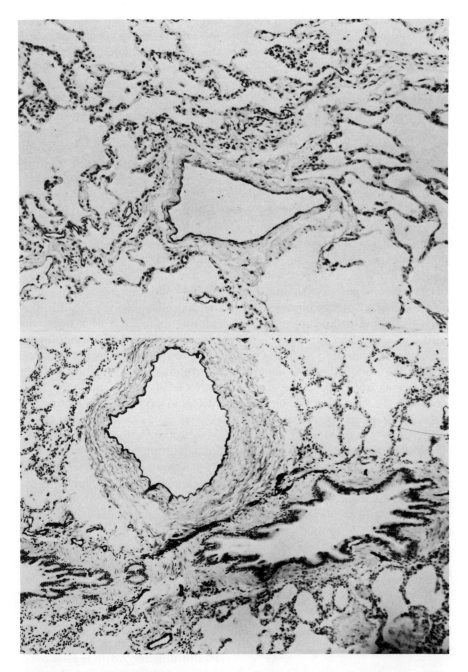

Figure 9. Lung biopsy section from a patient with pulmonary hypertension; thick-walled pulmonary artery with endothelium and deeply positive immunoperoxidase stain for von Willebrand factor. (×160)

branous bodies suggesting a degenerative process (Fig. 8).

Endothelial cells produce factor VIII (von Willebrand factor) and altered endo-thelial-platelet interaction has been impli-cated as part of the mechanism of increased pulmonary vascular reactivity and progres-sive pulmonary vascular disease. We applied immunocytochemical techniques to determine whether the apparent increase in metabolic function observed in pulmonary endothelial cells from thick-walled arteries may be resulting in increased production of the von Willebrand factor. Using an immunoperoxidase stain, we found that thick-walled pulmonary arteries stain densely for factor VIII, whereas normal vessels do not (Rabinovitch et al., 1986) (Fig. 9). Moreover, we found that most patients with pulmonary hypertension have elevated circulating levels of the von Willebrand factor. An increase in antigenic activity without an increase in biological activity is usually evident (Rabinovitch et al., 1986). The increase in antigenic activity is associated with an abnormal multimeric pattern showing loss of the high molecular weight components. If the factor VIII being produced lacks the high molecular weight components, there would be a tendency for decreased platelet endothelial adherence. Alternatively, the high molecular weight components of the molecule may be undetectable because they are consumed in platelet aggregates. This is being resolved in further studies.

Our most recent observations in lung biopsy tissue from patients with a ventricular septal defect suggest that a process of degradation and increased synthesis of connective-tissue proteins in the subendothelium and media may be important in the pathogenesis of pulmonary vascular disease. We speculate that abnormal distribution of elastin and collagen may decrease compliance of the arteries and result in fixed elevation in pulmonary vascular resistance.

Experimental Studies

Experimental in-vivo models, such as the creation of a ventricular septal defect in a newborn lamb (Boucek et al., 1985), will help greatly in elucidating the evolution of pulmonary vascular disease. In a collabora-

tive study, we have been able to correlate the early decrease in vascular compliance of the central pulmonary arteries with fragmentation of elastin. It will be interesting now to determine how this might disturb flow dynamics in distal vessels and affect the development of structural changes.

Newly developed techniques of harvesting pulmonary arterial endothelial and smooth-muscle cells from central pulmonary arteries and from microvessels (Ryan et al., 1978, 1982) will help greatly in answering basic questions related to endothelial-smooth-muscle interaction and endothelial-blood element (platelet, leukocyte) interaction.

We have devised a system whereby we are able to grow pulmonary arterial endothelial cells onto the flexible polyvinyl-chloride membrane of a transducer dome and then pulsate the monolayer at high pressure (100/60 mmHg), thus mimicking the condition of a ventricular septal defect with a left-to-right shunt (Fig. 10) (Rabinovitch et al., 1985). On ultrastructural analysis, we have observed features similar to those apparent in endothelial cells in patients with pulmonary hypertension. There is an increase in microfilament bundles and in rough endoplastic reticulum.

In our most recent studies, we have cultured smooth-muscle cells with the medium taken from endothelial cells that had been pulsated at high pressure. There was a decrease in the smooth-muscle incorporation of both ^{3}H-thymidine and ^{14}C-leucine, suggesting that pulsation had induced endothelial release of an inhibitor of smooth-muscle hypertrophy and hyperplasia. How this initial, perhaps protective, inhibition of smooth-muscle growth is later overcome to permit induction of medial hypertrophy will be the subject of further study.

We can also use cell and organ culture systems to determine whether heightened pulmonary vascular reactivity is due to increased release of an endothelial-derived contracting factor (DeMey and Vanhoutte, 1982) or decreased sensitivity of hypertro-

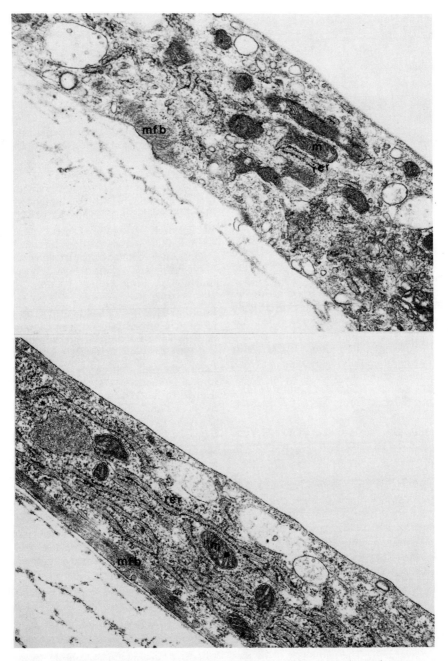

Figure 10. Electron photomicrographs from cells cultured on transducer domes; compared to (A) cell from a stationary dome, cell from a dome that was pulsated 100 times/minute at high pressure 100/60 mmHg for 48 hours (B) shows increased rough endoplasmic reticulum (rer) and microfilament bundles (mfb). (×34,000)

phied smooth muscle to a relaxing factor (Furchgott, 1983) or the effect of platelet activating factor (Tan et al., 1985).

Ultimately, experimental studies should lead to a better understanding of the basic biochemical systems and genetic control mechanisms important in causing heightened pulmonary vascular reactivity and in the development of pulmonary vascular disease.

References

Addonizio VP Jr, Smith JB, Strauss JF III, et al. Thromboxane synthesis and platelet secretion during cardiopulmonary bypass with bubble oxygenation. *J Thorac Cardiovasc Surg* 1980;79:91–96.

Boucek MM, Chang R, Synhorst DP. Hemodynamic consequences of inotropic support with digoxin and amrinone in lambs with ventricular septal defect. *Pediatr Res* 1985;19:887–891.

DeMey JG, Vanhoutte PM. Heterogeneous behaviour of the canine arterial and venous wall; Importance of the endothelium. *Circ Res* 1982;51:439–447.

DuShane JW, Krongrad E, Ritter DG, McGoon DC. The fate of raised pulmonary vascular resistance after surgery for inventricular septal defect. In Rowe RD, Kidd BSL (Eds): *The Child after Congenital Heart Surgery.* Mount Kisco, NY: Futura, 1976.

Friedli B, Kidd BS, Mustard WT, Keith JD. Ventricular septal defect with increased pulmonary vascular resistance. *Am J Cardiol* 1974;33:403–409.

Furchgott RF. Role of endothelium in responses of vascular smooth muscle. *Circ Res* 1983; 53:557–573.

Haworth SG, Reid L. A morphometric study of regional variation in lung structure in infants with pulmonary hypertension and congenital heart defect. A justification of lung biopsy. *Br Heart J* 1978;40:825–831.

Haworth SG. Pulmonary vascular disease in different types of congenital heart disease. Implications for interpretation of lung biopsy finding in early childhood. *Br Heart J* 1984;52:557–71.

Heath D, Edwards JE. The pathology of hypertensive pulmonary vascular disease. *Circulation* 1958;18:533–547.

Hislop A, Haworth SG, Reid L. Quantitative structural analysis of pulmonary vessels in isolated ventricular septal defects in infancy. *Br Heart J* 1975;37:1014–1021.

Hoffman JIE, Rudolph AM. The natural history of ventricular septal defect in infancy. *Am J Cardiol* 1965;16:634–653.

Jones ODH, Shore DF, Rigby ML, et al. The use of tolazoline hydrochloride as a pulmonary vasodilator in potentially fatal episodes of pulmonary vasoconstriction after cardiac surgery in children. *Circulation* 1981;64(Suppl11):134–139.

Meyrick B, Clarke SW, Symons C, et al. Primary pulmonary hypertension. A case report including electron microscopic study. *Br J Dis Chest* 1974;68:11–20.

Meyrick B, Reid LM. Ultrastructural findings in lung material from children with congenital heart defects. *Am J Pathol* 1980;101:527–537.

Rabinovitch M, Haworth SG, Castaneda AR, et al. Lung biopsy in congenital heart disease: A morphometric approach to pulmonary vascular disease. *Circulation* 1978;58:1107–1122.

Rabinovitch M, Keane JF, Fellows KE, et al. Quantitative analysis of the pulmonary wedge angiogram in congenital heart defects. Correlation with hemodynamic data and morphometric findings in lung biopsy tissue. *Circulation* 1981;63:152–164.

Rabinovitch M, Castaneda AR, Reid L. Lung biopsy with frozen section as a diagnostic aid in patients with congenital heart defects. *Am J Cardiol* 1981;47:77–84.

Rabinovitch M, Andrew M, Thom H, et al. Abnormal pulmonary vascular endothelial metabolism of factor VIII in patients with pulmonary hypertension. *Circulation* 1983;68:111–36 (abstract).

Rabinovitch M, Keane JF, Norwood WI, et al. Vascular structure in lung biopsy tissue correlated with pulmonary hemodynamic findings after repair of congenital heart defects. *Circulation* 1984;69:655–667.

Rabinovitch M, Bothwell T, Hayakawa BN, et al. Pulmonary vascular endothelial abnormalities in patients with congenital heart defects and pulmonary hypertension. A correlation of scanning and transmission electron with light microscopy. *Lab Invest* 1986 (in press).

Rabinovitch M, Mullen M, Watchurst T, Spicer P. Structural abnormalities in pulmonary artery endothelial cells pulsated at high pressure. An "in vitro" model of pulmonary hypertension. *Am Rev Resp Dis* 1985;131:A410 (abstract).

Ryan U, Clements E, Habliston D, Ryan JW. Isolation and culture of pulmonary artery endothelial cells. *Tissue and Cell* 1978;10:535–554.

Ryan US, White LA, Lopez M, Ryan JW. Use of microcarriers to isolate and culture pulmonary microvascular endothelium. *Tissue and Cell* 1982;14:597–606.

Tan EL, Snyder F. Metabolism of platelet activating factor by capillary enthothelial cells isolated from rat epididymal adipose tissue. *Thromb Res* 1985;38:713–717.

Ventricular Septal Defects: Overview of Management

Julien I. E. Hoffman

Management of ventricular septal defects is in the first instance conservative because of the relatively high incidence of spontaneous closure or diminution in size of these defects. If the defect is small, the incidence of spontaneous closure is very high, perhaps occurring in over 80–90% of cases (Alpert et al., 1979; Hoffman, 1968; Hoffman and Rudolph, 1965, 1970). Even bigger defects have about a 50% chance of closing or becoming smaller spontaneously, so that it is often worth waiting for spontaneous improvement in the evolution of these defects (Hoffman and Rudolph, 1965, 1970; Nouaille et al., 1967). How long one should wait and what considerations will lead to surgery depend on the size of the defect.

Small Defects

With most small defects in asymptomatic patients, the initial management is merely supervisory. The only specific therapy needed is antibiotic treatment of, or prophylaxis for, infections. Some cardiologists consider an episode of infective endocarditis in these patients to constitute a reason for surgical closure of the defect. They argue that such a patient is at risk of recurrent endocarditis. If this course of action is entertained, the possibility that the small defect is muscular in nature should be excluded by echocardiography or cardiac catheterization, since small muscular defects may be impossible to find at surgery. Not all cardiologists agree with this course of action. One study reported that, over one time period in the Toronto region, infective endocarditis developed in two adults with small ventricular septal defects that were managed conservatively but in three who had had surgical closure of similar defects (Shah et al., 1966). This risk of postoperative endocarditis disappears after six months. Better data on the risks of endocarditis in this population are needed.

The other exception to conservative therapy for small ventricular septal defects

Supported in part by Program Project Grant HL 25847 from the United States Public Health Service.
From: Anderson, RH, Neches, WH, Park, SC, Zuberbuhler, JR, eds: *Perspectives in Pediatric Cardiology*: Mount Kisco, New York, Futura Publishing Co., © 1988.

is if the defect is doubly committed and subarterial (supracristal). These defects are high in the right ventricular outflow tract and are roofed by the conjoined leaflets of the pulmonary and aortic valves (Goor et al., 1970; Kirklin and Barratt-Boyes, 1986; Nadas et al., 1964; Van Praagh and McNamara, 1968). The importance of the position of this defect is that, frequently, the right coronary or noncoronary leaflet of the aortic valve prolapses through the defect. This is probably because of lack of support of the leaflet at this site, and possibly because of negative pressures produced in this region by the jet of blood passing from the left ventricle through the defect (Tatsuno et al., 1973). Even if the defect appears small on echocardiography or angiography, and the shunt through it is small, there may be a large defect that is partly occluded by a prolapsing aortic valve leaflet (Kirklin and Barratt-Boyes, 1986; Nadas et al., 1964; Van Praagh and McNamara, 1968). These defects roofed by aortic-pulmonary continuity occur in about 5% of patients with ventricular septal defects in the Western world (Goor et al., 1970; Nadas et al., 1964), but make up as much as 35% of all ventricular septal defects in China and Japan (Tatsuno et al., 1975). As indicated above, the significance of these defects is that they are often associated with aortic incompetence. The aortic valve leaflets may be elongated and thickened, and there can be dilation of the aortic root or even an aneurysm of the sinus of Valsalva (Kirklin and Barratt-Boyes, 1986; Nadas et al., 1964; Van Praagh and McNamara, 1968). Aortic incompetence seldom appears before two years of age (Corone et al., 1977; Kirklin and Barratt-Boyes, 1986; Momma et al., 1984; Nadas et al., 1964), but, once it develops, it is thought to progress (Keane et al., 1977). Many cardiologists therefore consider the presence of a "supracristal" defect as reason for surgical closure in the hope of preventing the aortic valve lesion. If there is already aortic incompetence or prolapse, there may be more reason to close the defect.

Large Defects

There is a completely different set of considerations if the defect is large and the patient has marked congestive heart failure. Although spontaneous closure of large defects is less common than of small defects, enough of them close or become smaller and hemodynamically insignificant to make medical management initially the approach of choice (Hoffman and Rudolph, 1965; Nouaille et al., 1967). Specific therapy in such a protocol includes restriction of salt intake, giving diuretics, digitalizing the patient, and if necessary, using afterload-reducing agents such as hydralazine, prazosin, or angiotensin-converting enzyme inhibitors like Captopril or Enalapril. Maintaining a hematocrit above 40% is important, not only to increase systemic oxygen transport but also to keep an adequate blood viscosity (Lister et al., 1982). During anemia, the lowered blood viscosity lowers pulmonary vascular resistance and leads to an increased pulmonary blood flow for any given sized ventricular septal defect and aortic pressure. Conversely, raising blood viscosity in the presence of these defects helps to minimize the pulmonary blood flow. Pulmonary vascular resistance can also be kept quite high if the patient breathes low oxygen mixtures. Giving such mixtures by mask or oxygen tent is not often done therapeutically, but the same effect is achieved naturally in those who live at high altitude. Thus, infants with large ventricular septal defects have pulmonary-to-systemic flow ratios that average 3.3:1 at sea level but 2.3:1 in Denver, which is about one mile above sea level (Blount, 1977; Vogel et al., 1967).

If, during medical management, the defect becomes smaller, the patient will improve until all medication can be stopped. Eventually, if the child is lucky, the defect will close completely. On the other hand, in many children the defect remains large for a long time, so that surgery will have to be considered under certain circumstances.

Early surgery is needed on those rare occasions when medical treatment fails to control congestive heart failure and the child seems likely to die unless the volume load is removed. Although the cause of refractoriness to medical management is often not evident, two specific circumstances are recognized. Sometimes the reason for the lack of response to medical treatment is an associated secundum atrial septal defect (not just a stretched oval foramen). With a large atrial septal defect, the left atrium is decompressed. It is impossible, therefore, for the left ventricle to develop a large enough end-diastolic ventricular volume to maintain both an adequate systemic blood flow as well as the huge left-to-right ventricular shunt, or it can do so only at the expense of massive congestion. Another cause of refractoriness to treatment is prematurity. The myocardium in the prematurely born infant is not as efficient as in later childhood. It has more water and fewer myofibrils per unit mass of muscle (Friedman, 1973). It is also stiffer and less able to respond to changes in stroke volume (Rudolph, 1985). Furthermore, the pulmonary vascular resistance may not be maintained as high in prematurely born infants as in those born at term. A large left-to-right shunt consequently develops more rapidly in the infant born prematurely. Thus, a heart that in itself has relatively low efficiency in handling excessive loads is called upon to handle such loads before compensatory hypertrophy has had time to develop. The resultant congestive heart failure may be severe and difficult if not impossible to control medically.

Some infants respond well enough to medical treatment to avoid early surgery but may require it in the next few months. Our criteria for postponing early surgery are that the infant should be able to be fed at home by the parents and should gain weight, even though the weight gain is subnormal. If treatment achieves this result, then the infant can be sent home but will need frequent medical evaluation. This conservative management may have to be abandoned relatively early for one of three reasons. The first reason is that, frequently, congestive heart failure becomes worse, necessitating many readmissions to adjust medications. These episodes may be precipitated by upper respiratory tract infections, minor aspiration secondary to gastroesophageal reflux, electrolyte imbalance due to poor dietary intake or diuretics, or to incorrect administration of the multiple drugs by the parents. Whatever the cause, it becomes clear that the infant is barely managing to survive and is in jeopardy of dying. Surgery thus becomes necessary. The second reason is seen when congestive heart failure is moderately well controlled, even though the infant is still ill, but socioeconomic factors make continued medical treatment unwise. Inadequate parental care sometimes jeopardizes the infant. Sometimes the strain of looking after the infant is too much for the family. These infants often require two-hourly feeding. In essence, they need continuous nursing around the clock. Moreover, they are usually very fussy and thus unsatisfying to look after. Consequently, the parents become tired and irritable, other children in the family are neglected, and quite often marriages break up. Sometimes, an infant who might be able to be managed by a family living near a medical center may not do as well in a remote rural area where emergency care or advice is not readily available. In all of these circumstances, the issue is not whether surgery is compulsory for strict medical reasons, but whether conservative medical management is too costly for the family or impossible to monitor because of distance or social circumstances. The third and final reason is that a few children come to surgery without any of the preceding causes but because of growth failure. No infants with large ventricular septal defects grow well. Indeed, if the infant is not below the third percentile for weight and the tenth percentile for height, there is some reason to doubt the diagnosis of severe congestive heart failure due to a large left-to-right shunt. These growth deficits are not a good reason for surgery, because once the shunt is reduced spontaneously or surgically, there is a strong tendency for the child to catch up to a normal weight and height (Cartmill et al., 1966; Clarkson, 1973; Feldt et al., 1969). What may be more important is failure of head growth. Most of the infants in severe congestive heart failure with a large left-to-right ventricular shunt maintain normal head growth despite poor growth of height and weight. In a few of them, however, the head circumference (which might have started off in the 50th percentile) gradually falls below the third percentile by three or four months of age (Clarkson, 1973). The brain is disproportionately large in newborn infants. It comprises about 15% of body weight, requires 30% of the resting cardiac output, uses about 70% of the resting total body oxygen consumption, and metabolizes over 95% of the glucose produced by the liver. It is, therefore, not surprising that in severe congestive heart failure, an increased metabolic rate due to increased work of breathing and increased sympathetic stimulation might divert some calories that should have gone to brain growth. The counterpart of this has been described in low birthweight infants kept at temperatures below thermoneutrality and with a relatively low caloric intake. They also have retarded head growth (Glass et al., 1975). Because over 50% of head growth is achieved by six months after birth, a longer delay in treating the cause of the growth failure results in a decrease in final brain size. This may be why, in one study, infants with large ventricular septal defects that were closed surgically at about two years of age tended to catch up to normal weight and height unless they had a small head circumference at the time of surgery. We do not know all the implications of a small head circumference but it seems unwise to allow failure of head growth to continue. Surgical closure of the ventricular septal defect in these infants under six months of age is followed by rapid head growth until a normal head circumference is reached (Fig. 1).

If medical treatment is not terminated for one of the above reasons, the infant can continue to be treated conservatively until about 12 months of age. Often at about this age there may be an improvement in the signs and symptoms of congestive heart failure. The child begins to grow better, has a better appetite, has less tachypnea and tachycardia, the liver becomes smaller and the heart less hyperactive. The doses of digoxin and diuretics can be seen to be lower per unit body weight than they were earlier. On x-ray, the heart is smaller and the pulmonary arterial markings indicate a smaller left-to-right shunt. All these features indicate that there is a reduced left ventricular volume load due to a decrease in the left-to-right shunt. Although this clinical improvement is very welcome to the child and the parents, it should be viewed with suspicion by the physician. A smaller left-to-right ventricular shunt may occur for one of three reasons. In about 5 to 10% of these children, infundibular stenosis develops. The increased obstruction to right ventricular outflow decreases the left-to-right shunt. In about 45 to 50% of these children, there is progressive pulmonary vascular disease, and in the other 45 to 50% the ventricular septal defect is becoming smaller. All three developments will reduce the left-to-right shunt and cause clinical improvement, but only the last of them—diminution in size of the defect—removes the need for surgery. Pulmonary vascular disease demands early surgery to prevent progression, and infundibular stenosis will almost certainly require surgical treatment at some future time.

Each of these three outcomes eventually produces a different combination of right ventricular wall thickness and intensity of the closure sound of the pulmonary valve. Spontaneous closure leads to a normal heart. Infundibular stenosis produces right ventricular hypertrophy and a soft pulmonary closing sound. Pulmonary vascular disease produces right ventricular hy-

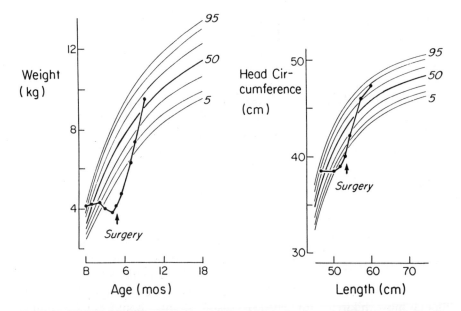

Figure 1. Effect of surgical closure of large ventricular septal defect on weight gain (left graph) and head growth (right graph). Although head circumference is plotted against body length rather than age, the final measurement of head circumference was made at the time of the last measurement of weight.

pertrophy and a loud pulmonary closing sound. Despite these clear-cut differences that exist when each of the three developments is complete, in the early stages of a reduced left-to-right shunt from one of these three causes, it is not possible to use these distinguishing features with safety. Right ventricular hypertrophy, always present with a big ventricular septal defect, may take several months to regress even after pulmonary arterial pressure has returned to normal. Gradations of intensity of the pulmonary second sound are impossible to evaluate by ear. What is essential is that, whenever there is evidence of a reduced left-to-right shunt in these children, they must be evaluated carefully to determine why the shunt has become smaller. Only by doing this can pulmonary vascular disease be detected soon enough for surgery to be curative. Initial evaluation is by echocardiography, and if the diagnosis is not clear-cut, then cardiac catheterization will be needed.

There are a few children who develop enough pulmonary vascular disease before one year of age that they will require early surgery. They will also show clinical improvement due to a reduced left-to-right shunt, and require the same type of investigation as do those whose clinical improvement occurs later. It is not the time at which the change occurs but rather the change itself that mandates further investigation. On the other hand, there are also children who, at one year of age, seem to have as large a left-to-right shunt as they did when younger. If the shunt really is still large, they cannot have much pulmonary vascular disease. Their management must be supervised with the realization that after one year of age the risks of severe pulmonary vascular disease begin to increase quite rapidly. For example, Blackstone et al. (1976) found that, by one year of age, the probability of surviving surgery and having a low pulmonary arterial pressure is at least 95%, whereas by two years of age it may be as low as 60% in those with significant pulmonary vascular disease. Furthermore, by two years of age, about one-third of children with large ventricular septal defects had irreversible pulmonary vascular disease (DuShane et al., 1972). Thus, even though it is still possible for large ventricular septal defects to get smaller spontaneously after one year of age, it becomes unwise to leave these defects open unless there can be very close observation of the child with repeated echocardiograms and cardiac catheterization.

Moderate-Sized Defects

Although most children with ventricular septal defects have defects that either are small from the outset or else are very large with high pulmonary blood flows and pulmonary arterial pressures, there are some children who have large left-to-right shunts but pulmonary arterial pressures that are below 50% of aortic pressures. The defect has enough resistance to produce a large pressure drop in systole between the left and right ventricles but not enough to restrict the left-to-right shunt significantly. These children usually develop congestive heart failure but this is, as a rule, easily controlled by medical treatment. There is a reasonable chance that the defect will become smaller. If it does not, the best form of treatment is uncertain. In the absence of a high pulmonary arterial pressure, these children are not at high risk of early pulmonary vascular disease. If, however, the defect does not become smaller, they may develop pulmonary vascular disease in late childhood or early adult life (Hoffman and Rudolph, 1970). This situation is comparable to that in which patient with large left-to-right shunts due to atrial septal defects develop late pulmonary vascular disease. Furthermore, even in the absence of severe symptoms, these children have dilated left ventricles and left ventricular hypertrophy.

Some studies in adults with moderate-sized ventricular septal defects have demonstrated subnormal ventricular function during exercise (Jablonsky et al., 1983; Otterstad et al., 1985). It is possible that if ventricular hypertrophy persists long enough (perhaps for only a few years), myocardial function may become permanently impaired. Indeed, the duration of a large left-to-right shunt may affect late ventricular function after surgery. This is because function appears to be better in those whose defects are closed in infancy than at 5 to 10 years of age (Cordell et al., 1976; Jarmakani et al., 1971; Maron et al., 1973). These considerations—pulmonary vascular disease and myocardial dysfunction—suggest that a conservative approach to these large shunts should not be continued for many years. More studies of this group are needed to define what time course of treatment should be followed.

Surgical Procedures

Primary closure of the ventricular septal defect in centers of excellence can today be done with a mortality that is below 5%. At one time, banding the pulmonary trunk was the method of choice, but this has been abandoned for all but certain problems because of its many disadvantages. The procedure has a substantial mortality in these very sick infants (Barratt-Boyes and Kirklin, 1986; Hoffman, 1976), and prior banding adds to the mortality and morbidity of subsequent surgical closure of the defect. The band may not stay in place on the pulmonary trunk. Instead, it may migrate distally and occlude one pulmonary artery, it may move proximally so that pulmonary valve motion is abnormal and the pulmonary valve may become thickened or deformed, or it may even slowly cut through the arterial wall until it lies loose inside the artery. There is also the problem of how tight to make the band at the time of surgery. If it is tight enough to make the left-to-right shunt small, then, as the child grows and cardiac output increases, the band will rapidly become too tight and a right-to-left shunt will develop. If, on the other hand, the band is deliberately made loose so that it will take longer to become too tight, then for a long time it will not control congestive heart failure. Furthermore, if there is some pulmonary vascular disease, then it will not be possible to place a tight band on the pulmonary trunk and the decrease in pulmonary arterial pressure will be suboptimal (Utley, 1973). In fact, judging how tight to make the band is difficult at the time of surgery. Despite all attempts to quantify the degree of tightness by measuring pressures and flows, the best bands are usually those which an experienced surgeon judges to be adequate. Given all these complications, banding of the pulmonary trunk is usually reserved for very small (preterm or small for gestational age) infants, for those with other diseases or anomalies that preclude cardiopulmonary bypass, and for infants with multiple muscular defects ("swiss cheese" septum) that carry a 50% mortality rate for surgical correction in infancy. For all others, closure of the defect during cardiopulmonary bypass can be done with a mortality rate usually of under 5%.

Although surgical mortality is low, there is some morbidity, and late complications do occur. About 20 to 40% of children, especially infants, have residual defects after surgery (Rein et al., 1977; Weidman et al., 1977). These are usually small and can even disappear spontaneously. If they persist, they will leave the patient susceptible to infective endocarditis. Furthermore, some patients have complete heart block that is present at the end of the operation or develops late, particularly in those who had transient heart block at the time of surgery or who were left with right bundle branch block and a left anterior hemiblock (Blake et al., 1982). Sudden death, presumably related to ventricular arrhythmias, has also occurred in several patients (Blake et al.,

1982). Surgical closure of ventricular septal defects is, therefore, not benign, despite a low mortality. This gives more force to the conservative approach to managing these lesions.

Management of Pulmonary Vascular Disease

If children have severe pulmonary vascular disease (with pulmonary vascular resistance of over 15 $mmHg/L/min/m^2$), then it is probably safer not to close the defect. Studies of such patients at the Mayo Clinic showed that, if operated on, about 70% would die within one year of surgery (Clarkson et al., 1968). On the other hand, patients with more severe pulmonary vascular disease who were not operated on usually lived comfortably into the third or later decades (Cartmill et al., 1966). Avoiding surgery is not the only management required for these patients. Because it is likely that pulmonary vascular disease will progress, and because current evidence implicates platelet aggregation as one of the important factors in this progression (Hoffman et al., 1981), it is worthwhile placing the patients on acetylsalicylic acid, dipyridamole, or both. Not only may this treatment prevent or retard the development of further pulmonary vascular disease, but it may also prevent the distressing episodes of hemoptysis that occur late in the course of the illness. If patients become polycythemic from their right-to-left shunts, then periodic phlebotomies are needed to keep the hematocrit below 55% together with supplemental iron administration to prevent iron deficiency anemia.

Although this management of established pulmonary vascular disease is used by many cardiologists, there is no proof of its efficacy. Nevertheless, it has a good pathophysiological rationale. What may be equally important is to treat patients who have a moderately raised pulmonary vascular resistance who have survived cardiac surgery. Many of these patients maintain a moderately high pulmonary vascular resistance or even get worse, quickly or slowly (Cartmill et al., 1966; Hallidie-Smith et al., 1977; Hoffman and Rudolph, 1966; Vogel et al., 1974). We have in the past assumed that such patients had irreversible anatomical changes, that they were past the age at which new pulmonary blood vessels would form and, therefore, that no specific therapy could or need be given. This attitude may not be correct. For all we know, the fact that pulmonary vascular resistance is elevated after surgery may lead to gradual progression of the pulmonary vascular disease. This progression is likely to be exacerbated if there is any element of vasoconstriction. It may therefore be prudent to minimize pulmonary vasoconstriction by the use of drugs such as hydralazine or nifedipine, and to give agents that prevent platelet aggregation. In this way we may be able to minimize the chances of progression of the pulmonary vascular disease.

References

Alpert BS, Cook DH, Varghese PJ, Rowe RD. Spontaneous closure of small ventricular defects: Ten-year follow-up. *Pediatrics* 1979;63:204–206.

Blackstone EH, Kirklin JW, Bradley EL, et al. Optimal age and results in repair of large ventricular septal defects. *J Thorac Cardiovasc Surg* 1976;72:661–679.

Blake RS, Chung EE, Wesley H, Hallidie-Smith KA. Conduction defects, ventricular arrhythmias, and late death after surgical closure of ventricular septal defect. *Br Heart J* 1982;47:305–315.

Blount SG Jr. Comparison of patients with ventricular septal defect at high altitude and sea level. *Circulation* 1977;56(Suppl I):79–82.

Cartmill TB, DuShane JW, McGoon DC, Kirklin JW. Results of repair of ventricular septal defect. *J Thorac Cardiovasc Surg* 1966;52:486–499.

Clarkson PM. Growth following corrective cardiac operation in early infancy. In Barratt-Boyes BG, Neutze JM, Harris EA (Eds): *Heart Disease in Infancy: Diagnosis and Surgical Treatment.* London: Churchill Livingstone, 1973;75–81.

Clarkson PM, Frye RL, DuShane JW, et al. Prognosis for patients with ventricular septal defect and severe pulmonary vascular obstructive disease. *Circulation* 1968;38:129–135.

Cordell D, Graham TP Jr, Atwood GF, et al. Left heart volume characteristics following ventricular septal defect closure in infancy. *Circulation* 1976;54:294–298.

Corone P, Doyon F, Gaudeau S, et al. Natural history of ventricular septal defect. A study involving 790 cases. *Circulation* 1977;55:908–915.

DuShane JW, Weidman WH, Ritter DG. Influence of the natural history of large ventricular septal defects on management of patients. *Birth Defects—Original Article Series* 1972;8:63–68.

Feldt RH, Stickler GB, Weidman WH. Growth of children with congenital heart disease. *Am J Dis Child* 1969;117:573–579.

Friedman WF. The intrinsic properties of the developing heart. In Friedman WF, Lesch M, Sonnenblick EH (Eds): *Neonatal Heart Disease.* New York: Grune and Stratton 1973;21–49.

Glass L, Lala RV, Jaiswal V, Nigam SK. Effect of thermal environment and calorie intake on head growth and low birth weight infants during the late neonatal period. *Arch Dis Child* 1975;50:571–573.

Goor DA, Lillehei CW, Rees R, Edwards JE. Isolated ventricular septal defects. Development basis for various types and presentation of classification. *Chest* 1970;58:468–482.

Hallidie-Smith KA, Wilson RSE, Hart A, Zeidifard E. Functional status of patients with large ventricular septal defect and pulmonary vascular disease 6 to 16 years after surgical closure of their defect in childhood. *Br Heart J* 1977;39:1093–1101.

Hoffman JIE. Natural history of congenital heart disease. Problems in its assessment with special reference to ventricular septal defects. *Circulation* 1968;37:97–125.

Hoffman JIE, Rudolph AM. The natural history of ventricular septal defects in infancy. *Am J Cardiol* 1965;16:634–653.

Hoffman JIE, Rudolph AM. The natural history of isolated ventricular septal defect, with special reference to selection of patients for surgery. *Adv Pediatr* 1970;17:57–79.

Hoffman JIE, Rudolph AM, Heymann MA. Pulmonary vascular disease with congenital heart lesions: Pathologic features and causes. *Circulation* 1981;64:873–877.

Jablonsky G, Hilton JD, Liu PP, et al. Rest and exercise ventricular function in adults with congenital ventricular septal defects. *Am J Cardiol* 1983;51:293–298.

Jarmakani JM, Graham TP Jr, Canent RV Jr,

Capp MP. The effect of corrective surgery on left heart volume and mass in children with ventricular septal defect. *Am J Cardiol* 1971;27:254–258.

Keane JF, Plauth WH Jr, Nadas AS. Ventricular septal defect with aortic regurgitation. *Circulation* 1977;56(Suppl I):72–77.

Kirklin JW, Barratt-Boyes BG. *Cardiac Surgery.* New York: John Wiley and Sons, 1986.

Lister G, Hellenbrand WE, Kleinman CS, Talner NS. Physiologic effects of increasing hemoglobin concentrations in left-to-right shunting in infants with ventricular septal defects. *N Engl J Med* 1982;306:502–506.

Maron BJ, Redwood DR, Hirshfield JW Jr. Postoperative assessment of patients with ventricular septal defect and pulmonary hypertension. Response to intense upright exercise. *Circulation* 1973;48:864–874.

Momma K, Toyama K, Takao A, Ando M, Nakazawa M, Hirosawa K, Imai Y. Natural history of subarterial ventricular septal defect. *Am Heart J* 1984;108:1312–1317.

Nouaille J, Gautier M, Lucet P, Mercier J-N, Kachaner J. Les communications interventriculaires du nourrisson et de l'enfant, à propos de 500 observations. I. Etude clinique et problèmes thérapeutiques. *Arch Mal Coeur* 1967;60:1138–1188.

Nadas AS, Thilenius OG, LaFarge CG, Hauck AJ. Ventricular septal defects and aortic regurgitation. Medical and pathologic aspects. *Circulation* 1964;29:862–873.

Otterstad JE, Simonsen S, Erikssen J. Hemodynamic findings at rest and during mild supine exercise in adults with isolated, uncomplicated ventricular septal defects. *Circulation* 1985; 71:650–662.

Rein JG, Freed MD, Norwood WI, Castenada AR. Early and late results of closure of ventricular septal defect in infancy. *Ann Thorac Surg* 1977;24:19–26.

Rudolph AM. Distribution and regulation of blood flow in the fetal and neonatal lamb. *Circ Res* 1985;57:811–821.

Shah P, Singh WSA, Rose V, Keith J. Incidence of bacterial endocarditis in ventricular septal defects. *Circulation* 1966;34:127–131.

Tatsuno K, Konno S, Ando M, Sakakibara S. Pathogenetic mechanism of prolapsing aortic valve and aortic regurgitation associated with ventricular septal defect. *Circulation* 1973; 48:1028–1037.

Tatsuno K, Ando M, Takao A, et al. Diagnostic importance of aortography in conal ventricular-septal defect. *Am Heart J* 1975;89:171–177.

Utley JR. Hemodynamic observations during and after pulmonary arterial banding. *Ann Thorac Surg* 1973;15:493–509.

Van Praagh R, McNamara JJ. Anatomic types of ventricular septal defect with aortic insufficiency. Diagnostic and surgical considerations. *Am Heart J* 1968;75:604–619.

Vogel JHK, Grover RF, Jamieson G, Blount SG Jr. Long-term physiologic observations in patients with ventricular septal defect and increased pulmonary vascular resistance. *Adv Cardiol* 1974;11:108–122.

Vogel JHK, McNamara DG, Blount SG Jr. Role of hypoxia in determining pulmonary vascular resistance in infants with ventricular septal defects. *Am J Cardiol* 1967;20:346–349.

Weidman WH, Blount SG Jr, DuShane JW et al. Clinical course in ventricular septal defect. *Circulation* 1977;56(Suppl I):56–69.

1.8

Ventricular Septal Defects: A Surgical Viewpoint

John W. Kirklin, James K. Kirklin, Benigno Soto, Eugene A. Blackstone, and Lionel M. Bargeron, Jr.

The cardiac surgeon probably looks at many more ventricular septal defects than does any other member of the group of people concerned with congenital heart disease. Unfortunately, usually he or she cannot view the defect from both left and right ventricular aspects. Most importantly, he can refresh his memory of a particular ventricular septal defect only by reviewing his operative note rather than by restudying the specimen. The surgeon works with ventricular septal defects not only as isolated lesions but also as a part of other congenital cardiac lesions which he is called upon to repair. He places sutures around their margins, locating them not only to provide a secure repair, but also in such a manner as to avoid damage to conduction tissues, atrioventricular and arterial valves, and coronary arteries. On occasions, he modifies a defect by enlarging its margins in one direction or another. These processes are safe only when the anatomical nature of the borders of the defect, and its relationship to surrounding structures, are well understood. It is natural, then, that the surgeon is attracted to a method of describing ventricular septal defects that is specific and basically anatomical, and takes cognizance of the margins of the defect; that describes relevant associated cardiac abnormalities; and that is applicable in all settings. Such a method has evolved, and its evolution has been the result of the interaction of surgeons with individuals from many other disciplines.

It has long been stated, and to a limited extent quite correctly, that from a surgical point of view, the name given to a cardiac anomaly is not important, but that what is important is accurate and complete understanding of the defect, its repair, and the survival of the patient (Table 1). This oversimplification of reality ignores the need to generalize surgical concepts and improve results, to investigate anatomical and surgical interrelations, to communicate with colleagues, and to transmit knowledge.

From: Anderson, RH, Neches, WH, Park, SC, Zuberbuhler, JR, eds: *Perspectives in Pediatric Cardiology*: Mount Kisco, New York, Futura Publishing Co., © 1988.

Table 1
"Who Cares?"

No one, when:
- Early mortality after cardiac surgery approaches zero (CL 0%–5%), function is normal, and late survival is not different from the general population.
- New knowledge is not needed or desired.
- Codes and translating devices ensure communication without confusion.

Characterization of Ventricular Septal Defects

Full understanding of a ventricular septal defect, whether it be an isolated defect or part of a more complex congenital cardiac anomaly, demands not only a description of the precise anatomical details of the defect (Table 2). It also requires a description of the commitment or relation of the ventricular septal defect to the great arteries (Lev et al., 1972). Related cardiac anomalies must be described. The position of the cardiac conduction system, and its relation to the margins of the defect, must be known.

Anatomical Location of Ventricular Septal Defects

The margins of a ventricular septal defect (whether it is an isolated [primary] con-

Table 2
Characterization of Ventricular Septal Defects

Anatomical location
Commitment to great arteries (Lev et al.)
Related anomalies
  Overriding great arteries
  Ventricular septal malalignment
  Atrial and ventricular septal malalignment
  Overriding atrioventricular valves
Conduction system

Table 3
Anatomical Location of Ventricular Septal Defects

Muscular	Inlet septum
	Outlet septum
	Trabecular septum
	Apical trabecular septum
	• anteriorly
	• centrally
	• superiorly
	• apically
	• multiple
Marginal	Perimembranous (juxtatricuspid)
	Juxtaaortic
	Juxtapulmonary
	Juxtaarterial
	Juxtatruncal
	Juxtacrux

Note: The description of the location in the interventricular septum of muscular defects is from the right ventricular aspect.

genital cardiac anomaly or part of a complex such as tetralogy of Fallot, complete or congenitally corrected transposition, double outlet right or left ventricle) may be completely *muscular*. Such defects are located in various parts of the interventricular septum (Table 3). (The phrase "interventricular septum" is used since part of the ventricular septum in normal hearts is not interventricular, and since the outlet septum is, for example, not interventricular in the Taussig-Bing heart.) Many ventricular septal defects are at *a margin* of the interventricular septum and are bordered only in part by muscle of the interventricular septum. The remainder of the border is then either an atrioventricular valve, a space over which is one or two arterial valves, or the crux cordis.

Commonly, a marginal ventricular septal defect abuts and is bordered by the tricuspid valve in the region of the commissural tissue between its septal and anterosuperior leaflets. Such defects are generally called *perimembranous* (Soto et al., 1980), although they could be termed juxtatricuspid defects. The ventricular septal defect in the tetralogy of Fallot is bordered in part by a space which the aortic valve overrides, and can be termed a juxtaaortic ventricular septal defect, or a marginal defect with overriding aorta. Such ventricular septal defects are usually perimembranous as well, but in about 20% of hearts with tetralogy of Fallot the posteroinferior border is muscular, due to fusion of the septal band (the septomarginal trabeculation) and the ventriculoinfundibular fold (Anderson et al., 1981), and the defect is described morphologically only by the term juxtaaortic. In the tetralogy of Fallot, the trabecular and outlet portions of the ventricular septum are again malaligned.

In the Taussig-Bing heart, the ventricular septal defect is marginal and juxtapulmonary, and the pulmonary valve overrides the space that forms one border of the defect. Such defects may be perimembranous, or they may have a muscular posteroinferior border. The ventricular septal defect in some hearts with double outlet right ventricle, whether it be perimembranous or have a muscular posteroinferior border, is bordered elsewhere completely by muscle but is located near the pulmonary valve. Lev (1972) has properly described such defects as being subpulmonary, meaning that they are committed to, or near, the pulmonary valve. Such ventricular septal defects are not, however, juxtapulmonary when they are not overridden by the attachments of the valve.

Both aortic and pulmonary valves may lie over the space above some marginal ventricular septal defect, and these defects are termed juxtaarterial. The two valves are contiguous in this situation. In the setting of a common arterial trunk (truncus arteriosus), the ventricular septal defect is juxtatruncal.

Rarely, a marginal ventricular septal defect is bordered by the crux cordis. Such defects exist because of malalignment of the atrial and ventricular septal structures. They are usually, if not always, also perimembranous. The location of the atrioventricular node and the penetrating atrioventricular conduction axis is abnormal because the interventricular septum does not reach to the crux cordis. This defect usually is accompanied by straddling and overriding of the atrioventricular valve (Rastelli et al., 1968). It is termed a juxtacrux defect.

Summary

A surgically helpful method for precise, concise, and complete description of ventricular septal defects, whether they occur as isolated congenital cardiac anomalies or as part of a more complex anomaly, has gradually evolved. Because it is specific, analyses presented in its terms can be readily translated into the terms of the systems used by others.

References

Anderson RH, Allwork SP, Ho SY, et al. Surgical anatomy of tetralogy of Fallot. *J Thorac Cardiovasc Surg* 1981;81:887–896.

Lev M, Bharati S, Meng CCL, et al. A concept of double-outlet right ventricle. *J Thorac Cardiovasc Surg* 1972;64:271–281.

Rastelli GC, Ongley PA, Titus JL. Ventricular septal defect of atrioventricular canal type with straddling atrioventricular valve and mitral valve deformity. *Circulation* 1968;37:816–825.

Soto B, Becker AE, Moulaert AH, et al. Classification of ventricular septal defects. *Br Heart J* 1980;43:332–343.

II

Ebstein's Malformation: Significance of the Anatomical Spectrum

2.1

Introduction

Robert H. Anderson

The history of Wilhelm Ebstein is most splendidly covered in the thorough review by Mann and Lie (1979). As they indicate, he was born on November 27, 1836 in the town of Jauer in Schiesen, Prussia. With the shift of boundaries in the turbulent times since then, his birthplace has now become Jawor in Silesia, Poland. His father was a merchant and Wilhelm attended the local town grammar school. In 1855, he enrolled for medical studies in the University of Breslau, the famous seat of learning for which Brahms wrote his "Academic Festival Overture" when receiving his honorary doctorate. Ebstein did not stay long in Breslau. Almost immediately he transferred to Berlin, where he came under the influence of Virchow. Ebstein graduated in 1859, presenting an undergraduate thesis of starches undergoing microscopic changes when mixed with saliva. In 1861 he returned to Breslau as assistant physician and remained there for nine years. After a short interruption for service in the Franco-Prussian war, he again returned to Breslau as medical officer to the state almshouses. In 1874 he became Professor of Medicine in Gottingen, and there he spent the rest of his life.

Although known today because of the cardiac malformation which bears his name, most of his research was devoted to other areas. His bibliography contains 237 items, of which only 12 are concerned with the heart and blood vessels. Ebstein died in Gottingen on October 22, 1912, having achieved the age of 76. As stated, his widespread fame now rests with his described cardiac lesion, although this publication was a mere case report in his overall corpus of work, was barely mentioned by his contemporaries and, indeed, was largely ignored until after his death.

Joseph Prescher was a 19-year-old laborer admitted to All-Saints Hospital, Breslau under the care of Dr. Julius de Pastau (born 1815). The presenting symptom was shortness of breath and the patient admitted to palpitations since childhood. On admission, Prescher was emaciated and had facial cyanosis and marked elevation of the jugular venous pulse. His heart was enlarged and multiple murmurs and heart sounds were audible. The attending physicians diagnosed a congenital cardiac malformation, but could do little for treatment and the patient died on July 6, eight days after admission. Ebstein performed the autopsy. It

From: Anderson, RH, Neches, WH, Park, SC, Zuberbuhler, JR, eds: *Perspectives in Pediatric Cardiology*: Mount Kisco, New York, Futura Publishing Co., © 1988.

was his full findings, together with two exquisite drawings, which formed the basis of his case report (Ebstein, 1866). He clearly described an anomalous formation of the anterosuperior leaflet of the tricuspid valve and noted abnormal downward displacement of the septal leaflet. His drawings depict what we would now term linear attachment of the anterosuperior leaflet (see Chap. 2.2), and he observed how the anomalous attachments converted the inlet component of the right ventricle to a sack. His drawings show the communication between this sack and the outlet component to be through the anticipated site of the anteroseptal commissure. He inferred from his observations that the lesion dated from the time of formation of the valve leaflets during gestation, and pointed out that, at that time, his finding was unique. His explanations of the hemodynamic and pathological consequences are remarkably accurate (see Mann and Lie, 1979, for a detailed account).

Recognition of further cases appeared slowly during Ebstein's lifetime; at least eight were described before he died (Mann and Lie, 1979). The eponym was used by Yater and Shapiro (1937). Nowadays, the lesion is relatively commonplace, although surgical treatment remains problematic. In this review, Zuberbuhler and I will first discuss the natural history and anatomical appearances of the "classic" lesion, namely, that occurring in patients with otherwise normally connected hearts (Chap. 2.2). In the next chapter, Silverman and Birk will consider the echocardiographic approach to diagnosis, an approach that has revolutionized recognition of the different forms of the lesion (Chap. 2.3). Thereafter, Freedom and Smallhorn (Chap. 2.4) will consider the more traditional approach using catheterization, an approach not without its dangers since Paul Wood, writing in 1962, observed that "I have personally catheterized seven cases of Ebstein's disease, but do not propose to catheterize another wittingly." In this chapter, the Toronto authors also describe Ebstein's malformation as it afflicts the morphologically tricuspid valve in pa-

tients with discordant atrioventricular connection (congenitally corrected transposition). Finally, Kirklin and his colleagues from Birmingham, Alabama, describe their results with replacement of the tricuspid valve. Ideally, our surgical section should also incorporate an account of reconstruction of the malformed tricuspid valve. We had hoped to include a description of the extensive experience of Danielson at the Mayo Clinic, but this proved impossible. The interested reader, nonetheless, should certainly read and study his technique. This is well described in the section of the Mayo Clinic Proceedings devoted to Ebstein's malformation (Danielson et al., 1979). Their paper is an excellent introduction to this alternative surgical procedure. At the Pittsburgh symposium, Danielson presented an account of over 80 patients operated with this technique, with excellent results.

Acknowledgments: The historical account of Ebstein is taken exclusively from the excellent paper by Mann and Lie (1979). If charges are laid against me of plagiarism, they are entirely justified. I recommend the original to all who are interested in historical aspects.

References

Danielson GK, Maloney JD, Devloo RAE. Surgical repair of Ebstein's anomaly. *Mayo Clin Proc* 1979;54:185–192.

Ebstein W. Über einen sehr seltenen Fall von Insufficienz der Valvula tricuspidalis, bedingt durch eine angeborene hochgradige Missbildung derselben. *Arch von Riechert Bois-Raymond* 1866;2:238–254.

Mann RJ, Lie JT. The life story of Wilhelm Ebstein (1836–1912) and his almost overlooked description of a congenital heart disease. *Mayo Clin Proc* 1979;54:197–204.

Wood P. *Diseases of the Heart and Circulation* (2nd ed). London: Eyre and Spottiswoode, 1962; 352–358.

Yater WM, Shapiro MJ. Congenital displacement of the tricuspid valve (Ebstein's disease): Review and report of a case with electrocardiographic abnormalities and detailed histologic study of the conduction system. *Ann Intern Med* 1937; 11:1043–1062.

Ebstein's Malformation of the Tricuspid Valve: Morphology and Natural History

James R. Zuberbuhler and Robert H. Anderson

The cardinal feature of Ebstein's malformation is a displacement of part of the origin of the tricuspid valve from the atrioventricular junction into the cavity of the right ventricle. The degree of this displacement is variable, and there are usually other abnormalities of the valve, including dysplasia of the leaflets and abnormal attachment of their distal margin. In previous communications, we and others have pointed out that the variable morphology of the tricuspid valve constitutes a spectrum, ranging from minimal displacement of the leaflet origin to complete division of the right ventricle via muscular partitions separating the inlet from the outlet and trabecular portions (Anderson et al., 1978, 1979; Zuberbuhler et al., 1979).

In addition to the valvular anomalies, there are often right and even left ventricular abnormalities as well, and other congenital cardiac malformations may be associated. The morphological features of Ebstein's malformation result in hemodynamic changes that determine presentation and clinical course. In this chapter we will review the morphology of a series of specimens with Ebstein's malformation existing in the cardiopathological collection at Children's Hospital of Pittsburgh. We will then relate this morphology to the clinical findings of 37 patients with this malformation who have been seen at Children's Hospital over the last 17 years. Cineangiographic and echocardiographic diagnosis and surgical repair of the lesion will be covered in the subsequent chapters of this section of the book. As an introduction to the morphology of Ebstein's malformation, however, we found it helpful to review the anatomy of the normal tricuspid valve.

During the course of this investigation, RHA was supported by the Patrick Dick Memorial Fund.

From: Anderson, RH, Neches, WH, Park, SC, Zuberbuhler, JR, eds: *Perspectives in Pediatric Cardiology*: Mount Kisco, New York, Futura Publishing Co., © 1988.

The Normal Tricuspid Valve

The leaflet structure of the normal tricuspid valve is more variable than that of the mitral. There are usually three recognizable leaflets: the septal, the anterosuperior (anterior), and the inferior (mural, posterior) (Fig. 1). The septal leaflet, as its name suggests, arises from the septum, demarcating the inferior margin of the atrioventricular septum (because it normally attaches more distally than does the mitral valve). It extends from the junction of the parietal wall with the septum inferiorly and crosses the membranous septum superiorly. The commissure between the septal and anterosuperior leaflets is supported by the medial papillary muscle complex, which takes origin from the posterior limb of the septomarginal trabeculation beneath the membranous septum. The commissure between the septal and inferior leaflets is supported by the inferior papillary muscle. Between these muscles a variable number of cords extend from the junction of the inlet and trabecular portions of the right ventricle to support the body of the septal leaflet. The anterosuperior and inferior leaflets originate along the parietal portion of the atrioven-

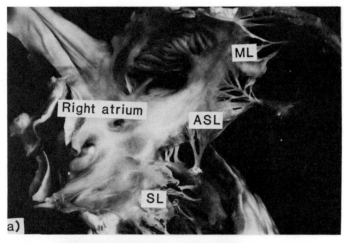

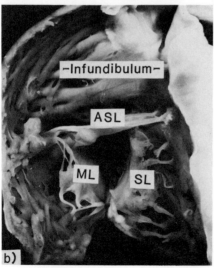

Figure 1. Inlet (a) and outlet (b) aspects of the normal tricuspid valve showing the arrangement of the septal (SL), anterosuperior (ASL), and mural or inferior (ML) leaflets.

tricular junction. There is usually a fairly well-defined commissure between these leaflets. This is supported by the anterior papillary muscle, which arises from the body of the septomarginal trabeculation in conjunction with the moderator band. The inferior leaflet usually receives further support from cords running to the parietal wall.

The right ventricular cavity itself has three zones. The inlet portion is bounded by the atrioventricular junction on one hand and the origin of the papillary muscle and cords supporting the tricuspid leaflets on the other. The area of septum thus delineated is usually termed the "inlet septum" but, because of the normal wedge position of the subaortic outflow tract (see Chapter 1.2), it separates in part the inlet of the right ventricle from the outlet of the left. The trabecular portion lies laterally and apically to the inlet portion. The outlet zone lies between the inlet and trabecular areas and the pulmonary valve. The impression is often gained of an extensive area of "septum" between the limbs of the septomarginal trabeculation. In reality, because the pulmonary leaflets are supported on a sleeve of outlet musculature, this "septum" is part of the outer wall of the heart (see Chapter 1.2).

The Tricuspid Valve in Ebstein's Malformation

Differing Abnormalities of the Leaflets

The abnormality of the valve leaflets is usually thought of in terms of "downward displacement," although several authors have emphasized that the original case described by Wilhelm Ebstein was probably characterized by dysplasia more than displacement. Dysplasia is now certainly recognized as an integral part of the lesion (Becker et al., 1971), but our recent observations, coupled with the review performed

specifically for this chapter, indicate that the distal attachment of the leaflets is at least as significant in determining clinical features as is the degree of displacement or dysplasia. In this section, therefore, we will account for all these features, namely displacement, distal attachment, and dysplasia.

Displacement of the Leaflets

Although displacement of the proximal origin of the leaflets is taken to be (and, indeed, is) the cardinal feature of Ebstein's malformation, not all the leaflets are displaced. In our experience, with rare exceptions (Zuberbuhler et al., 1984), the anterosuperior leaflet always retains its normal attachment to the underside of the ventriculoinfundibular fold (Fig. 2). Thus, it is the

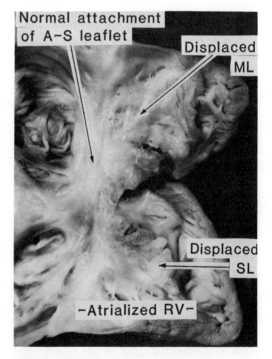

Figure 2. The inlet aspect of an example of Ebstein's malformation showing the displaced attachments of the mural (ML) and septal (SL) leaflets but a normal attachment of the anterosuperior (AS) leaflet. Note the thin-walled atrialized segment of the right ventricle (RV).

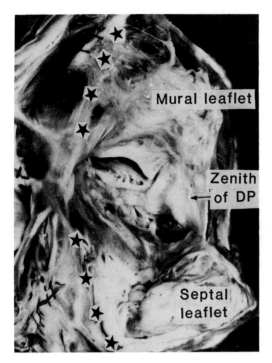

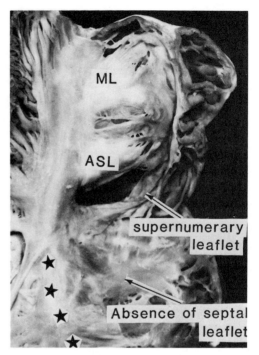

Figure 3. An example of Ebstein's malformation in which the zenith of displacement (DP) of the leaflets is at the commissure between the septal and mural leaflets. The stars indicate the level of the atrioventricular junction.

Figure 4. In this example of Ebstein's malformation, only the septal leaflet is displaced from the atrioventricular junction (marked by stars). The mural (ML) and anterosuperior (ASL) leaflets are attached proximally at the level of the junction.

septal and mural leaflets that exhibit displacement. Anderson et al. (1979) emphasized this feature, pointing out that the inferior commissure between these leaflets tended to mark the site of maximal displacement and, hence, the zenith of atrialization of the ventricular inlet component. While this arrangement pertains in many cases (Fig. 3), it is not universally present. Indeed, in some hearts with severe Ebstein's malformation, the mural leaflet retains its usual attachment to the parietal atrioventricular junction (Fig. 4). In such hearts, displacement is confined to the septal leaflet, although this displacement in itself can enclose a substantial area of atrialized right ventricle (Fig. 5). Displacement is not always the perfect term to describe the deformity of the septal leaflet. In some hearts there is no question that the entire leaflet has a septal origin well within the ventricu-

lar cavity, the leaflet tissue being heaped up at this site in cauliflower-like excrescences (Fig. 6a). In other hearts, the tissue of the septal leaflet may be virtually absent, represented only by scattered clumps of tissue along the anticipated line of displacement (Fig. 6b). In yet other hearts, the leaflet is more markedly deformed, extending as a supernumerary hammock-like structure to fuse with the anterosuperior or inferior leaflet (Fig. 7; see below). In summary, therefore, the origin of the anterosuperior leaflet is rarely displaced, that of the mural leaflet usually, but not always, while the leaflet tissue septally may sometimes be better considered virtually absent (or undelaminated) rather than displaced.

Irrespective of its extent, the major effect of displacement is "atrialization" of a portion of right ventricle. In hemodynamic terms, this means that an atrial pressure

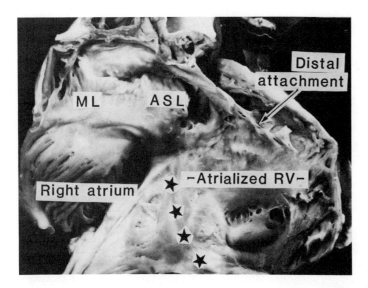

Figure 5. This aspect of the heart shown in Fig. 4 demonstrates the extensive atrialized portion of the right ventricle (RV) to be found even when only the septal leaflet is displaced.

zone lies within the inlet component of the morphologically right ventricle. This is "physiological" atrialization. It must be distinguished from "anatomical" atrialization. The latter term describes thinning of the pa- rietal wall which bounds the physiologically atrialized portion of the ventricle. Physiological atrialization is universally present in this anomaly (although not necessarily recognizable clinically). Anatomical atrializa-

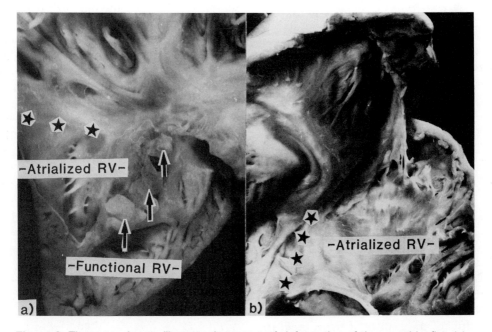

Figure 6. These two hearts illustrate the extent of deformation of the septal leaflet: (a) a mass of cauliflower excrescences (arrowed) forms the boundary between the atrialized and functional components of the right ventricle (RV); (b) in this heart, however, the septal leaflet is virtually absent. The stars mark the level of the atrioventricular junction.

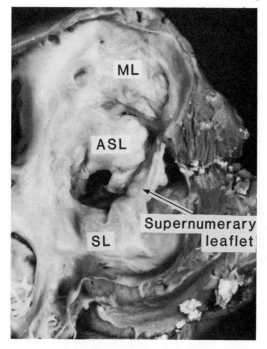

Figure 7. In other examples of Ebstein's malformation, seen from the inlet aspect, a supernumerary leaflet bridges between the displaced septal (SL) and the other leaflets (ASL, ML).

tion is variable. Still a third consequence of distal displacement is a reduction in size of the functional right ventricle. This functional component is, in essence, made up of the apical trabecular and outlet components. The greater the displacement, the larger the atrialized portion and the smaller the part of the right ventricle that has ventricular hemodynamic characteristics.

Distal Attachment

Although Ebstein's malformation is defined according to the abnormal origin of the leaflets, their anomalous distal attachments are particularly important in inducing hemodynamic abnormality. The supporting apparatus of the leaflets of the normal tricuspid valve consists of cords arising from the right ventricular myocardium. The attachments of these structures to the ventricular wall can be thought of as being focal.

Such focal attachments permit free flow of blood from the inlet to the trabecular and outlet portions of the ventricle under the leading edges of the leaflets. Some hearts with Ebstein's malformation display a more or less linear attachment of the anterosuperior and/or inferior leaflets to the junction between the inlet and trabecular zones (Fig. 8a). Others exhibit linear attachments of the septal leaflet together with a tongue of leaflet tissue which connects the apical part of the septum with the other leaflets (Fig. 7). In such hearts, these junctions are marked by a muscular ridge or shelf that extends inferiorly from the junction of the parietal wall and septum and runs in superior direction toward the outlet portion. There are often gaps in the attachments of the leaflets to this ridge which permit some blood to pass directly from the inlet to the trabecular zone. This can be conceptualized in terms of a hyphenated distal attachment (Fig. 9). Tags of leaflet tissue are often heaped up in cauliflower fashion along these hyphenations. If the attachment is completely "linear," the only exit from the inlet portion is through the commissure between the septal and anterosuperior leaflets. Hearts with linear attachment of the leaflets display a degree of tricuspid stenosis, since there can no longer be free flow of blood under the entire distal edges of the anterosuperior and inferior leaflets as is possible with focal attachment (Fig. 8b). Should the leaflet attachment be completely linear and the anterosuperior commissure absent, the result is an imperforate Ebstein's malformation (Fig. 10). In summary, the distal attachments of the leaflets show a spectrum of abnormality extending from focal through hyphenated and linear to imperforate arrangements.

Leaflet Dysplasia

The tricuspid valve leaflets usually display some degree of dysplasia in hearts with Ebstein's malformation and, in some, the dysplasia is extreme. The septal leaflet is

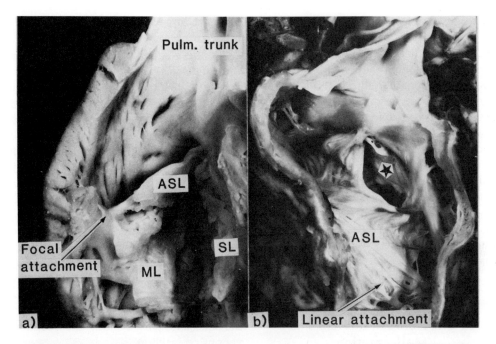

Figure 8. These outlet views show the difference between focal (a) and linear (b) attachment of the anterosuperior leaflets (ASL). With linear attachment (b), the commissure between the leaflets (starred) forms the communication between the components of the right ventricle.

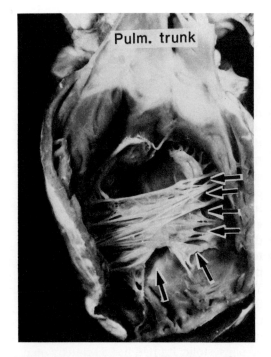

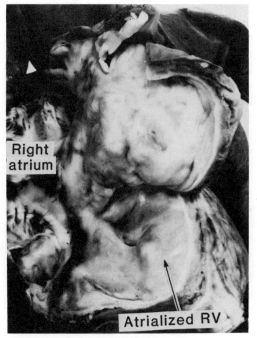

Figure 9. In this example of Ebstein's malformation, viewed from the outlet aspect, there is a hyphenated attachment of the septal leaflet and supernumerary tongue (arrowed).

Figure 10. This inlet view shows an imperforate example of Ebstein's malformation, resulting in the clinical picture of tricuspid atresia.

often thickened and may consist of clumps of dysplastic tissue confined to the superior border of the inlet zone. The anterosuperior and inferior leaflets may be filmy, fenestrated, and large and redundant (billowing). Both the anterosuperior and inferior leaflets sometimes have patchy attachments to the parietal wall. In some hearts, septal and inferior leaflet tissue is recognizable in the atrialized ventricle and is "plastered down" to the wall. In others, the septal wall appears bare and valve tissue is recognizable only near the displaced tricuspid orifice, which is effectively between the inlet component of the ventricle (physiologically atrialized) and its distal component, which has functional ventricular characteristics.

The Heart in Ebstein's Malformation

Right Ventricular Abnormalities

In the setting of "isolated" Ebstein's malformation (that is to say, cases not associated with pulmonary atresia or congenitally corrected transposition), the morphologically right ventricle may be normal in size or may be enlarged. As indicated above, there is usually, but not always, anatomical atrialization consisting of thinning of the inferior parietal wall. The right ventricular aspect of the inlet septum is often abnormally smooth and may be somewhat thin.

Left Ventricular Abnormalities

The left ventricle may be misshapen and have an abnormal contraction pattern. In a previously reported series from this institution (Monibi et al., 1978), 12 of 13 patients studied with cineangiography demonstrated both an abnormal contour and contraction pattern within the left ventricle. Five of these also had prolapse of the leaflets of the mitral valve.

Other Congenital Cardiac Anomalies

Ebstein's malformation is seen in about one-quarter of patients with pulmonary atresia with intact ventricular septum. It is also common with congenitally corrected transposition (the combination of discordant atrioventricular and ventriculoarterial connections). If such patients are excluded, the most commonly associated cardiac anomaly by far is an interatrial communication. An interatrial septal defect was found in 15 of 23 patients in our series who had cardiac catheterization at greater than one month of age, all being within the oval fossa ("secundum defects"). In this same series, four patients had a ventricular septal defect, three had pulmonary stenosis, and one each had valvular aortic stenosis, coarctation of the aorta, and partial anomalous pulmonary venous connection.

Functional Consequences of Ebstein's Malformation

Mild forms may not influence hemodynamics, but if the malformation is more severe, the net effect of the morphological abnormality is impairment of right heart function. The displacement of the origin of the leaflets of the tricuspid valve, their abnormal distal attachment, and their dysplasia can each have important hemodynamic consequences. Probably the most common hemodynamic abnormality is tricuspid regurgitation, which is due primarily to leaflet dysplasia. The regurgitation may be through fenestrations in the anterosuperior leaflet or may be due to poor coaptation of thickened and poorly mobile or thin and billowing leaflets. Since pressure in the functional right ventricle is usually low, the murmur of tricuspid regurgitation is soft and may not be pansystolic. It often has a scratchy quality. The murmur is frequently introduced by an unusually loud tricuspid component of the first heart sound (the so-called sail sound), presumably generated by a large mobile and billowing anterosuperior leaflet.

It is the linear nature of the distal attachment of the tricuspid valve that causes tricuspid stenosis. The murmur of tricuspid stenosis is always soft and subtle and is medium-pitched, certainly not a "rumble." If there is substantial tricuspid regurgitation, a similar diastolic murmur represents relative rather than organic tricuspid obstruction. Tricuspid stenosis is the dominant hemodynamic abnormality in an occasional patient. In the patient with an imperforate Ebstein's malformation, the hemodynamics are those of tricuspid atresia. As in tricuspid atresia, it is usual for a ventricular septal defect to be the portal to the distal components of right ventricle and, hence, to be the source of pulmonary blood flow.

The third functional abnormality, a small and restrictive functional right ventricle, is seen if there is marked distal displacement of the origin of the inferior and septal leaflets. As discussed, this is because there tends to be an inverse relationship between the size of the atrialized and functional portions of this ventricle.

The net result of the tricuspid regurgitation, tricuspid stenosis, and restriction of the right ventricle is impairment of forward flow from the right ventricle. This is enhanced if right ventricular pressure is high, as it will be if there is associated pulmonary stenosis, a large ventricular septal defect, or if pulmonary vascular resistance is elevated. Right-to-left shunting occurs if there is an interatrial communication and if any of the hemodynamic alterations, either singly or in combination, are sufficiently marked. The normal elevation of pulmonary vascular resistance in the newborn period explains the tendency shortly after birth for tricuspid regurgitation to be marked and cyanosis to be intense. The clinical picture usually improves markedly with the normal fall in pulmonary vascular resistance and right ventricular pressure and the concomitant increase in right ventricular compliance.

Natural History

To further define the presentation and course of patients with Ebstein's malformation followed in a single institution, we reviewed 37 cases seen at Children's Hospital of Pittsburgh between 1970 and 1985. Most patients were seen by one of the authors (JRZ). The diagnosis was made at catheterization and angiography in 31 of 37. In eight of these it was further confirmed at surgery or autopsy. The diagnosis was based on clinical and echocardiographic findings in the six patients who did not undergo cardiac catheterization.

Presentation

Nearly two-fifths of the patients were seen during the first week of life (Fig. 11) and nine presented during the first day. In each, the presence of congenital heart disease was suspected because of either a murmur or cyanosis. Most patients demonstrated both. The large number of patients seen during the neonatal period, together with the presenting findings of cyanosis and tricuspid regurgitation, are undoubtedly related to the normal neonatal elevation of pulmonary vascular resistance and right ventricular pressure along with the relatively low compliance of the neonatal right ventricle. Of the six patients first seen between one week and one year of age, four had a murmur, two were cyanotic, and one had supraventricular tachycardia. By far the most common presentation in the 17 patients seen at ages greater than one year was with the systolic murmur of tricuspid regurgitation (14 of 17). Only one of these patients presented with cyanosis, while the other two had supraventricular tachycardias.

Congestive heart failure was relatively uncommon, occurring in only six patients in the entire series. In three of these there was another reason for the failure. A ventricular

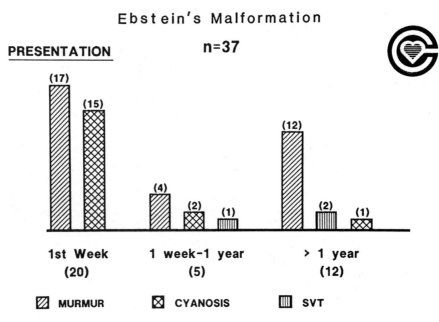

Figure 11. Signs at presentation in 37 infants and children with Ebstein's malformation. Numbers are in parentheses. SVT = supraventricular tachycardia.

septal defect coexisted in two while supraventricular tachycardia was present in one. The other three patients presented during the first week and each had both cyanosis and a murmur in addition to evidence of congestive failure. The infrequency of congestive heart failure in our series was in striking contrast to its incidence in the large multicenter series collected by Watson (1974) where nearly three-quarters of infants were in congestive heart failure.

The "classic" physical findings associated with Ebstein's malformation include the systolic murmur of tricuspid regurgitation, the diastolic murmur of tricuspid stenosis (both heard at the low left sternal border), and a widely split first heart sound with a loud and delayed tricuspid component (sail sound) (Fig. 12). Because of the commonly associated right bundle branch block, the second heart sound is also usually widely split. All but one of our patients had a systolic murmur heard on at least one examination at the low left sternal border which was consistent with tricuspid regurgitation. Seventy percent of the patients had

a murmur of tricuspid stenosis (either organic or relative) heard at some time, but this murmur was relatively rare during the first year of life, being heard in only one-quarter of these patients. Half of the patients demonstrated a sail sound, but only 40% had the triad of systolic and diastolic murmurs and a loud and delayed tricuspid component of the first heart sound. The diagnosis of Ebstein's malformation must be considered, therefore, in patients who do not have all of the classic physical findings, especially in the newborn period. Indeed, the diagnosis should be considered in any cyanotic newborn (especially if there is a murmur of tricuspid regurgitation) and in any older child with either a murmur of tricuspid regurgitation or unexplained cardiomegaly.

Cyanosis was present at some time in the course of 20 of the 37 patients. It was noted during the first day of life in 13, during the first week in an additional two and during the first two months of life in another four. In only one patient did cyanosis appear after the first year (at 18 months of

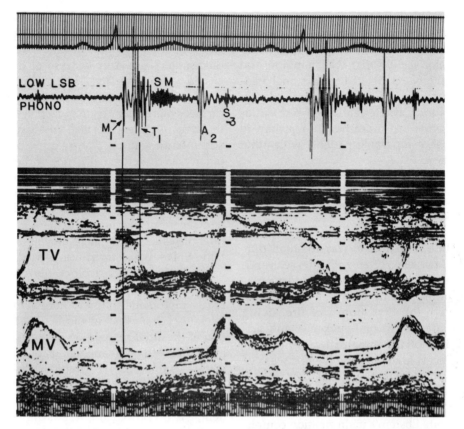

Figure 12. Phonocardiogram and echocardiogram showing a "sail sound," representing late tricuspid valve closure. A_2 = aortic valve closure; LSB = left sternal border; M_1 = mitral valve closure; MV = mitral valve; S_3 = third heart sound; SM = systolic murmur; T_1 = tricuspid valve closure; TV = tricuspid valve.

age). In 11 patients, the cyanosis persisted either until death or surgical repair, or was present at the last follow-up visit. In the remaining nine patients the cyanosis cleared, usually during the first week of life. Only one patient had early clearing of cyanosis with subsequent reappearance.

Cardiac Catheterization

Cardiac catheterization was done in 31 of the 37 patients. Many of these studies were done for diagnostic purposes prior to the advent of cross-sectional echocardiography. Others were performed so as to assess associated anomalies or in anticipation of surgical repair.

Right ventricular pressure was clearly related to age. Four of the six patients catheterized during the first day of life had right ventricular pressure in excess of 40% of left ventricular pressure. Only one of four undergoing invasive study from two to seven days of age had an elevated right ventricular pressure and only two patients studied at greater than one week of age had high right ventricular pressures. One of these had severe pulmonary stenosis while the other had a large ventricular septal defect.

The only mortality associated with catheterization occurred early in the series. This occurred in a newborn who was very cyanotic prior to catheterization and who became acidotic and died a few hours following the procedure. One very polycythemic patient suffered a cerebrovascular accident following catheterization but subsequently recovered completely. Supraventricular tachycardia was common and one patient experienced paroxysmal ventricular tachycardia which required cardioversion. Catheterization in our hands thus seemed no more hazardous than in otherwise comparable patients with other anomalies.

Clinical Course

While presentation was common during the first week, often with intense cyanosis, there was a striking tendency to spontaneous improvement. Only one infant failed to survive the first month of life, dying shortly after birth of hypoxemia and acidosis. Two of the three patients with congestive heart failure during the first week of life responded to the usual therapeutic measures and failure did not recur when digoxin was discontinued. The third had an imperforate Ebstein's malformation complicated by severe subvalvular aortic stenosis and died in congestive failure. Cyanosis cleared in half of those demonstrating it. In general, growth and development were normal unless there were important associated anomalies.

Cardiac Surgery

Cardiac surgery was carried out in 10 patients. In four, only associated anomalies were corrected. A large ventricular septal defect was closed in one infant, severe valvular pulmonary stenosis repaired in another infant and severe valvular aortic stenosis in a three-year-old. In the fourth, an infant with coarctation and ventricular septal defect, the coarctation was repaired and the pulmonary trunk banded. Recoarctation occurred and the child died at three and one-half months of age with pneumocystis

infection. In none of these four cases did the Ebstein's malformation seem hemodynamically important. Six patients underwent cardiac surgery primarily because of their tricuspid valve anomaly. Two patients with severe tricuspid regurgitation and marked cardiac enlargement were judged at surgery to have relatively normal anterosuperior and inferior leaflets. The tricuspid regurgitation was related to deficiency of the septal leaflet. In each, an annuloplasty eliminated the tricuspid regurgitation and neither patient is currently symptomatic. Two patients had severe displacement of the septal and inferior leaflets with linear attachment distally. Valve replacement was carried out in each. Complete heart block necessitated permanent artificial pacing in one, but both are asymptomatic and have normal exercise tolerance. One five-year-old boy had plication of the atrialized portion of the ventricle and repair of partial anomalous pulmonary venous connection. He continues to have moderate cardiomegaly at age 17 but is without symptoms. The sixth operated patient, a five-year-old girl, was asymptomatic until she presented with a large pericardial effusion following upper respiratory infection. The effusion recurred following pericardiocentesis and a pericardial window was surgically created to relieve tamponade. She suddenly became hypotensive several hours following surgery and did not respond to the usual supportive measures. An emergency annuloplasty and ventricular plication was undertaken but she failed to survive.

Mortality

Seven patients died during the period covered by this study. Death was sudden and unexpected in three, who were aged 9, 11, and 12 years, respectively. None of these children had been symptomatic or had evidence of ventricular ectopy. One had a Wolff-Parkinson-White syndrome and the

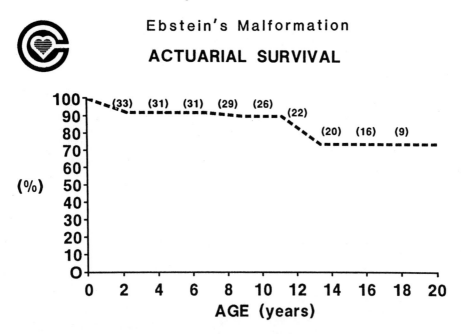

Figure 13. Actuarial survival curve of children with Ebstein's malformation. The numbers of patients surviving to each age are in parentheses.

left ventricle was found to be hypertrophied and dilated at autopsy. No autopsy was done in the other two. The five-year-old girl with pericardial effusion has already been mentioned, as has the $3\frac{1}{2}$-month-old with coarctation and ventricular septal defect who underwent coarctation repair and banding of the pulmonary trunk and died of pneumocystis infection, and the one-day-old who died of hypoxemia and acidosis. The final infant, with an imperforate Ebstein's malformation and severe subvalvular aortic stenosis, died in congestive heart failure.

The actuarial survival curve of our series is shown in Figure 13. Survival was 78% at age 13 (21 patients) and no further deaths were noted in those followed until age 19 (six patients).

An attempt was made to assess the clinical status of the 30 survivors. Exercise treadmill tests were done in 11 patients. This study was considered normal in eight (including one patient following valve replacement who had been able to exercise

for only one and one-half minutes prior to surgery). Exercise tolerance was severely limited in another cyanotic unoperated patient and mildly reduced in two further individuals.

Paroxysmal supraventricular tachycardia occurred in 9 of the 37 patients (24%). Onset was before one year of age in two and from 7 to 15 years in the remaining five. Wolff-Parkinson-White syndrome occurred in six (16%), three of whom also had supraventricular tachycardia. Overall, 21 patients were completely without cardiovascular symptoms at last follow-up and had normal exercise tolerance. Three were cyanotic, four continued to have episodes of ventricular tachycardia, and two had some degree of exercise intolerance.

Our study confirms some findings of previous reports, but is at variance with others. Like Watson (1974), we found that most patients who survived early infancy did relatively well. Our incidence of Wolff-Parkinson-White syndrome and supraventricular tachycardia was similar to his. Unlike Watson's findings of a very high incidence of congestive heart failure in infancy, only three of our uncomplicated patients had congestive failure, which was transient in two of the three. It seems clear that the great majority of symptomatic newborns will improve as pulmonary arterial and right ventricular pressures fall and as compliance of the right ventricle increases. Surgical intervention is not indicated in this age group. Our surgical experience in older children is limited, but suggests that a procedure should be chosen in light of the morphology and its hemodynamic consequences. If the major abnormality is tricuspid regurgitation and if the distal tricuspid leaflet attachment is focal, annuloplasty with or without plication of the atrialized ventricle seems appropriate. If there is linear attachment of the margins of the leaflets, there will be an element of tricuspid stenosis and tricuspid regurgitation tends to be less severe. Valve replacement is probably the surgical procedure of choice in these patients.

References

Anderson KR, Lie JT. Pathologic anatomy of Ebstein's anomaly of the heart revisited. *Pediatr Cardiol* 1978;41:739–745.

Anderson KR, Zuberbuhler JR, Anderson RH, et al. Morphologic spectrum of Ebstein's anomaly of the heart. *Mayo Clinic Proc* 1979;54:174–180.

Becker AE, Becker MJ, Edward JE. Pathologic spectrum and dysplasia of the tricuspid valve: Features in common with Ebstein's malformation. *Arch Pathol* 1971;91:167–178.

Monibi AA, Neches WH, Lenox CC, et al. Left ventricular anomalies associated with Ebstein's malformation of the tricuspid valve. *Circulation* 1978;57:303–306.

Watson H. Natural history of Ebstein's anomaly of tricuspid valve in childhood and adolescence. An international co-operative study of 505 cases. *Br Heart J* 1974;36:417–427.

Zuberbuhler JR, Allwork SP, Anderson RH. The spectrum of Ebstein's anomaly of the tricuspid valve. *J Thorac Cardiovasc Surg* 1979;77:202–211.

Zuberbuhler JR, Becker AE, Anderson RH, Lenox CC. Ebstein's malformation and the embryological development of the tricuspid valve. *Pediatr Cardiol* 1984;5:289–296.

Ebstein's Malformation of the Tricuspid Valve: Cross-Sectional Echocardiography and Doppler

Norman H. Silverman and Einat Birk

Ebstein's malformation consists of a spectrum of several morphological abnormalities of the tricuspid valve that are readily identifiable by echocardiography. The echocardiographic technique, when augmented by Doppler ultrasound and injection of contrast material into a peripheral vein, provides an assessment comparable with or superior to that obtained by angiography and cardiac catheterization while avoiding the dangers of producing serious arrhythmias and other life-threatening complications (Broadbent et al., 1953).

Because of the great variability of pathological expression, it is better to consider the anomaly as a spectrum of abnormalities with considerable variability (Anderson et al., 1979; Zuberbuhler et al., 1979). We shall describe the echocardiographic abnormalities by categories. These include displacement of the proximal attachments of the leaflets, displacement of their distal attachments, and dysplasia.

Technique and Findings

Our echocardiographic description of this anomaly is based on our analysis of records of 41 fetuses, infants, and children (see Table 1).

Echocardiographic Method

A complete echocardiographic examination was performed on all patients, using M-mode and cross-sectional techniques as well as pulsed and continuous-wave Doppler ultrasound. We used a large complement of views for cross-sectional imaging, including parasternal, apical, and subcostal views (Lundstrom, 1973; Ports et al., 1978). The parasternal short-axis plane displays the anterosuperior and septal leaflets of the tricuspid valve, as well as the size and function of the right ventricular outflow

From: Anderson, RH, Neches, WH, Park, SC, Zuberbuhler, JR, eds: *Perspectives in Pediatric Cardiology*: Mount Kisco, New York, Futura Publishing Co., © 1988.

Table 1
Ebstein's Malformation

	Sex	Dx done at the newborn period	Death	Cath	Surgery	Type of surgery	Associated findings
1	M	+					SVT
2	M	Prenat	+				
3	F	+	+				
4	F	+	+	+			
5	M						Mild PS, PI
6	F						
7	M	+		+	+	Coarc, PDA, ASD	Coarc AS, ASD MS
8	F	Baby		+			VSD, ASD, PS
9	M	+		+			SVT
10	M						
11	M	+					
12	M	+		+	+	Glenn; ASD; annuloplasty	AV dissociation
13	M						
14	F	+					
15	F	+	+	+	+	Annuloplasty	
16	F				+		
17	F			+	+	PAD	PAD
18	F			+	+	Annuloplasty	
19	M	+					
20	F	+					
21	M						SVT
22	F						
23	F	+		+			SVT, VSD, ASD
24	M						
25	F						
26	F	+	+				Premie; Liver dis
27	F						
28	M	+		+			
29	F						
30	F	Prenat	+				
31	F	+		+	+	BT shunt Glenn, RA	SVT
32	M	+	+	+			PAD
33	F						
34	M	+	+	+	+	PAD	
35	M	+					
36	M	+					
37	M			+	+	BT shunt, Aop shunt	SVT, Mild PS, ASD
38	M			+			
39	F						
40	F	Prenat	+				
41	F		+				Valvular pulmonary atresia

AS = aortic stenosis; ASD = atrial septal defect; Coarc = coarctation of aorta; MS = mitral stenosis; PS = pulmonary stenosis; PAD = patent arterial duct; SVT = supraventricular tachycardia; VSD = ventricular septal defect.

tract. The distal attachment may also be examined from this plane (Fig. 1). The apical four-chamber view displays the displacement of the septal and anterosuperior leaflets, including the morphology of their distal attachment (Fig. 2). The subcostal coronal and sagittal views display the motion and distal attachment of the anterosuperior leaflet, as well as the distal displacement of the attachment of the inferior (mural) leaflet (Fig. 3). The subcostal sagittal image obtained in the plane orthogonal to the coronal plane provides views that augment and complement those obtained in the coronal plan (Fig. 4). These views enable us to assess the size of the functional right ventricle, as well as the pulmonary and infundibular areas.

Displacement of the Leaflets

The most characteristic and readily recognizable echocardiographic feature of this lesion is the displacement of the atrioventricular junctional attachment of the septal

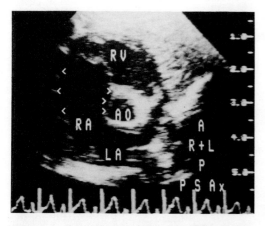

Figure 1. Parasternal short-axis (PSAx) view from a patient with Ebstein's malformation. The anterosuperior and septal leaflets of the tricuspid valve are displaced toward the right ventricular outflow tract (RV), and are tethered to the right ventricular free wall and septum, respectively. The right atrium (RA) is dilated. A = anterior; AO = aorta; L = left; LA = left atrium; P = posterior; R = right.

and inferior leaflets of the tricuspid valve (Fig. 5). This displacement, together with anomalous attachment of the anterosuperior leaflet, produces a bipartite right ventricle with functional and atrialized portions. The junction between the right atrium and the atrialized portion of the right ventricle is guarded by the atrioventricular groove which, for most of its circumference, is devoid of mobile attachment to the leaflets of the atrioventricular valve. The displacement, however, does not usually involve the anterosuperior leaflet. Rather, it forms a spiral, with the inferior and septal leaflets being more displaced than the anterosuperior leaflet, which usually has a normal attachment (Schiebler et al., 1968; Zuberbuhler et al., 1979).

The first echocardiographic description of displacement of the septal leaflet was observed from the parasternal windows but it is better seen from the apical four-chamber view (Fig. 2) (Ports et al., 1978). Displacement of the septal leaflet is caused by the adherence of the leaflet to the underlying ventricular septum. The posterior apical four-chamber view shows the position of the septal leaflet of the tricuspid valve relative to the mitral valve and the central fibrous body. In a normal heart, there is only a slight distal displacement of the septal leaflet relative to the septal attachment of the leaflets of the mitral valve. The ratio of the distances between the apex and the mitral and tricuspid septal insertions, respectively, does not exceed 1.3:1 (Ports et al., 1978). In Ebstein's malformation, in contrast, it has been noted that the displacement can be so severe as to extend to the junction of the inlet and trabecular zones of the ventricle (Zuberbuhler et al., 1984). Unlike in the normal heart, the septal leaflet of the tricuspid valve becomes liberated at a point that is distant from the mitral insertion to the central fibrous body. The septal leaflet may be thickened and immobile, diminutive, or absent. The leaflet, as observed by cross-sectional echocardiography, may be distally displaced from its nor-

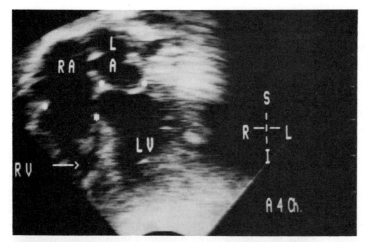

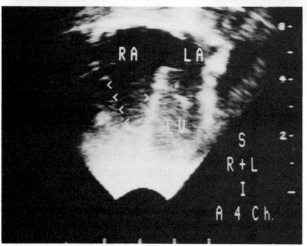

Figure 2. Top: An apical four-chamber view (A4Ch) shows the displacement of the tricuspid valve leaflets toward the cardiac apex, as compared with the normal attachment of the mitral leaflets (∗). The tethering of the leaflets is outlined with arrows. The atrialized right ventricle is located between the atrioventricular groove (∗) and the displaced effective orifice of the tricuspid valve. The moderator band can be seen in the apex of the right ventricle (RV). Bottom: This frame shows an example of more severe distal displacement of the tricuspid valve leaflets. I = inferior; LV = left ventricle; S = superior.

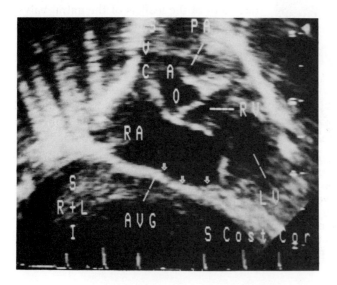

Figure 3. The subcostal coronal view (SCostCor) displays the distal attachment of the anterosuperior leaflet and the distal displacement of the inferior (mural) one relative to the atrioventricular groove (AVG). The tethering of the leaflet is outlined by arrows. PA = pulmonary artery; RA = right atrium; SVC = superior caval vein.

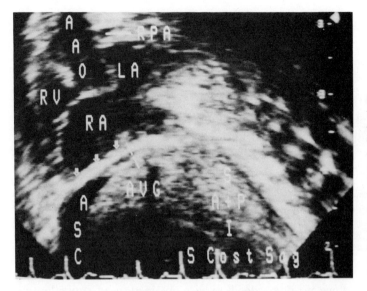

Figure 4. The subcostal sagittal view (SCostSag) shows the distal attachment of the anterosuperior leaflet and the degree of tethering of the mural leaflet (arrows). The size of the functional right ventricle is diminished. A small amount of ascites is seen, caused by the intrauterine congestive heart failure. AAO = ascending aorta; ASC = ascites; AVG = atrioventricular groove; RPA = right pulmonary artery.

mal position, and its motion is diminished or even absent. These features are best seen in the posterior apical four-chamber cut passing through the central fibrous body and the septal attachment of the mitral valve. Although the displacement of the septal leaflet may be more marked anteriorly, its quantitation may be impeded due to interposition of the aortic root between the ventricular septum and the mitral valve.

In the four-chamber apical view, the echo arising from the atrioventricular valve groove can be displayed, thus marking the atrioventricular junction. This is helpful for delineating the separation between the atrialized right ventricle and right atrium as well as providing the posterior limit of the atrialized right ventricle. It is also useful for displaying the position of the anticipated normal insertion of the leaflets of the tricuspid valve. The degree of distal displacement of the septal leaflet, however, is unrelated to the severity of symptoms or the success of surgical treatment (Shiina et al., 1983,

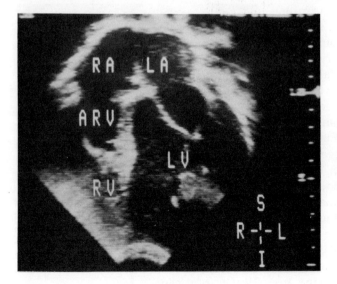

Figure 5. An apical four-chamber view in a teenager with severe hypoplasia of the right ventricle (RV) shows the displaced septal attachment of the tricuspid valve which produces a bipartite right ventricle with an atrialized portion (ARV) and a functional one. The junction between the right atrium (RA) and the ARV is marked by the atrioventricular groove.

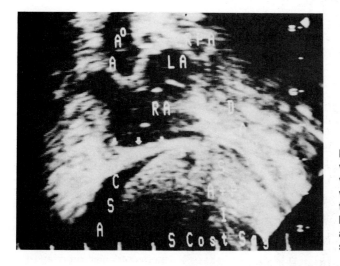

Figure 6. In the subcostal sagittal view (S Cost Sag), the Eustachian valve (EV) can be imaged together with the inferior caval vein (IVC). The tethering of the mural leaflet is outlined by arrows. A small amount of ascites (ASC) is present. DAO = descending aorta.

1984). This is not surprising since no one single plane provides the opportunity for observation of the entire displacement of the leaflets of the tricuspid valve together with the volume of the atrialized right ventricle. The dimensions of the atrialized portion of the right ventricle and its volume, therefore, must be synthesized from observations in several planes before the overall degree of valvular displacement can be adequately defined. The atrialized portion of the right ventricle may consist of attenuated musculature. In severe forms of the anomaly, it may exhibit paradoxical expansion during systole.

The inferior (mural) leaflet of the tricuspid valve is also displaced. In some subjects, it too has been reported to be diminutive or absent. We have recently observed that subcostal imaging in parasagittal planes allows an evaluation of the inferior leaflet as well as the septal and anterosuperior ones (Fig. 4). With the transducer plane in the subcostal sagittal location, the Eustachian valve (which is frequently large in this anomaly) can be imaged together with the inferior caval vein (Fig. 6). Once these structures are located, the plane may be directed further to the left, where the anterosuperior and mural leaflets can be imaged. The position of the atrioventricular groove as well as the distal tethering of the leaflets may also be demonstrated in this plane. In-

deed, images obtained in an equivalent ultrasound plane in fetal life have been valuable in establishing the diagnosis of Ebstein's malformation (Figs. 7–10). If this tethering of the leaflets is extreme, no motion of the leaflets can be observed.

Subcostal imaging in the coronal plane (Figs. 3 and 9) demonstrates the degree of displacement of the mural leaflet. The displacement can be judged relative to the location of the Eustachian valve, the latter lying close to the atrioventricular junction. It is the attachment of the mural leaflet on the

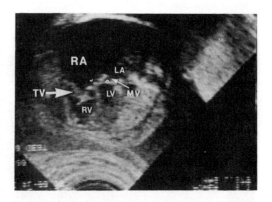

Figure 7. A four-chamber plane from a 26-week fetus with Ebstein's malformation shows a right atrial enlargement as well as displacement of the thickened tricuspid valve leaflets toward the cardiac apex. The arrows indicate the insertion of the tricuspid and mitral valves. MV = mitral valve; TV = tricuspid valve.

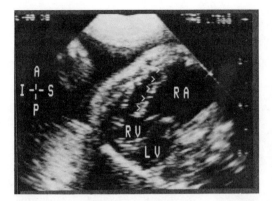

Figure 8. A subcostal sagittal view from a 32-week fetus with Ebstein's malformation displays the apical displacement of a thickened anterosuperior leaflet (indicated by arrows).

diaphragmatic surface, coupled with the appearance of the echo from the inferior aspect of the right atrioventricular groove,

that provides the characteristic image observed from cineangiograms profiled in posteroanterior projections (Figs. 3, 4, and 6). With more anterior angulation of the transducer, all three valve leaflets can be identified and the relationship of the leaflets to the right ventricular outflow area and the pulmonary valve can be assessed.

The anterosuperior leaflet, which is the largest one, is easily identified in many planes. This leaflet is the primary contributor to the competence of the tricuspid valve. In the apical four-chamber plane, the large leaflet is usually seen to be normally attached to the atrioventricular junction. (Figs. 2 and 5) In this plane, therefore, there is usually no observable displacement of the leaflet. Although anatomical examination might suggest that the leaflet observed from this plane might be the mural one, there are

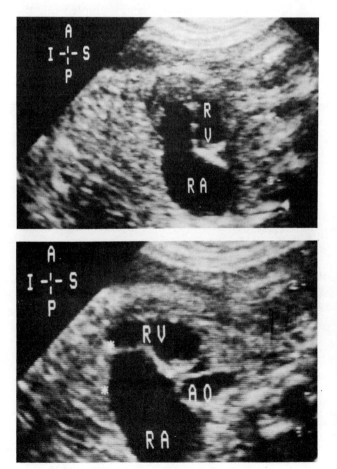

Figure 9. Top: An angulated subcostal taken during diastole in a coronal plane from the fetus shown in Fig. 8 showing the atrialized portion of the right ventricle bounded by the tricuspid valve and the atrioventricular groove. Bottom: The same view in systole shows the insertions of the leaflets in relation to the atrioventricular groove (all indicated by *). AO = ascending aorta.

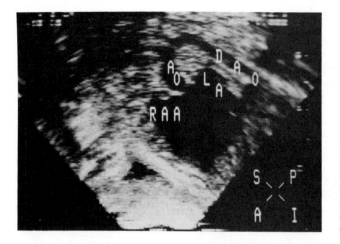

Figure 10. An oblique subcostal plane (between the coronal and sagittal ones) shows a marked enlargement of the right atrium and its appendage (RAA). A normal aortic arch as well as head and neck vessels are demonstrated.

several reasons to suggest this is the antero-superior leaflet. First, there is often clockwise rotation of the heart, resulting from the right heart enlargement. Second, the observed leaflet is large and its excursion, as observed with cross-sectional as well as M-mode echocardiography, is quite marked. It is the redundancy of this leaflet which is responsible for producing the "sail" sound or nonejection clicks frequently audible in Ebstein's malformation (Fontana et al., 1972). The anterosuperior leaflet can also be imaged in the parasagittal long-axis (Fig. 11), the parasternal short-axis (Fig. 1), and in subcostal coronal and sagittal views (Figs.

4, 12, and 13). The excursion of the leaflet, however, can be best appreciated from parasternal and apical long-axis views.

By using a combination of planes, the area of the atrialized right ventricle may be better appreciated than by simply using the apical four-chamber view. Previous studies were unable to correlate the measurements of displacement in the four-chamber view with the degree of severity of the lesion as indicated by symptoms or final outcome (Shiina et al., 1983). The displacement alone, therefore, is only one of the factors that may determine the outcome. This suggests a need for additional information as

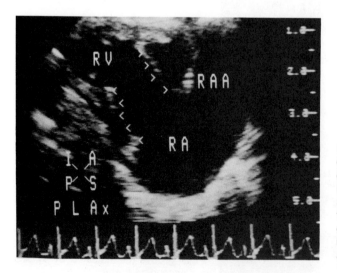

Figure 11. The parasternal long-axis (PLAx) through the right ventricle (RV) shows the large anterosuperior leaflet of the tricuspid valve, as well as the smaller mural leaflet and its tethering to the underlying myocardium. The right atrium (RA) is enlarged. RAA = right atrial appendage.

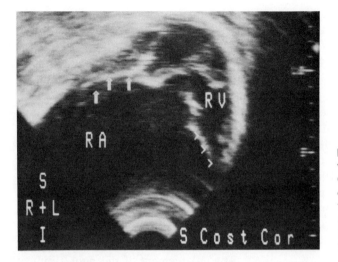

Figure 12. The subcostal coronal view with left anterior angulation (S Cost Cor) shows a linear attachment of the anterosuperior leaflet of the tricuspid valve, as outlined by arrows. The right atrium (RA) is enlarged at the expense of the functional right ventricle (RV).

outlined above. This crucial information can be obtained from the subcostal and the parasternal planes.

Distal Attachment

An important point in determining the appropriate surgical approach is the degree of tethering of the large sail-like anterosuperior leaflet as well as the presence of cordal attachments of this leaflet to the free wall of the right ventricle (Figs. 8 and 9). Linear attachment in this position, together with formation of a supernumerary tongue between the septal and anteroseptal leaflets, produces a degree of obstruction between the inlet and outlet portions of the right ventricle. Since its introduction, the reconstructive surgical approach (Hardy et al., 1964), which is aimed at restoring the atrioventricular junction by plicating the atrialized portion of the right ventricle, has been widely used. The existence of linear attachment and tethering may preclude this form of surgery. The ability to detect it is thus significant. The degree of tethering may be observed from several planes of examination. The degree of obstruction, however, may be more difficult to assess. This is because the entry of blood into the right ventricle may occur only through the commis-

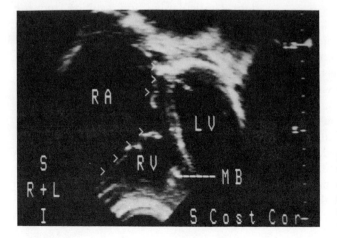

Figure 13. The subcostal coronal view (S Cost Cor) shows the anterosuperior leaflet as well as the distal displacement of the mural one. The right atrium is markedly enlarged. MB = moderator band.

sures of the abnormally constricted valve and through perforations at the area along the linear distal attachment. Some indication as to whether there is major obstruction, nonetheless, can be ascertained from observing the mobility of the leaflets. Contrast echocardiography, with agitated saline injected into a peripheral vein, is also helpful in assessing whether or not there is a major obstruction. Rapid appearance of intense ultrasonic contrast in the functional right ventricle suggests that the stenosis is not marked. Little contrast appearance with a large degree of right-to-left atrial shunting suggests that there is a significant obstruction of the inflow.

Dysplasia

Dysplasia of the valve is the third feature of this malformation. The myriad deformities demonstrated pathologically are usually expressed echocardiographically by dense echoes arising from the valve. They can be observed from almost every plane of examination. The variation of thickening of the valve on echocardiography is similar to that observed in the mitral valve with prolapse and mucinous degeneration of the thickened leaflets.

Size of the Functional Right Ventricle

A characteristic feature of Ebstein's malformation is the diminution in size of the functional right ventricle. This may vary from minimal diminution in size to an almost complete absence of the cavity when associated with pulmonary atresia. The size of this part of the right ventricle may be assessed from the various echocardiographic planes, but no studies to date have provided volumetric data. Right ventricular cavity size can be appreciated from many views, but the most important are the apical four-chamber and the subcostal views.

(Figs. 2, 3, and 5) The parasternal short-axis view was the first view used to describe the echocardiographic findings of Ebstein's malformation. This view is useful because it allows the appreciation of the outflow portion of the right ventricle, this component making up the larger part of the functional right ventricle. This portion is bounded by the septal leaflet of the tricuspid valve, the walls of the right ventricular outflow tract and the pulmonary valve (Fig. 1).

Right Atrial Enlargement

The enlargement of the right atrium is also a characteristic feature. This may be observed in the fetus and may be a prominent feature leading to the diagnosis of Ebstein's malformation as early as 20 weeks gestation (Figs. 7–10). The right atrium is almost always markedly enlarged (Fig. 10), regardless of the severity of the malformation.

Associated Lesions

We have detected numerous associated lesions in our patients. Patency of the arterial duct is a common association and has been present in almost all of our small infants. The patent duct permits the aortic pressure to be transmitted into the pulmonary arterial system. Coupled with the poor right ventricular ejection resulting from the tricuspid regurgitation and the decreased size of the functional right ventricle, there may be diminution or even elimination of the flow of blood from the right ventricle into the pulmonary trunk. The pharmacological manipulation of the duct in the early neonatal period is thus of critical importance in the survival of these infants beyond the neonatal period. The situation in which such an infant becomes dependent on left-to-right shunting at the ductal level to maintain pulmonary blood flow is often associated with an unfavorable outcome.

At the time of closure of the duct, either spontaneously or therapeutically, the infant may survive on forward flow into the pulmonary arteries from the right ventricle. Whether this results from an improvement in the right ventricular function or lowering of pulmonary arterial pressure and decreased right-to-left atrial shunting has yet to be determined.

In infants with Ebstein's malformation and ductal patency, the increased transmitted pressure into the pulmonary circuit may hold the pulmonary valve in the closed position. It may therefore be difficult to differentiate between the situation mentioned above and the situation where the pulmonary valve leaflets are held in the closed position because of pulmonary stenosis or valvular pulmonary atresia, both of which are also found in conjunction with Ebstein's malformation. One way of differentiating these different situations is to demonstrate the presence of pulmonary regurgitation, which excludes pulmonary atresia. We have been able to use Doppler interrogation of the right ventricular outflow tract or retrograde injection of saline contrast from an umbilical arterial catheter to determine pulmonary insufficiency. If this is found, the pulmonary valve is obviously not imperforate.

Valvular and/or infundibular pulmonary stenosis can also appear in conjunction with Ebstein's malformation. In such patients, obstruction of the right ventricular outflow may be detected at various levels. For example, in its most severe expression, the adhesion of the leaflets of the tricuspid valve to the right ventricular wall may lead to pulmonary atresia.

In one of the fetuses we examined with ultrasound, valvular pulmonary atresia was noted at autopsy. This lesion may be extremely difficult to differentiate from the situation where the valve is held closed by the high pressure in the fetal pulmonary arteries. The elevated pressure holding the pulmonary valve closed during fetal development may contribute to the development of valvular atresia. When there is right ventricular outflow obstruction, the infants may not be able to survive unless duct patency is maintained by prostaglandin E_1, or a surgical shunt is created.

An atrial septal defect may be an obligatory component of the malformation. Certainly, the fact that right-to-left atrial shunting in fetal life is augmented by tricuspid regurgitation may cause right atrial dilation and an increase of its pressure. This may in turn cause the oval foramen to become larger than normal. We have not encountered patients with Ebstein's malformation who do not have some shunting at the atrial level. Although mild right-to-left interatrial shunting may be difficult to determine from clinical examination, contrast echocardiography has been valuable for demonstrating this feature.

In a previous series from our institute, two patients with ventricular septal defects were reported (Ports et al., 1978). One of these defects was in the inlet portion of the ventricle (perimembranous) and was proximal to the atrioventricular valve; in other words, it communicated with the atrialized right ventricle. The other was located distally and opened into the outlet component of the functional right ventricle.

Doppler Findings in Ebstein's Malformation

Tricuspid regurgitation has been found in all the patients with Ebstein's malformation we examined with Doppler ultrasound. We have detected tricuspid regurgitation in a fetus at 20 weeks of gestation even before it was possible accurately to demonstrate the displacement of the valve leaflets. The relationship of regurgitation to the temporal development of displacement and abnormal valve function remains speculative. Another feature of tricuspid regurgitation during intrauterine life is that its velocity is low, even in the presence of pulmonary atresia. The velocity of the regurgitation jet through the tricuspid valve in two of the fetuses that we followed was only $2\frac{1}{2}$ m/sec (equivalent to a 20–30 mmHg pressure gradient across the valve). The right ventricle, therefore, does not develop high pressure prior to delivery. We have suggested that the elevation of atrial pressure and concurrent elevated venous pressure may interfere with the delicate relationship at capillary level and result in fetal hydrops (Silverman, et al., 1985).

The Doppler findings show that regurgitation usually occurs over the entire orificial area of the tricuspid valve. The regurgitation can also be detected across the leaflets well into the area of the atrialized right ventricle. Thus, tricuspid regurgitation can occur in the area normally occupied by the right ventricle. This finding is analagous to those obtained with an electrode tip catheter which records right atrial pressure while right ventricular electrical potentials are being recorded in the atrialized right ventricle.

Doppler ultrasound may underestimate the degree of obstruction at the tricuspid valve because of the low pressure generated proximal to the obstruction. The latter is partly due to the right-to-left atrial shunting. With regard to the Doppler interrogation of the pulmonary valve, a retrograde signal is frequently found in infants, suggesting that the blood flow into the pulmonary arteries is derived from the arterial duct in the early postnatal period. Detecting forward flow across the pulmonary valve when it is patent has been consistent with a more favorable outcome.

Outcome

Seven of the infants in our series, as well as all the fetuses we have examined prenatally, have died. This is a death incidence of 70% in neonates with Ebstein's malformation. Two of the fetuses we examined were referred for examination because of fetal hydrops and a third developed this ominous prognostic sign later in the course of the pregnancy. We have previously reported that nonimmune hydrops may be the result of fetal cardiac failure, itself caused by tricuspid regurgitation (Silverman et al., 1985). This is caused by the elevated venous pressure and concomitant increased capillary hydrostatic oncotic pressure relationships. One of these three fetuses died prior to delivery at 34 weeks of gestation, and the other two in the first few days of life. The fetuses who present to us for clinical examination are usually symptomatic, either with nonimmune fetal hydrops or fetal arrhythmia, indicating that they are more severely affected by virtue of their symptoms. We have also examined 10 neonates, of whom 7 have died. The presence of associated lesions seems to make the prognosis worse. This seems to be a higher incidence than reported by Giuliani et al. (1979) but is similar to the incidence reported by Watson and his colleagues (1974). It appears that the infant group is at a greatest risk of dying in our series, but that once the infant has survived this period, the prognosis is improved. It is this group of survivors that may require surgical correction later in life. There is, therefore, a high attrition rate in the more severe forms of Ebstein's malformation. Only the less severely affected patients survive gestation and the neonatal period and continue to live into adolescence and adult life.

References

Anderson KR, Zuberbuhler JR, Anderson RH, et al. Morphologic spectrum of Ebstein's anomaly of the heart. A review. *Mayo Clin Proc* 1979;54:174–180.

Broadbent JC, Wood EH, Burchell HB, Parker RL. Ebstein's malformation of the tricuspid valve: Report of J cases. *Proc Staff Meet Mayo Clin* 1953;28:79–88.

Fontana ME, Wooley CF. Sail-sound in Ebstein's

anomaly of the tricuspid valve. *Circulation* 1972;46:155–164.

Giuliani ER, Fuster V, Brandenburg RO, Mair DD. Ebstein's anomaly. The clinical features and natural history of Ebstein's anomaly of the tricuspid valve. *Mayo Clin Proc* 1979;54:163–173.

Hardy KL, May IA, Webster CA, Kimball KG. Ebstein's anomaly: A functional concept and successful definitive repair. *J Thorac Cardiovasc Surg* 1964;48:927–940.

Lundstrom NR. Echocardiography in the diagnosis of Ebstein's anomaly of the tricuspid valve. *Circulation* 1973;47:597–605.

Ports TA, Silverman NH, Schiller NB. Two-dimensional echocardiographic assessment of Ebstein's anomaly. *Circulation* 1978;58:336–343.

Schiebler GL, Gravenstein JS, Van Mierop LHS. Ebstein's anomaly of the tricuspid valve. Translation of original description with comments. *Am J Cardiol* 1968;22:867–873.

Shiina A, Seward JB, Edwards WD, et al. Two-dimensional echocardiographic spectrum of Ebstein's anomaly: Detailed anatomic assessment. *J Am Coll Cardiol* 1984;3:356–370.

Shiina A, Seward JB, Tajik AJ, et al. Two-dimensional echocardiographic-surgical correlation in Ebstein's anomaly: Preoperative determination of patients requiring tricuspid valve plication vs replacement. *Circulation* 1983;68:534–544.

Silverman NH, Kleinmann CS, Rudolph AM, et al. Fetal atrioventricular valve insufficiency associated with nonimmune hydrops. *Circulation* 1985;72:825–832.

Watson H. Natural history of Ebstein's anomaly of tricuspid valve in childhood and adolescence. *Br Heart J* 1974;36:417–427.

Zuberbuhler JR, Allwork SP, Anderson RH. The spectrum of Ebstein's anomaly of the tricuspid valve. *J Thorac Cardiovasc Surg* 1979;77:202–211.

Zuberbuhler JR, Becker AE, Anderson RH, Lenox CC. Ebstein's malformation and the embryological development of the tricuspid valve. With a note on the nature of "clefts" in the atrioventricular valves. *Pediatr Cardiol* 1984;5:289–296.

2.4

Ebstein's Malformation of the Morphologically Tricuspid Valve: A Consideration of Regurgitant and Obstructive Forms in Patients with Concordant and Discordant Atrioventricular Connections

Robert M. Freedom and Jeffrey F. Smallhorn

While the classic (but mild) expression of Ebstein's malformation of the morphologically tricuspid valve may be compatible with a long life, some severely afflicted patients will succumb as neonates (Adams and Hudson, 1956; Watson, 1974). Some babies may demonstrate profound hypoxemia, with a pulmonary circulation that is seemingly duct-dependent (and thus responsive to an E-type prostaglandin) (Bharati et al., 1977; Freedom et al., 1978; Newfeld et al., 1967) (Fig. 1). In some of these babies, right ventricular angiography will suggest pulmonary atresia with no forward pulmonary blood flow. Whether such pulmonary atresia is organic or functional must be determined clinically because of the obvious clinical implications (Freedom et al., 1978) (Fig. 2).

There is less evidence that, in individuals with discordant atrioventricular and ventriculoarterial connections (congenitally

From: Anderson, RH, Neches, WH, Park, SC, Zuberbuhler, JR, eds: *Perspectives in Pediatric Cardiology*: Mount Kisco, New York, Futura Publishing Co., © 1988.

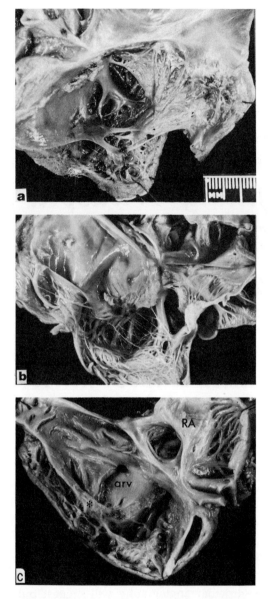

Figure 1. Severe forms of Ebstein's malformation of the tricuspid valve in left-sided hearts with concordant atrioventricular connection. (a) Note both the displacement and the sheet-like dysplasia of the severely enlarged anterior leaflet; (b) a terribly disorganized displaced and dysplastic tricuspid valve; (c) a nearly unguarded tricuspid orifice with just a small rim of displaced, dysplastic atrioventricular valvular tissue.

corrected transposition), mild forms of the Ebstein-like malformation of the left-sided morphologically tricuspid valve will be well tolerated. (Huhta et al., 1985). One obvious

reason for this could be the presence of other clinically significant intracardiac malformations (de Albuquerque et al., 1984; Sutherland et al., 1983). Yet, functional and organic aortic atresia have been documented in patients with congenitally corrected transposition in the setting of a severely distorted systemic atrioventricular valve and grossly abnormal right ventricular myocardium (Brenner et al., 1978; Craig et al., 1986; Deanfield et al., 1981; Muster et al., 1985). Thus, whether the atrioventricular connection is concordant or discordant, Ebstein's malformation of the morphologically tricuspid valve embraces a continuum of functional and structural abnormalities. We will explore this continuum in this chapter.

Associated Cardiac Malformations

Concordant Atrioventricular Connections

Perhaps the most common anomaly associated with Ebstein's malformation is an atrial septal defect within the oval fossa ("secundum" defect), be it large or restrictive. But one must remember that Ebstein's malformation has been found in hearts exhibiting pulmonary valvular stenosis of varying severity; pulmonary valvular atresia; congenital pulmonary regurgitation; ventricular septal defect; atrioventricular septal defect; tetralogy of Fallot; complete transposition; mitral valve prolapse; and overriding of the deformed tricuspid valve (Anderson and Lie, 1978, Caruso et al., 1978; Gussenhoven et al., 1984; Lev et al., 1970; Monibi et al., 1978; Roach et al., 1984).

Discordant Atrioventricular Connections

Assuming usual atrial arrangement (solitus) and a discordant atrioventricular con-

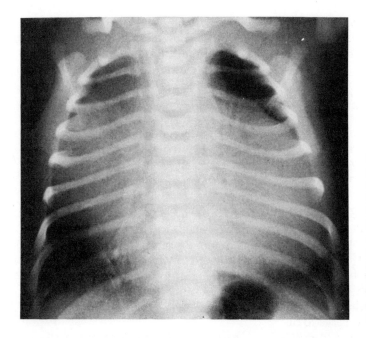

Figure 2. Massive cardiomegaly in a neonate with the classic, severe expression of the right-sided Ebstein's deformity. This chest radiograph is indistinguishable from the neonate with functional aortic atresia and a severe Ebstein-like deformity of the morphologically tricuspid but systemic atrioventricular valve in discordant atrioventricular connection.

nection, it is the left-sided or morphologically tricuspid valve which exhibits the Ebstein-like distorsion. The left-sided variety may show considerable morphological departures when compared to the classic anomaly (as seen in usual atrial arrangement with concordant atrioventricular connections). The proximal valve attachment will be displaced from the atrioventricular junction, but the left-sided variant rarely exhibits severe displacement (Anderson et al., 1978; Attie et al., 1980; Jaffe, 1976; Losekoot et al., 1983). Rather, substantial dysplasia is more common, with displacement and morphological atrialization being less conspicuous. The anterosuperior leaflet is usually small, not sail-like, and it rarely obstructs the outflow tract of the morphologically right ventricle.

The Ebstein-like malformation can occur in "isolation" with congenitally corrected transposition, or it may coexist with a ventricular septal defect or with ventricular septal defect and associated left ventricular outflow tract obstruction (subpulmonary outflow tract obstruction). This malformation may occur in hearts exhibiting some form of obstruction to systemic blood flow,

either at the ventricular (subaortic) or the aortic arch (aortic coarctation atresia or interruption) level (Craig et al., 1986). Rarely, aortic valve atresia can occur in the setting of discordant atrioventricular and ventriculoarterial connections. (Brenner et al., 1978; Craig et al., 1986; Deanfield et al., 1981; Matsukawa et al., 1983; Muster et al., 1985). Such patients exhibit a markedly distorted left-sided tricuspid valve which permits massive regurgitation. The resulting extreme cardiomegaly may produce a chest radiograph that is virtually indistinguishable from that seen in the neonate with the classic severe form of Ebstein's malformation with concordant atrioventricular connection (Fig. 2). Both the atrialized and functional components of the morphologically right ventricle may be considerably dilated despite the aortic valve atresia. The left-sided variant of Ebstein's malformation may also be identified in patients exhibiting so-called isolated atrioventricular discordant connection (Arciprete et al., 1985; Hazan et al., 1977; Quero Jimenez and Raposo-Sonnenfield, 1975; Snider et al., 1984). It is this unusual combination of connections that hemodynamically has the potential for producing the physiology of complete transposition in the patient with a discordant atrioventricular connection.

Functional Correlates

Perhaps the most common perception of the classic Ebstein's malformation (with usual atrial arrangement and a concordant atrioventricular connection) is that this anomaly results in tricuspid regurgitation of varying severity. Yet there is now an increasing awareness that the displaced right-sided atrioventricular valve may be obstructive, with a continuum from mild to severe obstruction (Anderson et al., 1979; Freedom et al., 1984; Zuberbuhler et al., 1979). Such obstructive lesions serve to demarcate the right ventricular inlet from the apical trabecular zone (and thus the outlet zone as well). Such examples lend support to the tripartite concept of ventricular organization (Anderson et al., 1978; Restivo et al., 1984; Zuberbuhler et al., 1979, 1984).

Not infrequently, morphological elements responsible for 'tricuspid' regurgitation and obstruction coexist. This may take place at the junction of the inlet and trabecular zones, but on occasion, the sail-like anterosuperior leaflet may have an anomalous insertion in the infundibulum, thus producing obstruction of the right ventricular outlet. In the continuum of varying obstruction, the free margin of the displaced tricuspid valve may be virtually sealed, resulting in an imperforate form of Ebstein's malformation. This is one form of imperforate atrioventricular valve that can be diagnosed by angiocardiography performed in the right atrium (Freedom et al., 1984; Rao et al., 1973). In the absence of an interventricular communication, the imperforate variant of Ebstein's malformation is also associated with pulmonary atresia (and an intact ventricular septum).

Angiocardiography (Figs. 3–7)

With Usual Atrial Arrangement and Concordant Atrioventricular Connections

There is a very extensive literature devoted to the angiocardiography of the classic Ebstein's malformation that is reviewed

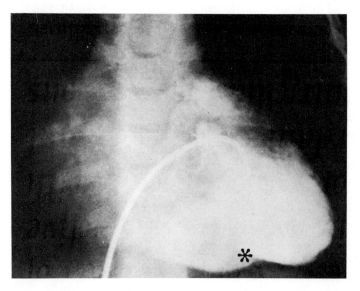

Figure 3. Classic Ebstein's malformation of the tricuspid valve with moderate displacement producing a notch (asterisk) on the diaphragmatic surface of the right ventricle. RA = right atrium; ARV = atrialized portion of right ventricle.

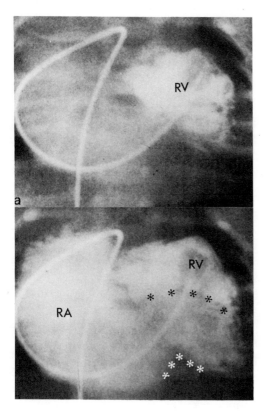

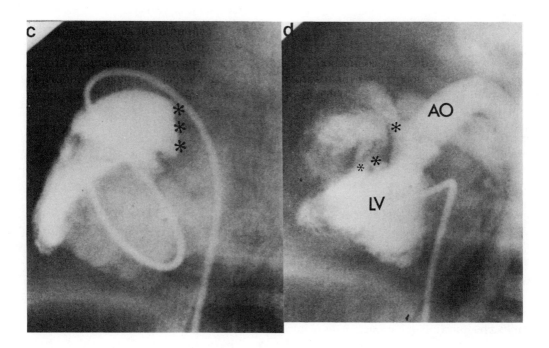

Figure 4. Severe neonatal expression of Ebstein's malformation of the tricuspid valve. (a) Injection into the infundibular portion of right ventricle (RV); (b) the severe notching of the diaphragmatic surface of the right ventricle (white asterisk) is observed. The sail-like anterosuperior leaflet (black asterisk) is evident. There is massive regurgitation into the gigantic right atrium; (c) no forward pulmonary blood flow is present (asterisk); (d) the left ventricular (LV) angiogram demonstrates a normal ascending aorta (AO) and multiple ventricular septal defects (asterisk).

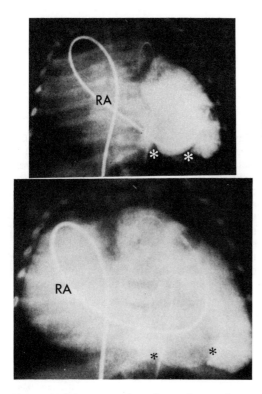

Figure 5. Other examples of massive cardiomegaly with extreme Ebstein's malformation. In both neonates, the angiography demonstrates massive regurgitation into right atrium (RA) and displacement of the tricuspid valve manifested as notching of the floor of the right ventricle (asterisk).

in our recent textbook (Freedom et al., 1984). Selective injection of contrast material into the morphologically right ventricle should demonstrate so-called "notching" of the diaphragmatic surface of the right ventricle. This notch corresponds to the insertion of displaced mural and septal leaflets of the valve (Becker et al., 1971). The degree of atrioventricular valve regurgitation reflects both the magnitude of displacement and disorganization of the valve. It has been suggested that angiographic definition of the various components of the tricuspid valve (and thus the right ventricle) is enhanced by injection of contrast material into the infundibular or immediately subarterial portion of the right ventricle (Elliott and Hartman, 1967). We endorse this sugges-

tion, but would point out that, at times, it may be difficult to place the catheter in the desired position (Freedom et al., 1984).

Differentiation of Organic from Functional Pulmonary Atresia

In patients with florid right-sided tricuspid regurgitation, the right ventricular myocardium may be deficient (as in the anomaly described by Uhl, 1952). More significantly, in the neonate whose pulmonary vascular bed is relatively muscularized and constricted, the right ventricle may be unable to generate enough systolic pressure to open a normally formed pulmonary valve. Yet, some patients with a nearly identical tricuspid valve and right ventricular morphology will have true organic (anatomical) atresia of the right ventricular outflow tract. In both groups of patients, right ventricular systolic pressure is often subsystemic. Indeed, it may be frankly low in the severely affected neonate, reflecting the massive tricuspid regurgitation and disordered right ventricle (Freedom et al., 1978; Newfeld et al., 1967). How, then, does one differentiate functional from organic pulmonary atresia? Such differentiation has obviously important clinical ramifications. Some years ago, we advocated prostaglandin-enhanced aortography to resolve this dilemma. In those patients with an anatomically normal pulmonary valve but with *no* forward flow from the right ventricle to the pulmonary trunk, aortography performed opposite the prostaglandin-dilated arterial duct demonstrated dense opacification of the pulmonary root, with subsequent regurgitation of contrast into the outlet of the right ventricle. The presence of contrast in the infundibulum of the right ventricle is unequivocal evidence for patency of the pulmonary valve (Freedom et al., 1978) (Fig. 8). While in our experience such pulmonary valves have usually proved to be normal, dysplasia producing congenital pulmonary regurgitation

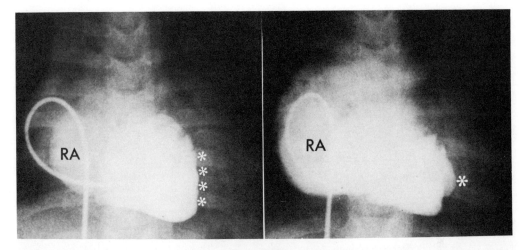

Figure 6. The imperforate form of Ebstein's anomaly in a neonate with an intact ventricular septum and, thus, pulmonary atresia. Note the angiography opacifies the small inlet of the right ventricle. In the left panel, there is clear separation of the inlet (white asterisk) from the apical trabecular zone. The displaced membranous imperforate valve is seen (solitary white asterisk) in the right panel.

or varying degrees of obstruction has been noted on occasion.

Today, retrograde aortography is not invariably required to differentiate the organic from the functional form of atresia. We have published elsewhere the role of cross-sectional echocardiography combined with Doppler interrogation as a relatively noninvasive methodology for making this assessment (Smallhorn et al., 1984).

Echocardiographic Evaluation of Ebstein's Malformation with a Concordant Atrioventricular Connection

Ebstein's malformation of the tricuspid valve presents as a spectrum, from the asymptomatic patient with a supraventricu-

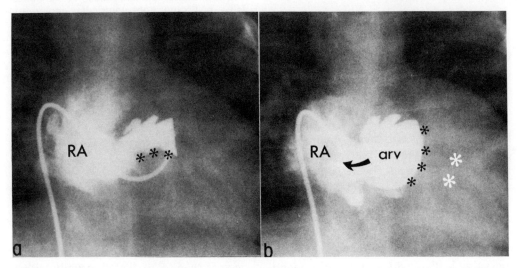

Figure 7. Another patient with pulmonary atresia and intact ventricular septum with an imperforate Ebstein's valve. a. The black asterisk note the imperforate valve; b. The forward margin (black asterisk) of the valve is noted. The apical trabecular zone (white asterisks) does not opacify.

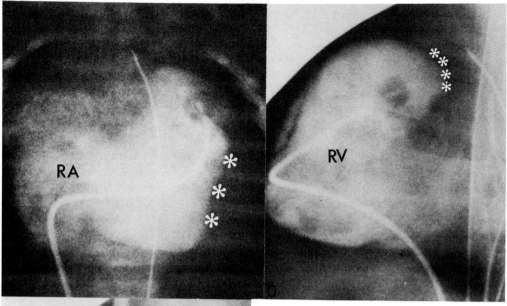

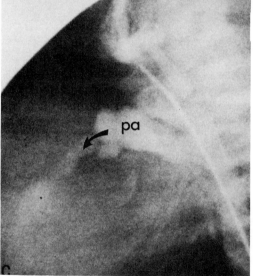

Figure 8. Functional pulmonary atresia in a neonate with Ebstein's malformation of the tricuspid valve. a. Frontal right ventricular angiography showing the level of the displaced valve (white asterisk) with regurgitation into the right atrium; b. No forward flow (white asterisk) is seen; c. Regurgitation (black arrow) from the pulmonary artery (PA) into the right ventricular infundibulum is evident.

lar rhythm disturbance or insignificant murmur to the newborn who presents with severe cyanotic heart disease. We will first address the issue of the newborn with Ebstein's malformation and associated cyanosis.

Characteristically, these infants have significant displacement and dysplasia of the valve leaflets which are readily identified by echocardiography. In the subcostal and precordial four-chamber view, it is pos-

sible to identify the displacement of the septal and mural leaflets (Kambe et al., 1980; Seward et al., 1979; Shiina et al., 1984) (Fig. 9). The atrioventricular junction is readily identified and usually the displacement is so severe that there is only a small remnant of functionally right ventricular cavity. The right atrium in both of these views is seen to be dilated, usually with an atrial defect with evidence of right-to-left shunting displayed by Doppler techniques.

The anterosuperior leaflet is displayed with superior and anterior angulation of the transducer. It usually appears as a large sail-like structure (Fig. 9b), but occasionally it may also be tethered to the wall of the right ventricle (Fig. 9c). This has important implications at a later age if surgical repair using this leaflet as a monocusp is to be undertaken.

Doppler interrogation of the tricuspid valve provides important information regarding its patency and if present, the degree of valvular regurgitation (Fig. 10). The degree of regurgitation can be ascertained by flow mapping in the right atrium or by the evaluation of the amount of reversed flow in the inferior caval and hepatic veins (Diebold et al., 1983; Garcia-Dorado, 1982).

The next step is to determine patency of the right ventricular outflow tract. This is best achieved by combining a subcostal long-axis view of the right ventricular outflow tract with a high precordial short-axis view. In this way both the infundibular and valvular regions can be evaluated. Obstruction may occur in the subvalvular region due to anomalous insertion of the anterosuperior leaflet (Fig. 11a). This division of the right ventricle into two cavities can be readily identified by this approach. Doppler interrogation of the subvalvular region then provides important information regarding the severity of obstruction, provided there is no associated obstruction at the level of the pulmonary valve.

Stenosis or atresia at the pulmonary valvular level can be encountered (Fig. 11b). Invariably the severity of stenosis can be evaluated using combined imaging and Doppler interrogation (Oliveira-Lima et al., 1983). Care must be taken during the first few days of life prior to a reduction in the pulmonary arterial pressure since a falsely low gradient may be recorded. With repeated evaluations over time, this issue can be resolved. Further clues can be elicited from the pressure drop as measured across the tricuspid valve by Doppler echocardiography. Thus, by measuring the pulmonary valvular gradient and combining this

with the right ventricular pressure, the precise pulmonary arterial pressure can be calculated.

The issue of anatomical versus functional pulmonary valvular atresia may at first produce a greater diagnostic challenge. Because of significant dysfunction of the right ventricle, there may be functional pulmonary valvular atresia such that the pulmonary arterial pressure is higher than that in the ventricle. This results in the inability of the pulmonary valve to open during systole. Fortunately, there is usually associated regurgitation in this situation, which can be detected by contrast or by Doppler echocardiography (Smallhorn et al., 1984) (Fig. 12). Care must be taken to interrogate both above and below the pulmonary valve with the direction of flow being toward the transducer and the timing occurring during ventricular systole (Fig. 12). If interrogation is performed only above the valve, then confusion may occur between ductal left-to-right shunting and true regurgitation.

In the absence of regurgitation, the diagnosis should be that of anatomical atresia, which requires management with a systemic to pulmonary arterial shunt. Functional atresia, in contrast, should be treated conservatively. The issue of anatomical versus functional atresia arises only when the valve leaflets and their attachments appear normal. In other cases, the valve and the subpulmonary infundibulum are clearly hypoplastic, making the diagnosis of anatomical atresia more certain.

Only mild displacement and dysplasia may be seen in the older asymptomatic patient with minimal tricuspid valvular incompetence (Gussenhoven et al., 1984). Significant right ventricular outflow tract obstruction is unusual in these patients.

Associated Anomalies

Ebstein's malformation may involve the right-sided component of the common valve in an atrioventricular septal defect, ei-

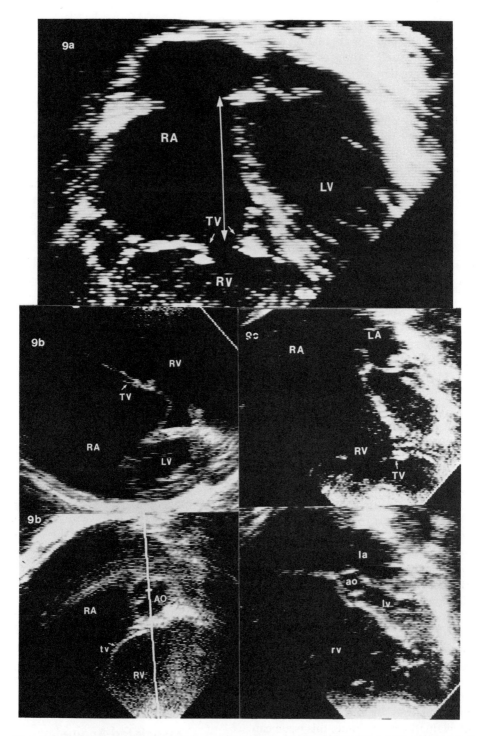

Figure 9. (a) This precordial four-chamber view demonstrates the significant displacement of the mural and septal leaflets of the tricuspid valve. Note the atrioventricular junction as indicated by the upper arrow. (b) This precordial short-axis cut (upper panel) from a case with severe Ebstein's malformation of the tricuspid valve shows the large sail-like anterosuperior leaflet. The lower panel is from the same patient with the transducer angled superiorly from a

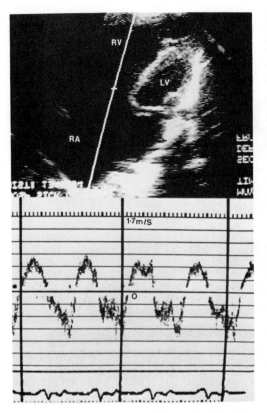

Figure 10. The upper panel is an apical four-chamber view in Ebstein's malformation of the tricuspid valve, showing the Doppler sample volume inserted in the right atrium. The lower panel reveals the forward diastolic and reversed systolic regurgitant flow.

ther in the presence of partitioned or common orifice. When there is a common orifice with potential for a large ventricular shunt, it is usually the inferior bridging leaflet that is displaced. Thus, when one is evaluating patients with an atrioventricular septal defect, attention should be paid to the inferior bridging leaflet from the subcostal four-chamber view. Ebstein's malformation may

also be associated with a hypoplastic morphologically right ventricle in association with pulmonary atresia and an intact ventricular septum (Fig. 13). In other patients the displaced tricuspid valve seals off a ventricular septal defect with the leaflet appearing to billow back and forth during the cardiac cycle. Finally, the tricuspid valve may be severely stenotic or imperforate. While Doppler interrogation may provide some clues to feature, care must be taken if there is a large interatrial communication which permits decompression of the right atrium.

Left-sided abnormalities are seen in approximately 10% of cases (Castaneda-Zuniga et al., 1982). The associated lesions range from a cleft mitral valve to stenosis of the pulmonary veins. They should be excluded in each case by combined imaging and Doppler interrogation.

Left-sided Ebstein's Malformation in Congenitally Corrected Transposition (Figs. 14–17)

Jaffe and others have reported the cardinal angiographic features of the left-sided variant of Ebstein's anomaly (Anderson et al., 1978; Attie et al., 1980; Freedom et al., 1984; Jaffe, 1976; Losekoot et al., 1983). As in the more common right-sided form, it is necessary to identify the level of the left-sided atrioventricular junction (by the course of the morphologically right coronary artery), and to assess those displaced and thickened components of the left-sided tricuspid valve. Notching of the diaphrag-

four-chamber view. Again note the large anterosuperior leaflet. (c) The upper picture is a precordial four-chamber cut in Ebstein's malformation demonstrating a case with a tethered anterosuperior leaflet. Note the severe displacement of the septal and mural leaflets in the upper panel. The lower panel is with superior angulation of the transducer. Note that a large anterosuperior leaflet is not seen. Ao = aorta; LA = left atrium; LV = left ventricle; RA = right atrium; RV = right ventricle; TV = tricuspid valve.

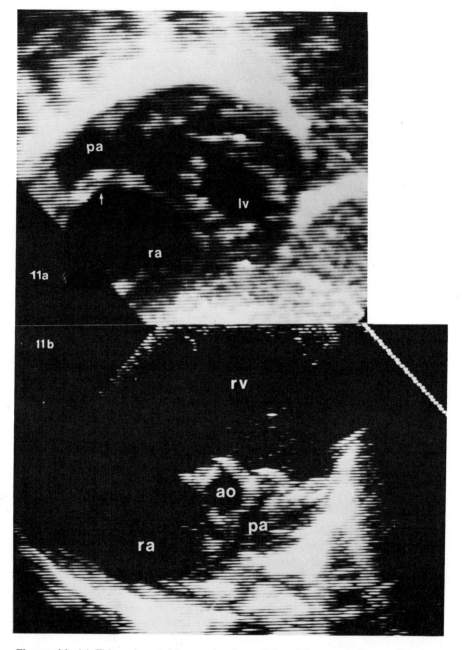

Figure 11. (a) This subcostal long-axis view of the right ventricular outflow tract demonstrates obstruction caused by the insertion of the anterosuperior leaflet (arrow). (b) The lower picture from a different patient shows obstruction occurring at the valvular level in the form of atresia. Note the associated small pulmonary trunk (pa).

matic surface of the morphologically right ventricle in this setting is suggestive of displacement of the valve. Regurgitation may range from relatively mild to very severe, again reflecting the same functional spectrum as seen in the right-sided variant.

In severely affected patients, the right ventricular outlet or infundibulum may be

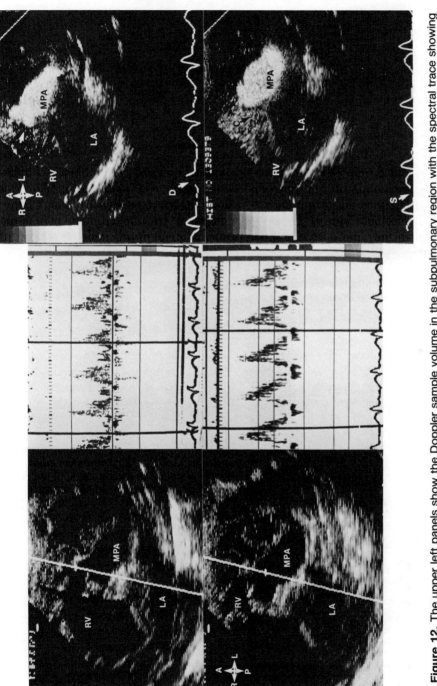

Figure 12. The upper left panels show the Doppler sample volume in the subpulmonary region with the spectral trace showing regurgitation during systole. The lower left panels with the sample volume distal to the pulmonary valve show systolic flow toward the valve, secondary to patency of the arterial duct. The right panels were taken following injection of contrast into the duct via the aorta. Note the regurgitation again occurring mainly during systole. C = contrast; MPA = pulmonary trunk. (Reprinted from Smallhorn et al.: *Am J Cardiol* 54:925–926, 1984.

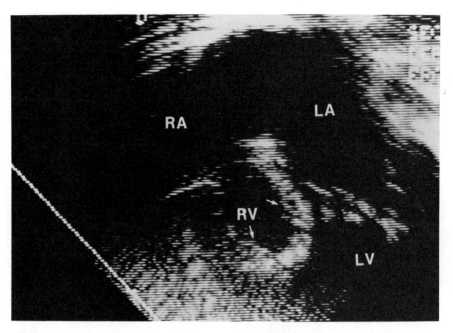

Figure 13. Precordial four-chamber cut in Ebstein's malformation of the tricuspid valve and associated hypoplasia of the right ventricle. Note that the tricuspid valve leaflets are plastered down to the walls of the right ventricular cavity.

narrowed, thus producing subaortic stenosis. The mechanisms responsible for this narrowing are usually muscular (or fibromuscular) but may represent dysplastic tissue of the atrioventricular valve (Craig et al., 1986). The muscular abnormalities include hypertrophy of free-wall muscle bundles, fibromuscular obstruction at the mouth of

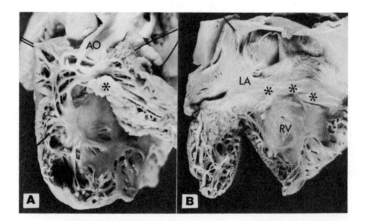

Figure 14. Dysplasia and displacement of the left-sided, systemic, morphologically tricuspid valve in the setting of discordant atrioventricular and ventriculoarterial connections. (a) Internal view of systemic right ventricle and aorta (AO). Note the severely dysplastic left AV valve (asterisk); (b) much of the left atrioventricular junction is unguarded.

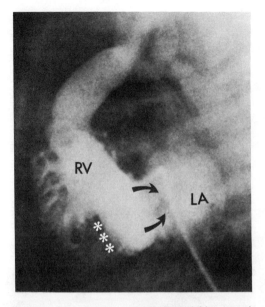

Figure 15. A displaced (white asterisk) systemic atrioventricular valve in congenitally corrected transposition. The right ventriculogram (RV) shows the regurgitation (black asterisk) into the left atrium.

the subaortic infundibulum, or wedging of the aortic outflow tract between a malaligned outlet septum and a prominent ventriculoinfundibular fold.

We have recently described the entire range of obstructive anomalies of the aortic arch complicating patients with discordant atrioventricular and ventriculoarterial connections (Craig et al., 1986). A nearly consistent finding in these patients was an Ebstein-like malformation of the systemic atrioventricular valve. Both functional and anatomical aortic atresia has been recognized in patients with massive regurgitation through this valve (Brenner et al., 1978; Craig et al., 1986; Deanfield et al., 1981; Matsukawa et al., 1983; Muster et al., 1985). As described above, the hearts are gigantic, with extensive dilation of the atrialized portion of the right ventricle. The left atria functions as a tremendously dilated reservoir. In at least one such patient, both the branch pulmonary arteries and the lungs themselves were hypoplastic, perhaps re-

flecting intrauterine molding by the massively dilated heart (Craig et al., 1986) (Fig. 16).

The association of the left-sided Ebstein-like malformation in the setting of a discordant atrioventricular and a concordant ventriculoarterial connection has been mentioned earlier in this chapter. Abnormalities of the left-sided morphologically tricuspid valve (atresia, stenosis, hypoplasia, etc.) are particularly common in this setting, and it is not surprising to encounter an Ebstein-like malformation (Arciprete et al., 1985; Calabro et al., 1980; Hazan et al., 1977; Quero-Jimenez and Raposo-Sonnenfeld, 1975; Snider et al., 1984). In our two recently studied patients, the morphologically right ventricle was modestly underdeveloped, but obstruction to the pulmonary outlet was not recognized. Similarly, a ventricular septal defect was identified in both patients. We have not examined, or at least have not recognized, a severely obstructive form of Ebstein's malformation in patients with a discordant atrioventricular connection. This is not surprising when one remembers that severe displacement is uncommon.

We must remember that, in the rare patient with a concordant atrioventricular connection, the morphologically mitral valve may be displaced and produce an atrialized portion of the morphologically left ventricle in the setting of mitral regurgitation (Actis-Dato and Milocca, 1966; Ruschhaupt et al., 1976).

In Ebstein's malformation with corrected transposition, echocardiography will display an element of dysplasia with some plastering down of the septal leaflet in the majority of cases. Others, however, commonly encountered in the newborn period, have significant displacement with thinning and dilation of the ventricular inlet portion (Fig. 18). The four-chamber cut from either the subcostal or precordial view provides optimal imaging of the valve. The tricuspid nature of the valve can be appreciated in this view, as can the septal attachments. The

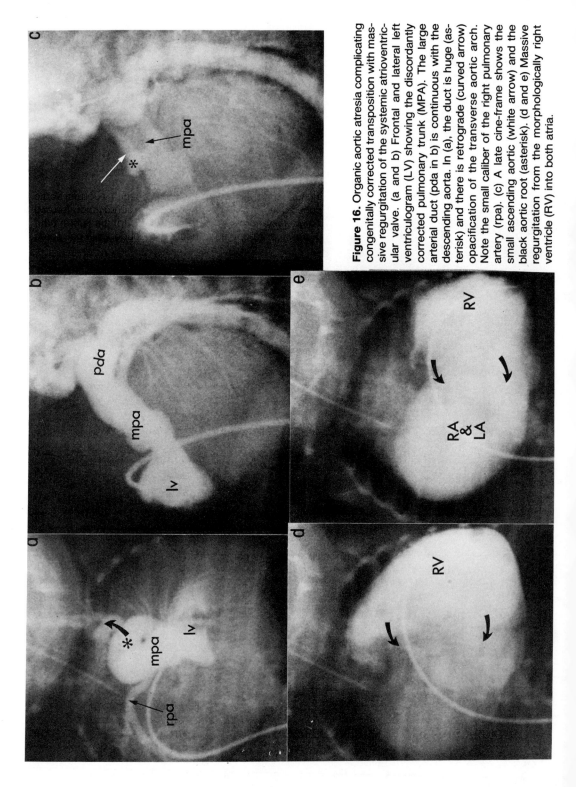

Figure 16. Organic aortic atresia complicating congenitally corrected transposition with massive regurgitation of the systemic atrioventricular valve. (a and b) Frontal and lateral left ventriculogram (LV) showing the discordantly corrected pulmonary trunk (MPA). The large arterial duct (pda in b) is continuous with the descending aorta. In (a), the duct is huge (asterisk) and there is retrograde (curved arrow) opacification of the transverse aortic arch. Note the small caliber of the right pulmonary artery (rpa). (c) A late cine-frame shows the small ascending aortic (white arrow) and the black aortic root (asterisk). (d and e) Massive regurgitation from the morphologically right ventricle (RV) into both atria.

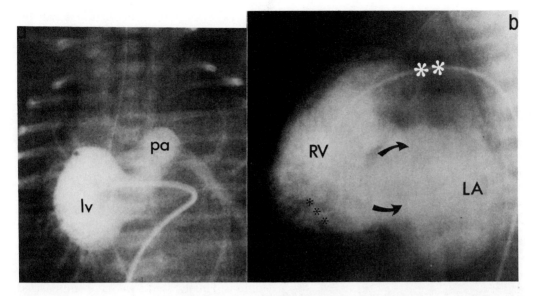

Figure 17. Functional aortic atresia in an infant with a right-sided heart and congenitally corrected transposition. (a) Frontal left ventriculogram (lv) shows the pulmonary trunk (pa); (b) the lateral right ventriculogram (RV) shows the displaced tricuspid valve (asterisk), the severe regurgitation (arrow) into the left atrium (LA). The ascending aorta (white asterisk) does not opacify despite a normal aortic valve at autopsy.

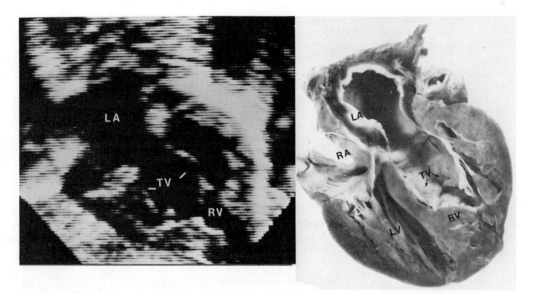

Figure 18. The picture on the left is an apical four-chamber view in severe Ebstein's malformation of the tricuspid valve in the setting of congenitally corrected transposition. Note the significant displacement and dysplasia of the valve with shortened cords. The picture on the right is the specimen from the same case and demonstrates the echocardiographic features. TV = tricuspid valve.

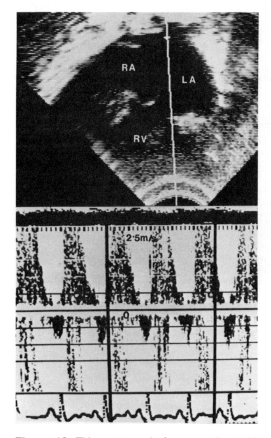

Figure 19. This montage is from a patient with severe Ebstein's malformation of the tricuspid valve and significant tricuspid valve regurgitation. Note the systolic regurgitant jet is detected at the most proximal portion of the left atrium. On flow mapping the jet was also broad as well as deep.

In conclusion, we have summarized the functional and anatomical spectrum of the dysplastic and displaced morphologically tricuspid valve in patients with both concordant or discordant atrioventricular connections. Organic or functional atresia of the arterial outlet reflects the severe distortion of the atrioventricular junction and ventricular myocardium. The atrioventricular junction itself in either type of atrioventricular connection may be nearly devoid of valve leaflet tissue (Brenner et al., 1978; Craig et al., 1986; Kanjuh et al., 1964). In this setting the underlying myocardial matrix may also be severely distorted. We have not identified obstructive anomalies of the coronary circulation in these unusual conditions. Finally, while we have emphasized the angiographic features in these conditions, cross-sectional echocardiography is probably the ideal modality for assessing the atrioventricular junction in these patients (de Albuquerque et al., 1984; Gussenhoven et al., 1984; Shiina et al., 1984).

degree of displacement of the septal and mural leaflets can be observed in those cases with a more severe malformation. Other cases studied in the newborn period and early infancy may have severe dysplasia with tethering of the leaflet by shortened cords but without appreciable associated plastering-down of the leaflets. These patients almost always have significant valvular regurgitation.

Doppler interrogation provides important physiological information regarding valvular function. With flow mapping, the severity of the regurgitation can be graded as mild, moderate, or severe (Fig. 19).

References

Actis-Dato A, Milocco I. Anomalous attachment of the mitral valve to the ventricular wall. *Am J Cardiol* 1966;17:278–281.

Adams JCL, Hudson REB. A case of Ebstein's anomaly surviving to age 79. *Br Heart J* 1956;18:129–132.

Anderson KR, Danielson GK, McGoon DC, Lie JT. Ebstein's anomaly of the left-sided tricuspid valve. Pathologic anatomy of the valvular malformation. *Circulation* 1978;53(Suppl I):87–91.

Anderson KR, Lie JT. Pathologic anatomy of Ebstein's anomaly of the heart revisited. *Am J Cardiol* 1978;41:739–745.

Anderson KR, Zuberbuhler JR, Anderson RH, et al. Morphologic spectrum of Ebstein's anomaly of the heart. A review. *Mayo Clin Proc* 1979;54:174–180.

Anderson RH, Wilkinson JL, Becker AE. The bulbus cordis—A misunderstood region of the developing human heart: Its significance to the classification of congenital cardiac malformation. In Rosenquist GC, Bergsma D (eds): *Morphogenesis and Malformation of the Cardiovascular Sys-*

tem. National Foundation, March of Dimes. Birth Defects: Original Article Series, vol. 14 (no. 7): pp. 1–28, 1978.

Arciprete P, Macartney FJ, DeLeval M, Stark J. Mustard's operation for patients with ventriculoartrerial concordance. Report of two cases and a cautionary tale. *Br Heart J* 1985;53:443–450.

Attie F, Soni J, Ovseyevitz J, Munoz-Castellanos L, et al. Angiographic studies of atrioventricular discordance. *Circulation* 1980;62:407–415.

Becker AE, Becker MJ, Edwards JE. Pathologic spectrum of dysplasia of the tricuspid valve. Features in common with Ebstein's malformation. *Arch Path* 1971;91:167–178.

Bharati S, McAllister HA, Chiemmongkoltip P, Lev M. Congenital pulmonary atresia with tricuspid insufficiency: Morphologic study. *Am J Cardiol* 1977;40:70–75.

Brenner JI, Bharati S, Winn WC Jr, Lev M. Absent tricuspid valve with aortic atresia in mixed levocardia (atrial situs solitus, L-loop). A hitherto undescribed entity. *Circulation* 1978;57:836–840.

Calabro R, Marino B, Marsico F. A case of isolated atrioventricular discordance. *Br Heart J* 1982;47:400–403.

Caruso G, Losekoot TG, Becker AE. Ebstein's anomaly in persistent common atrioventricular canal. *Br Heart J* 1978;40:1275–1279.

Castaneda-Zuniga W, Nath HP, Moller JH, Edwards JE. Left sided anomalies in Ebstein's malformation of the tricuspid valve. *Pediatr Cardiol* 1982;3:181–185.

Craig BG, Smallhorn JF, Rowe RD, et al. Severe obstruction to systemic blood flow in congenitally corrected transposition (discordant atrioventricular and ventriculo-arterial connexions): An analysis of 14 patients. *Int J Cardiol* 1986;11:205–217.

de Albuquerque AT, Rigby ML, Anderson RH, et al. The spectrum of atrioventricular discordance. A clinical study. *Br Heart J* 1984;51:498–507.

Deanfield JE, Anderson RH, Macartney FJ. Aortic atresia with "corrected transposition of the great arteries" (atrioventricular and ventriculoarterial discordance). *Br Heart J* 1981;46:683–686.

Diebold B, Touati R, Blanchard D, et al. Quantitative assessment of tricuspid regurgitation using pulsed Doppler echocardiography. *Br Heart J* 1983;50:443–449.

Elliott LP, Hartmann AF Jr. The right ventricular infundibulum in Ebstein's anomaly of the tricuspid valve. *Radiology* 1967;89:694–700.

Freedom RM, Culham JAG, Moes CAF. *Angiocardiography of Congenital Heart Disease.* New York: Macmillan, 1984;111–125.

Freedom RM, Culham G, Moes F, et al. Differentiation of functional and structural pulmonary atresia: Role of aortography. *Am J Cardiol* 1978;41:914–920.

Garcia-Dorado D, Falzgraf, Almazan A, et al. Diagnosis of functional tricuspid insufficiency by pulsed-wave Doppler ultrasound. *Circulation* 1982;66:1315–1321.

Gussenhoven EJ, Essed CE, Bos E, de Villeneuve VH. Echocardiographic diagnosis of overriding tricuspid valve in a child with Ebstein's anomaly. *Pediatr Cardiol* 1984;5:209–212.

Gussenhoven EJ, Stewart PA, Becker AE, et al. "Offsetting" of the septal tricuspid leaflet in normal hearts with Ebstein's anomaly. *Am J Cardiol* 1984;54:172–181.

Hazan E, Baillot F, Rey C, Dupuis C. Isolated ventricular discordance and complete atrioventricular canal in situs inversus. Report of successful surgical repair. *Am J Cardiol* 1977;40:403–466.

Hirschklau MJ, Sahn DJ, Hagan AD, et al. Cross-sectional echocardiographic features of Ebstein's anomaly of the tricuspid valve. *Am J Cardiol* 1977;40:400–404.

Huhta JC, Danielson GK, Ritter DG, Ilstrup DM. Survival in atrioventricular discordance. *Pediatr Cardiol* 1985;6:57–60.

Huhta JC, Edwards WD, Tajik AJ, et al. Pulmonary atresia with intact ventricular septum, Ebstein's anomaly of hypoplastic tricuspid valve, and double-chamber right ventricle. Two-dimensional echocardiographic-anatomic correlation. *Mayo Clin Proc* 1982;57:515–519.

Jaffe RB. Systemic atrioventricular valve regurgitation in corrected transposition of the great vessels. Angiographic differentiation of operable and nonoperable valve deformities. *Am J Cardiol* 1976;37:395–402.

Kambe T, Ichimiya S, Toguchi M, et al. Apex and subxiphoid approaches to Ebstein's anomaly using cross-sectional echocardiography. *Am Heart J* 1980;100:53–59.

Kanjuh VI, Stevenson JE, Amplatz K, Edwards JE. Congenitally unguarded tricuspid orifice with coexisting pulmonary atresia. *Circulation* 1964;30:911–917.

Lev M, Liberthson RR, Joseph RH, et al. The pathologic anatomy of Ebstein's disease. *Arch Path* 1970;90:334–343.

Losekoot TG, Anderson RH, Becker AE, et al. *Congenitally corrected transposition.* Edinburgh: Churchill Livingstone, 1983;130–137.

Matsukawa T, Yoshi S, Miyamura H, Eguchi S. Aortic atresia with Ebstein's and Uhl's anomaly in corrected transposition of the great arteries:

Clinicopathologic findings. *Jpn Circ J* 1983; 49:325–328.

Muster AJ, Idriss FS, Bharati S, et al. Functional aortic valve atresia in transposition of the great arteries. *J Am Coll Cardiol* 1985;6:630–634.

Newfeld EA, Cole RB, Paul MH. Ebstein's malformation of the tricuspid valve in the neonate. Functional and anatomic pulmonary outflow tract obstruction. *Am J Cardiol* 1967;19:727–731.

Oliveira Lima C, Sahn DJ, Valdes-Cruz LM, et al. Noninvasive prediction of transvalvular pressure gradient in patients with pulmonary stenosis by quantitative two-dimensional echocardiographic Doppler studies. *Circulation* 1983;67:866–871.

Quero-Jimenez M, Raposo-Sonnenfeld I. Isolated ventricular inversion with situs solitus. *Br Heart J* 1975;37:292–304.

Rao PS, Jue KL, Isabel-Jones J, Ruttenberg HD. Ebstein's malformation of the tricuspid valve with atresia. Differentiation from isolated tricuspid atresia. *Am J Cardiol* 1973;32:1004–1009.

Restivo A, Cameron AH, Anderson RH, Allwork SP. Divided right ventricle: A review of its anatomical varieties. *Pediatr Cardiol* 1984;5:197–204.

Roach RM, Tandon R, Moller JH, Edwards JE. Ebstein's anomaly of the tricuspid valve in persistent common atrioventricular canal. *Am J Cardiol* 1984;53:640–642.

Ruschhaupt DG, Bharati S, Lev M. Mitral valve malformation of Ebstein type in absence of corrected transposition. *Am J Cardiol* 1976;38:109–112.

Seward JB, Tajik AJ, Feist DJ, Smith HC. Ebstein's anomaly in an 85 year old man. *Mayo Clin Proc* 1979;54:193–196.

Shiina A, Seward JB, Edwards WD, et al. Two-dimensional echocardiographic spectrum of Ebstein's anomaly. Detailed anatomic assessment. *J Am Coll Cardiol* 1984;3:356–370.

Smallhorn JF, Izukawa T, Benson L, Freedom RM. Noninvasive recognition of functional pulmonary atresia by echocardiography. *Am J Cardiol* 1984;54:925–926.

Snider AR, Enderlein MA, Teitel DF, et al. Isolated ventricular inversion: Two-dimensional echocardiographic findings. A review of the literature. *Pediatr Cardiol* 1984;5:27–33.

Sutherland GR, Smallhorn JF, Anderson RH, et al. Atrioventricular discordance. Cross-sectional echocardiographic morphologic correlative study. *Br Heart J* 1983;50:8–20.

Uhl HSM. A previously undescribed congenital malformation of the heart. Almost total absence of the myocardium of the right ventricle. *Bull Johns Hopkins Hosp* 1952;91:197–205.

Watson H. Natural history of Ebstein's anomaly of tricuspid valve in childhood and adolescence. An international cooperative study of 505 cases. *Br Heart J* 1974;36:417–424.

Zuberbuhler JR, Allwork SP, Anderson RH. The spectrum of Ebstein's anomaly of the tricuspid valve. *J Thorac Cardiovasc Surg* 1979;77:202–211.

Zuberbuhler JR, Becker AE, Anderson RH, Lenox CC. Ebstein's malformation and embryological development of the tricuspid valve with a note on the nature of "clefts" in the atrioventricular valves. *Pediatr Cardiol* 1984;5:289–296.

2.5

Tricuspid Valve Replacement in Ebstein's Malformation

John W. Kirklin, Eugene H. Blackstone, and Lionel M. Bargeron, Jr.

The Controversy

The matter of repair or replacement of the tricuspid valve in patients with Ebstein's malformation and important tricuspid incompetence is likely to remain controversial for a very long time. In part, this is because Ebstein's malformation is uncommon, occurring in less than 1% of patients with congenital heart disease, and thus there is little opportunity to make formal comparisons between protocols of valve replacement as opposed to repair. In part, the persistence of this controversy is related to the fact that documentation of the results and advantages of atrioventricular valve repair in general, contrasted with those of valve replacement, has been difficult. In part also, the controversy persists because of the difficulties inherent in making comparisons between two treatment techniques of any kind in order to determine which is superior. These difficulties stem from the comparison of nonconcurrent experiences with possibly different and selected patient subsets of the conditions being studied, analyzed, and reported with differing standards.

Technique of Tricuspid Valve Replacement

The technique of tricuspid valve replacement and repair of the atrial septal defect in patients with Ebstein's malformation is straightforward (Fig. 1), and is based on the original description of the procedure by Barnard and Schrire (1963). In most patients requiring valve replacement for Ebstein's malformation, we currently prefer the St. Jude valve as the replacement device.

From: Anderson, RH, Neches, WH, Park, SC, Zuberbuhler, JR, eds: *Perspectives in Pediatric Cardiology*: Mount Kisco, New York, Futura Publishing Co., © 1988.

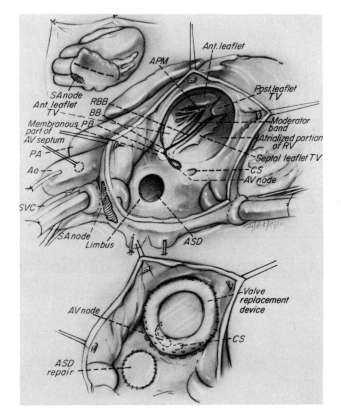

Figure 1. Replacement of the tricuspid valve and closure of the atrial septal defect in Ebstein's malformation. The upper left insert shows the siting of the atriotomy incision well anterior to the sinus node. The upper drawing shows the anatomical details seen by the surgeon and indicates the position of the conduction tissue and its vulnerability to damage. The lower drawing shows closure of the atrial septal defect and a method of insertion of the tricuspid prosthesis when the septal leaflet is absent or severely displaced into the right ventricle. Interrupted sutures may be used throughout. APM = anterior papillary muscle; AV node = atrioventricular node; BB = branching bundle; Cos = coronary sinus; PA = pulmonary artery; PB = penetrating bundle; RBB = right bundle branch; SA = sinoatrial. (Reproduced with permission from Bharati S, Lev M, Kirklin JW: *Cardiac Surgery and the Conduction System.* New York, Wiley, 1983.)

Results of Operation

Survival out to a mean time of four years after tricuspid valve replacement and repair of the atrial septal defect is 88%, including hospital deaths, in patients who preoperatively were in NYHA class II or III (Table 1). None who were preoperatively in NYHA class IV survived that long. Twelve (86%) of the 14 surviving patients currently are in NYHA class I, and 2 (14%) are in NYHA class II. Complete heart block developed in only one patient who was operated on 15 years ago.

Good function of the implanted valve resulted in all patients and none needed reoperation. Despite this, 10–20% of patients continue to have a troublesome supraventricular tachycardia which is *not* the Wolff-Parkinson-White syndrome (Westaby et al., 1982).

Some symptomatic patients with Ebstein's malformation who require surgical treatment do not require surgery to the tricuspid valve (Table 2). These are individuals who appear to have mild or no tricuspid valve incompetence. Some require the surgery because of a large left-to-right shunt, and others because of severe cyanosis from a right-to-left shunt. If indeed little or no tricuspid incompetence was present, the results have been good following closure of the atrial septal defects, with 6 (60%) of the 10 surviving patients in NYHA class I and the remaining 4 in Class II. Two patients died, both because of severe tricuspid incompetence developing or persisting after the operation. Thus, when surgical treatment without tricuspid valve surgery is contemplated for patients with Ebstein's malformation, there must be a high degree of certainty that the tricuspid valve is rea-

Table 1
Death after Tricuspid Valve Replacement and Repair of Atrial Septal Defect in Patients with Ebstein's Malformation Undergoing Surgery at the University of Alabama in Birmingham, USA and Green Lane Hospital, Auckland, New Zealand.

Preoperative NYHA class	n	Hospital deaths				Total deaths				II, III vs. IV			
		No.	%	CL	No.	%	CL	n	No.	%	CL		
I	—	—		—	—		—			—			
II	4	1	25%	3%–63%	1	25%	3%–63%	16	2	12%	4%–27%		
III	12	—	0%	0%–15%	1	8%	1%–26%		—				
IV	4	3	75%	37%–97%	4	100%	62%–100%	4	4	100%	62%–100%		
Total	20	4	20%	10%–33%	6	30%	19%–44%	20	6	30%	19%–44%		
p (Fisher)											.003		

CL-70% confidence limits; NYHA-New York Heart Association.
Note: Entry into series ended 1/1/81; follow-up ended 1/1/84, with follow-up varying between 0.5 and 9 years, mean 3.8 years.
Based on data from Kirklin JW, Barratt-Boyes BG: *Cardiac Surgery*. New York, Wiley, 1986, Chap. 27.

Table 2
Deaths After Surgery Without Repair of the Tricuspid Valve for Ebstein's Malformation in Operations Performed at the University of Alabama in Birmingham and Green Lane Hospital, Auckland, New Zealand

Operation	n	Hospital deaths			All deaths		
		No.	%	CL	No.	%	CL
Repair ASD	9	0	0%	0%–85%	1[a]	11%	1%–33%
Repair ASD + VSD	1	0	0%	0%–85%	0	0%	0%–85%
Repair ASD + PS	1	0	0%	0%–85%	0	0%	0%–85%
Repair ASD + tricuspid valvotomy	1	0	0%	0%–85%	1[b]	100%	15%–100%
Total	12	0	0%	0%–15%	2	17%	6%–35%

ASD = atrial septal defect; CL = 70% confidence limits; PS = pulmonary stenosis; VSD = ventricular septal defect.
Note: Entry into series ended 1/1/81; follow-up ended 1/1/84, with follow-up varying between 0.5 and 9 years, mean 3.8 years.
[a] Preoperatively in NYHA class IV. Death after later tricuspid valve replacement (elsewhere).
[b] Severe tricuspid incompetence present after operation; death two weeks after hospital dismissal.

sonably competent before and after the operation.

Summary

Successful repair of an incompetent tricuspid valve in patients with Ebstein's malformation is preferable to valve replacement. Coexisting congenital cardiac anomalies (atrial septal defects, ventricular septal defects, pulmonary stenosis, and accessory atrioventricular conduction pathways) are treated at the same operation. At the University of Alabama in Birmingham, because of uncertainty as to the long-term results of repair of the tricuspid valve, and because of the good results of valve replacement, most patients in this setting receive replacement rather than repair. The possibility that the morphology of the tricuspid valve will allow successful repair, however, is sought in each patient.

References

Barnard CN, Schrire Y. Surgical correction of Ebstein's malformation with a prosthetic tricuspid valve. *Surgery* 1963;54:302–308.

Westaby S, Karp RB, Kirklin JW, et al. Surgical treatment in Ebstein's malformation. *Ann Thorac Surg* 1982;34:388–395.

III

Tetralogy of Fallot with Pulmonary Atresia

Introduction: Pulmonary Atresia with Ventricular Septal Defect

Julien I. E. Hoffman

Pulmonary atresia with ventricular septal defect is regarded as an extreme example of tetralogy of Fallot, with which it indeed shares many features: a large ventricular septal defect, a large and overriding aorta and well-formed inlet and apical trabecular portions of the right ventricle. Both lesions, too, have a hypoplastic right ventricular outflow tract which, to be sure, is at its most extreme when there is pulmonary atresia. The two lesions also resemble each other in their pulmonary arterial anatomy. Pulmonary atresia typically has small right and left pulmonary arteries, and these are also found at times in tetralogies of Fallot, especially those with a very small annulus of the pulmonary valve. It is these small arteries that are often responsible for the poor results of surgery in these lesions. The one major difference between the two lesions is the high incidence of a dual blood supply to the lungs in pulmonary atresia. Some of the lung is supplied by the central pulmonary arteries and some is supplied by large aortopulmonary collateral arteries arising directly from the aorta. Sometimes the aortopulmonary collateral and the central pulmonary arterial branches join near the hilum of the lung, so that blood from both sources is then delivered to the lung through what appears to be a normal pulmonary vascular bed. At other times there is no overlap between these two blood supplies, so that some of the lung is supplied by central pulmonary arteries and the remainder of the lung is supplied from the aorta, as in a sequestration. The branching pattern of intrapulmonary arteries may be abnormal when the blood supply comes from these aortopulmonary collaterals, and in over 50% there are one or more stenotic regions in these arteries.

Some of the alterations in anatomy are secondary to known embryologic changes. The normal anatomy of inflow and body portions of the right ventricles in both lesions follows from the fact that, in both, the right ventricles eject blood into the aorta,

Supported in part by Program Project Grant HL 25847 from the United States Public Health Service.
From: Anderson, RH, Neches, WH, Park, SC, Zuberbuhler, JR, eds: *Perspectives in Pediatric Cardiology*: Mount Kisco, New York, Futura Publishing Co., © 1988.

and so are stimulated to grow. The small pulmonary arteries indicate lack of pressure stimulation during development. Because of the outflow tract obstruction, pressure in the pulmonary arteries depends on flow into them through the arterial duct (ductus arteriosus) which, being long and thin, allows perfusion of the lungs only at low pressures. In addition, because the total ventricular output is ejected into the ascending aorta, the flow through the aortic isthmus is greater than normal and no isthmic narrowing occurs. This probably explains the rarity of aortic coarctation in these two lesions. What is as yet unexplained is the formation of the large aortopulmonary collaterals which are only rarely found when there is severe tetralogy of Fallot, and hardly ever in pulmonary atresia with an intact ventricular septum. Because it is likely that the abnormal development leading to pulmonary atresia with a ventricular septal defect occurs much earlier than the abnormality that leads to pulmonary atresia with

an intact ventricular septum, it is likely that, in the former lesion, the developing intrapulmonary arteries are not stimulated to join the sixth arch (which gives rise to the right and left pulmonary arteries). Instead, they attach to the nearby descending aorta. When the pulmonary atresia occurs later, after closure of the interventricular communication, the central pulmonary arteries coming from the sixth arch are better formed and therefore connect with the intraparenchymal pulmonary arterial branches.

There is an urgent need to understand why the pulmonary arteries do not always grow after various types of surgical repair or palliation of pulmonary atresia. Are some arteries incapable of growing after a shunt is placed because of some structural abnormality, or are better methods of connecting shunts to these small arteries required? If we could answer these questions, we would be able to achieve much better results than can now be obtained in this challenging lesion.

Clinical Identification of the Pulmonary Blood Supply in Pulmonary Atresia

Jane Somerville

In pulmonary atresia with ventricular septal defect, the heart exhibits two basic abnormalities: a large subaortic ventricular septal defect (as in tetralogy of Fallot), and a complete obstruction between the right ventricular outflow tract and central pulmonary arteries. Indeed, the latter structures may be present in part or in total. When blood cannot pass directly from the right ventricle to the pulmonary arteries, the essential blood flow needed for oxygenation must be derived in other ways. The variation in systemic arterial saturation (Fig. 1) reflects the considerable differences in pulmonary blood supply which can originate from several sources (Table 1). In reality, this congenital heart anomaly should be considered and managed as a pulmonary vascular disease. For ease of understanding, the basic forms of pulmonary blood supply are described separately, although often they exist in combination.

The Pulmonary Arteries

When considering true pulmonary arterial blood supply, it is necessary to study both the central (intrapericardial) arteries and the full complement of lobar branches. The arrangement of the central pulmonary arteries has been classified according to what is present beyond the atretic right ventricular outflow (Fig. 2). This is basic knowledge required prior to any consideration of radical reparative surgery. The extent of central arteries present is dependent upon intrauterine development. Their size, in contrast, depends on their postnatal perfusion. Central right and/or left branch pulmonary arteries may be present in the absence of segmental or lobar arteries.

The growth and size of both the central and distal pulmonary arteries depend upon the source and size of systemic supply. This

From: Anderson, RH, Neches, WH, Park, SC, Zuberbuhler, JR, eds: *Perspectives in Pediatric Cardiology*: Mount Kisco, New York, Futura Publishing Co., © 1988.

PULMONARY ATRESIA
Arterial Oxygen Saturation at Rest

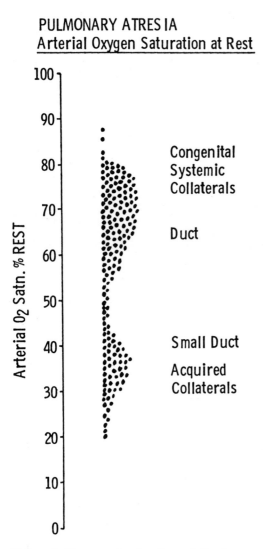

Figure 1. Diagram showing the variation in oxygen saturation according to the source of pulmonary supply in a large group of patients with pulmonary atresia and ventricular septal defect.

can be a duct (which exceptionally may be bilateral), can be through acquired systemic collateral arteries, through congenital major aortopulmonary collateral arteries, through fistulas from the coronary arteries, or via man-made shunts.

The Arterial Duct

When the duct remains open beyond the neonatal period in pulmonary atresia

Table 1
Sources of Pulm. Blood Flow—Pulm. Atresia

Pulmonary Arteries
Duct
Congenital Systemic Collaterals
Acquired Collaterals
Man-Made Shunts

Coronary Arteries ⟨ Acquired / Congenital

with ventricular septal defect, it is often an unusual looking structure, being long and horn-like, more vertical than those associated with coarctation, and appearing to perfuse one or another branch pulmonary artery (Fig. 3). Despite the apparent narrowing of the pulmonary arterial end of the duct seen at the time of study, this arrangement may be associated with unsuspected pulmonary hypertension which may show after a normal or increased flow is established. In exceptional cases, patients with duct-dependent arterial supply survive to late adolescence or early adult life. They may then develop an aneurysm of the duct (Fig. 4). An arterial duct may supply only the right or left pulmonary artery when it is separate and not connected to its contralateral artery (nonconfluent pulmonary arteries, so-called type 2) (Fig. 2). This arrangement may give the appearance of absence of the contralateral pulmonary artery before acquired collaterals have time to form (Fig. 5). It is vital in this setting that a thoracotomy be performed early in order to establish a shunt and pulmonary perfusion on that side. This must be done even if perfusion on the side supplied by the arterial duct is clinically adequate. When there is persistence of an arterial duct, stenosis at its site of insertion to the pulmonary artery is the rule.

When the duct persists with confluent central pulmonary arteries, the arteries themselves and their peripheral branches are usually well developed and ramify to supply all segments. In a small proportion of cases (7% of complex pulmonary atresia), an arterial duct coexists with congenital sys-

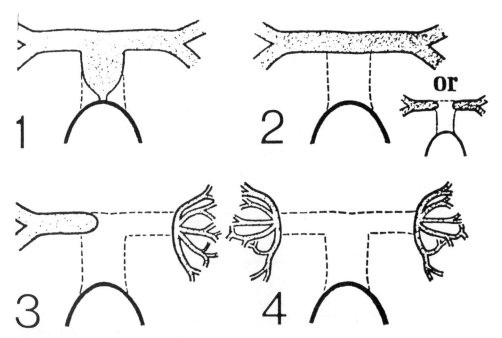

Figure 2. The system of classification of the pulmonary arterial pathways used at the National Heart Hospital in London.

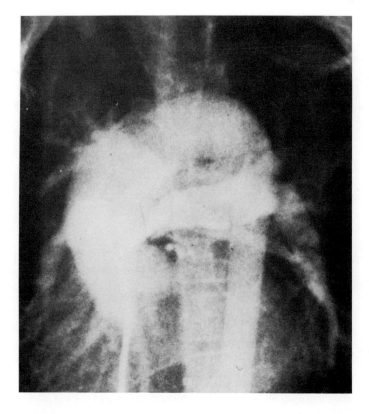

Figure 3. A long, horn-like arterial duct supplying confluent pulmonary arteries in a case of pulmonary atresia with ventricular septal defect.

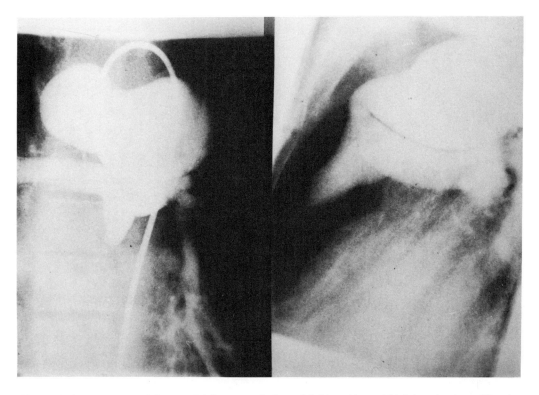

Figure 4. An aneurysm of the arterial duct seen in frontal (left) and lateral (right) projections. The duct was the source of pulmonary arterial supply in a patient with pulmonary atresia and ventricular septal defect.

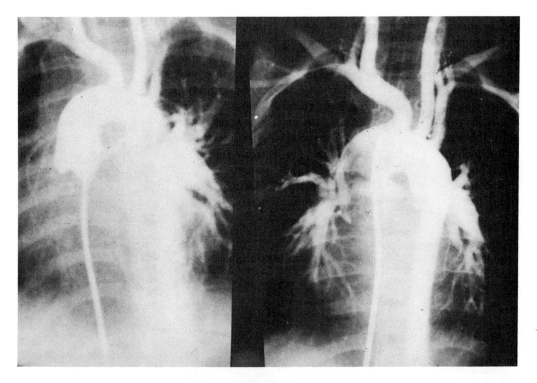

Figure 5. In this patient with nonconfluent pulmonary arteries, the arterial duct supplies the left artery (left panel), giving the impression of absence of the right artery. With the passage of time, and the development of acquired collateral arteries, the right pulmonary artery fills (right panel) and is seen to be of good size.

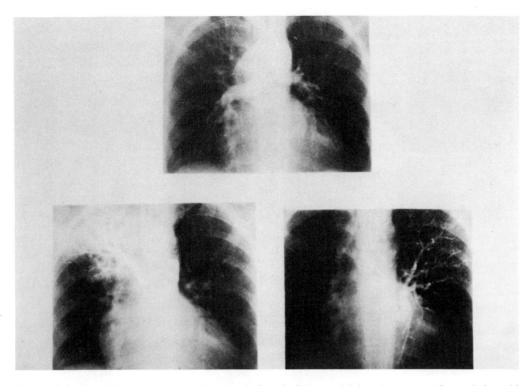

Figure 6. In this patient, the unusual situation is found of an arterial duct (upper panel) coexisting with congenital systemic-pulmonary collateral arteries (lower panels).

temic-pulmonary collateral arteries supplying some of the lung segments (Fig. 6). When this occurs, segmental arteries may be missing from some of the pulmonary arterial branches while sometimes there is a complete and separated dual blood supply to one or two lobes of the lung. Bilateral ducts, each supplying a separate nonconfluent pulmonary artery, do exist but are rare.

Acquired Systemic Pulmonary Collateral Arteries

These are numerous, uncountable, spidery, thin-walled, and tortuous small arteries that grow larger with the passage of time. They originate from arteries arising from the aorta within the thorax. They take time to develop an adequate size and connection with the pulmonary arteries and thus are not able to provide adequate perfusion if the duct closes abruptly in early life. They follow the bronchi (Fig. 7), become grotesquely large as intercostals after a thoracotomy, and effectively oxygenate even (and particularly) when no shunt has been established, they may perfuse the ipsilateral pulmonary artery (Fig. 8). It is these acquired but thin-walled large intercostal vessels which notch the ribs on the side of the thoracotomy and may rupture with infection, and prolonged intubation. It takes time (years) to develop them and they are not seen under age five years.

If a chronic granuloma such as that caused by tuberculosis develops in the lung, the resultant acquired collaterals enlarge further with improvement in the patient's color. Unfortunately, there is the danger of rupture, with death from hemoptysis, a sinister symptom in such a setting. Emboliza-

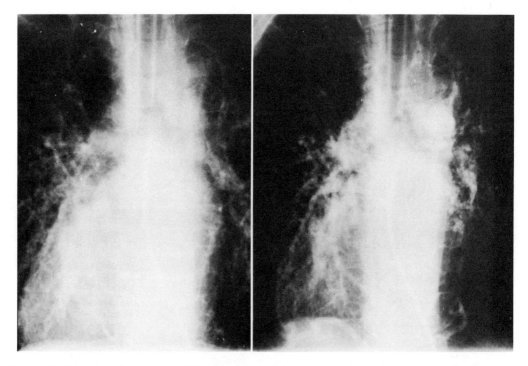

Figure 7. These injections show multiple acquired systemic-pulmonary collateral arteries in a patient with pulmonary atresia and ventricular septal defect.

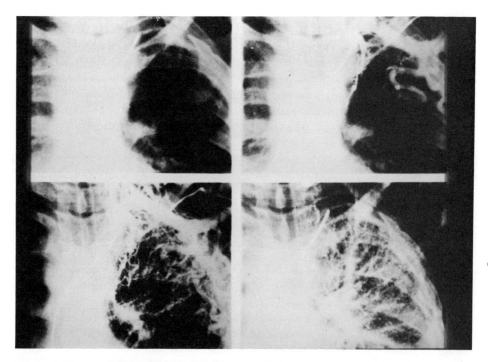

Figure 8. This sequence of panels shows the multiple acquired systemic-pulmonary collateral arteries which perfuse the pulmonary artery pathways to the left lung.

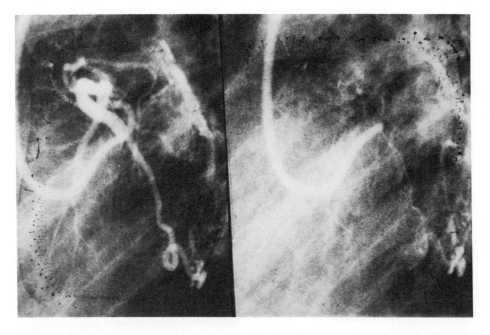

Figure 9. These injections show acquired systemic-pulmonary collateral arteries that are derived from the coronary arteries.

tion or lobectomy with a shunt to other pulmonary vessels may be the only solution.

In adults there is evidence that the coronary arteries can contribute acquired collateral vessels to the mediastinum with pulmonary atresia (Fig. 9), particularly if there has been earlier exploration of the mediastinum. They may then produce a coronary "steal" effect with resultant angina.

When acquired collateral arteries are developed prior to a thoracotomy, it usually means that there is a central pulmonary artery present on the side of the collaterals. They give the appearance of speckled lung fields on a routine chest x-ray which can be seen by one to two years of age.

Congenital Systemic Collateral Arteries

These are large arteries that are present at birth. They are countable (usually there are one to six), tortuous, and arise from the subclavian arteries or from the descending aorta at or below the isthmus (Fig. 10). When pulmonary atresia with subaortic ventricular septal defect is associated with congenital systemic collateral arteries, it is described as "complex pulmonary atresia"; the complex refers to the complexity and variation of the pulmonary blood supply and not to the intracardiac lesions, which are almost constant. A right aortic arch is present in 40% of patients; no other congenital heart disease has such a high incidence of this associated anomaly.

Each patient must be considered individually since there is no uniform or constant pattern of development of the collateral arteries. There are, however, several basic forms (Table 2). The large artery, which arises from the midportion of the thoracic aorta and curls up to give off vessels to one lung before crossing the midline to supply the opposite lung without obstruction, is rare. It occurs in only 3 to 4% of complex pulmonary atresias (Fig. 11). Such a vessel may arise from a right or left de-

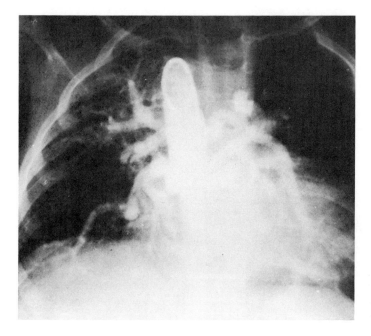

Figure 10. This descending aortogram in frontal projection shows the typical appearance of multiple congenital systemic-pulmonary collateral arteries.

scending aorta. A more uncommon variant of this pattern is when the collateral artery supplies one lung and the other pulmonary artery arises from the ascending aorta. With both types the blind, atretic outflow tract can be identified within the right ventricle and it is more appropriate to consider these patients as having complex pulmonary atresia rather than variants of common

Table 2
Congenital Systemic Collaterals— Pulmonary Atresia

From thoracic aorta or subclavian
  usually from below isthmus

One huge vessel from mid. thor. aorta
  supplies all parts lung

One to segment or lobe
  may join P.A.'s—(rare)
  or be end arteries

1–6 large, stenosed
  end arteries
  or one may enter true P.A.'s
  or fill them retrogradely

trunk. To be strictly accurate, nonetheless, it is more correct to describe the ascending arterial trunk arising from the heart as a solitary arterial trunk when the intrapericardial pulmonary arteries are completely absent.

These congenital systemic collateral arteries may be end arteries to lung lobes or may connect to the intrapericardial pulmonary arteries either centrally or at the hilar level. They may be stenotic at their origin or within the hila (Fig. 12). Before embarking on surgery, the anatomy, course, distribution to the lung, connection to intrapericardial pulmonary arteries, and extent of pulmonary arterial development must all be displayed. An aberrant right subclavian may look like, and contribute flow to, the pulmonary arteries and mimic a man-made shunt (Fig. 13). It is more common, however, to find a single vessel going to the lower lobe, and another curling up to the upper lobes. Less frequently, collateral arteries curl down to the lungs and look like horns. When aortopulmonary collateral arteries are present, the central pulmonary arteries are infrequently large (8%), more

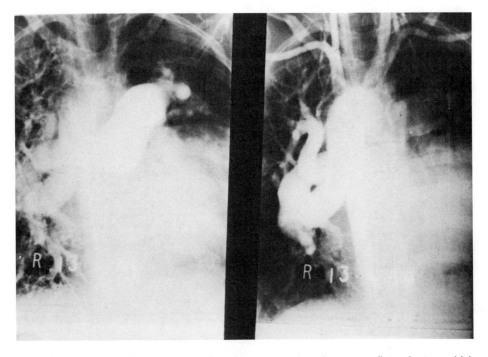

Figure 11. These injections reveal a solitary large systemic-pulmonary collateral artery which supplies branches to both lungs.

usually hypoplastic (82%) (Fig. 14), and less often completely absent (10%). The true central pulmonary arteries, when hypoplastic, are recognized by their "seagull" (gaviota) appearance in the central mediastinum (Fig. 15). Very frequently, there are deficiencies in the segmental branching pattern (Figs. 14 and 15b), particularly when a large aortopulmonary collateral artery supplies that part of the lung. The central pulmonary arteries can be so small and have so few branches that they are barely recognizable (Fig. 16).

A single ascending or descending aortopulmonary collateral artery may connect to one or another branch pulmonary artery at the level of the hilum (Fig. 15) or there may be several proximal connections. Each must be identified. Distal connections within the lung substance may also be found but these are less frequent with this form of collateral arterial supply. Those with a large communication to the pulmo-

nary arteries have good-sized pulmonary arteries but, in those with hypoplastic "seagulls," connections are usually small and from the periphery. Shunts, particularly when centrally placed, increase the size of the vessels and may disclose stenotic segments. Where the right pulmonary artery passes behind the ascending aorta, it usually develops a long narrow segment if perfusion is not large. The size of the central pulmonary arteries depends on the amount of blood flow carried, rather than the source which dictates the maintenance of this flow. The natural history and changing form of these various sources differs.

Coronary Artery Fistulas

A congenital fistula from the left coronary artery may effectively supply the pul-

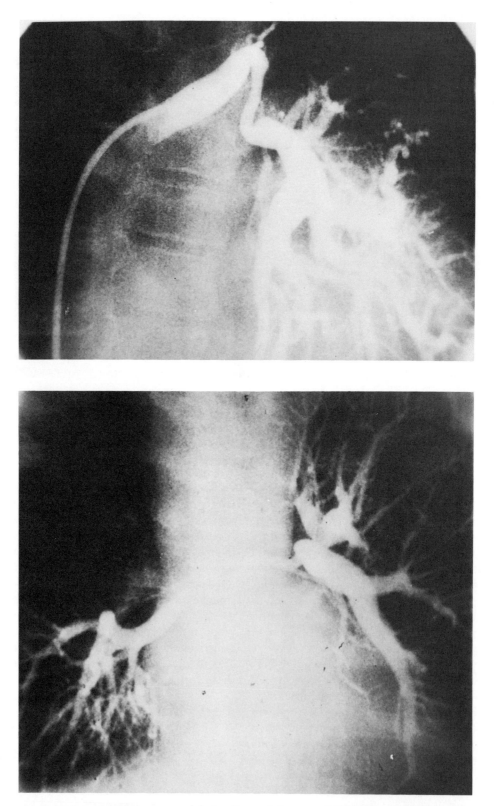

Figure 12. These selective injections show stenosis at the origin of the congenital systemic-pulmonary collateral artery (upper panel) and within the lung hilum (lower panel).

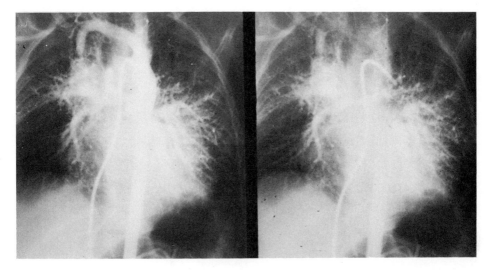

Figure 13. These selective injections show pulmonary blood flow to the lungs derived from an aberrant right subclavian artery (left panel) that resembles a man-made shunt.

monary circulation in 3% of patients with pulmonary atresia and ventricular septal defect (Fig. 17). If the pulmonary arteries are well developed, this implies a "steal" from the left ventricle which is an important consideration at complete repair and influences the long-term results since serious left ventricular dysfunction may develop. In excep-

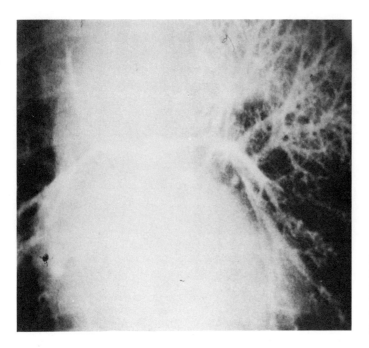

Figure 14. In this patient with multiple congenital systemic-pulmonary collateral arteries, the central pulmonary arteries are confluent but grossly hypoplastic.

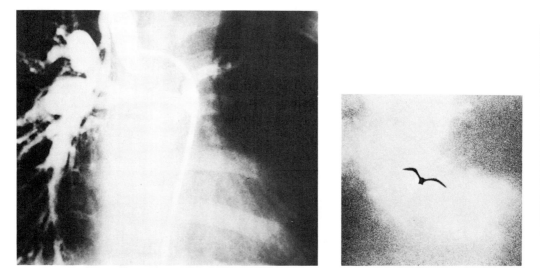

Figure 15. This selective injection into a systemic-pulmonary collateral artery (left) fills the central pulmonary arteries, which resemble a seagull in flight (right).

tional cases, a fistula occurs between a branch of the right coronary artery and the pulmonary circulation.

Adult patients with complex pulmonary atresia who have survived with or without surgical attempts commonly develop pulmonary hypertension, lose continuous murmurs, and appear with the Eisenmenger reaction in late second and third decades (Fig. 18).

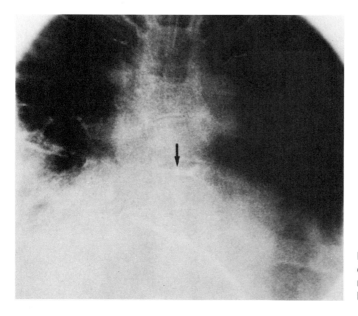

Figure 16. In this patient, the central pulmonary arteries (arrowed) are so small as to be barely recognizable.

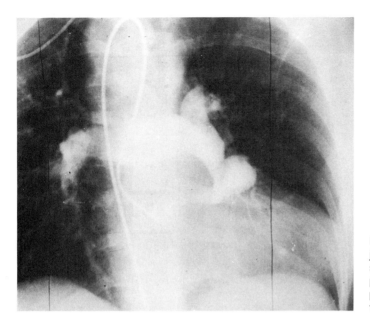

Figure 17. This selective injection in a coronary artery shows the rare pattern of supply of the pulmonary arterial pathway via a coronary arterial fistula.

Summary

The blood supply to the lungs in complex pulmonary atresia takes many forms (Fig. 19) that can be adversely and beneficially modified by man-made shunts. To increase the size of hypoplastic central pulmonary arteries may not be enough to provide a good result for radical repair with a valved conduit. An unsatisfactory result may occur, however, not only because lobar pulmonary artery branches are missing but also because pulmonary arterial stenoses are present.

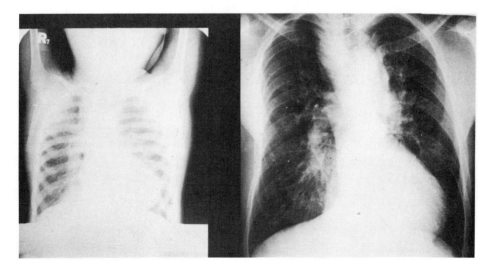

Figure 18. The progression from overfilled lungs (left) in childhood to the Eisenmenger situation (right) in an adult with pulmonary atresia and ventricular septal defect.

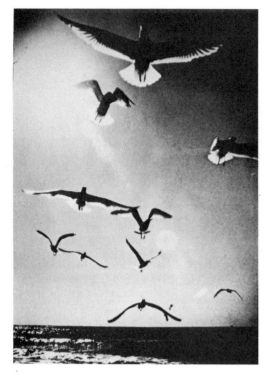

Figure 19. The potential variability of the pulmonary arterial pathways is well illustrated by this photograph of a flock of seagulls in flight.

Perhaps more important is that the walls of the central pulmonary arteries must be abnormal and, despite increase in size of the vessels or growth, they remain rigid, causing pulmonary hypertension. This topic requires more study. It is as important to long-term management and survival as are the gross anatomical malformations upon which attention is focused. Until now, anatomical definition of the pulmonary blood flow has relied on angiography. Now, magnetic resonance imaging has been shown to give useful information and since it is a noninvasive technique, it can be repeated without discomfort to assess vessel growth.

Each patient born with pulmonary atresia and ventricular septal defect should be considered individually. Until every anatomical variant of pulmonary blood supply is demonstrated, management cannot be correctly planned or outcome predicted. Many patients with complex pulmonary atresia and a generous pulmonary blood supply might live longer without surgical attempts to correct their anatomy.

Intrapulmonary Connections and Nonconnections in Tetralogy of Fallot with Pulmonary Atresia

Marlene Rabinovitch

In patients with tetralogy of Fallot and pulmonary atresia, it is important to elucidate the nature, the presence, and the size of communications between systemic collateral arteries, intrapulmonary arteries, and true central pulmonary arteries prior to planning the type and timing of surgical intervention. This chapter will discuss the embryology of the various connections, the nature of the anastomotic narrowing and its potential for occlusion, and the determinants of central and peripheral pulmonary artery growth.

Embryologic Considerations

During the first month of gestation, the lung buds receive blood supply from primitive pulmonary arteries derived from the sixth aortic arch and from a single pair of arteries from the dorsal aorta. Arrest in development at this stage has been observed (Goldstein et al., 1979) and results in an infant with persistent pulmonary hypertension (Fig. 1).

By the fifth week of gestation, a vascular plexus forms within the lung buds and this plexus communicates with many paired dorsal intersegmental arteries (Congdon, 1922). Between the fifth and seventh weeks of gestation, the plexus joins the central pulmonary arteries at the hilum and the dorsal communications with the intersegmental arteries begin to involute. These communications may, however, persist abnormally when there is hypoplasia of the pulmonary arteries and atresia of the pulmonary valve which cause decreased forward pulmonary blood flow during fetal life. The bronchial arteries, in other words, those vessels that arise from the underside of the aorta in the third and fourth thoracic segments and supply the bronchi, do not form until the

From: Anderson, RH, Neches, WH, Park, SC, Zuberbuhler, JR, eds: *Perspectives in Pediatric Cardiology*: Mount Kisco, New York, Futura Publishing Co., © 1988.

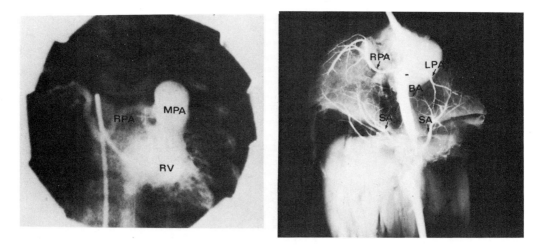

Figure 1. Postmortem pulmonary arteriogram in an infant who died on the first day of life with persistent pulmonary hypertension of the newborn. Structural abnormalities suggest an "arrest in development" at the fifth week of gestation. Primitive pulmonary arteries supply the upper lobes of the lung while systemic collateral arteries supply the lower lobes. (Reproduced with permission from Goldstein et al., 1979.)

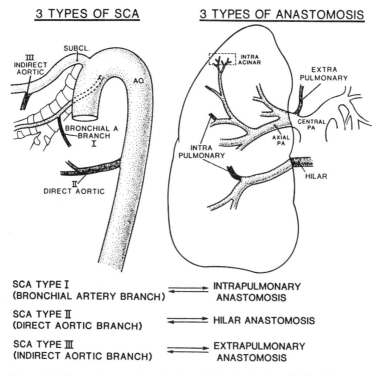

Figure 2. Three types of systemic collateral arteries (SCA) (direct and indirect aortopulmonary collateral arteries and bronchial collaterals) and three types of anastomoses with the pulmonary artery (PA) (hilar, intrapulmonary and extrapulmonary). SUBCL = subclavian; AO = aorta. (Reproduced with permission from Rabinovitch et al., 1981.)

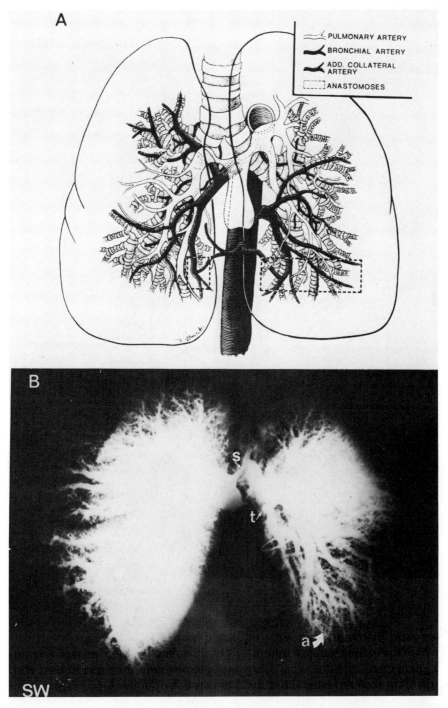

Figure 3A. *Top:* Intrapulmonary connections in a patient with tetralogy of Fallot plus pulmonary atresia. Direct aortic branches become pulmonary arteries of the right upper and right lower lobe anteriorly and the left lower lobe and lingula. A smaller direct aortic branch crosses the midline and joins with the larger direct aortic branches. Intrapulmonary anastomoses are present in the left lung between vessels originating from direct aortic branches and pulmonary arteries from neighboring segments of lobes. *Bottom:* The postmortem arteriogram shows a direct aortic branch(s) just below the subclavian artery. Another direct aortic branch (t) is from the descending thoracic aorta and supplies the left upper and left lower lobes. Intrapulmonary anastomoses (a) between these vessels and pulmonary arteries of remaining lobes are present.

171

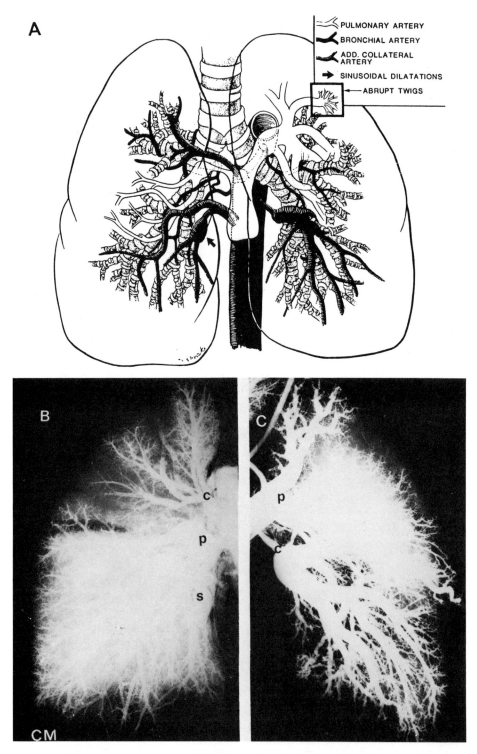

Figure 3B. Features in another patient with tetralogy of Fallot plus pulmonary atresia (*top*). Direct aortic branches become pulmonary arteries to right upper lobe, right lower lobe, and left lower lobe. There are no intrapulmonary anastomoses between branches of these vessels and branches from the pulmonary arteries of the right middle or left upper lobe. *Bottom; left:* The postmortem arteriogram of the right lung. c = collateral to right upper lobe; p = pulmonary artery to right middle lobe; s = poststenotic sinusoidal dilatation of collateral branch to right lower lobe. *Bottom, right:* Postmortem arteriogram of left lung. c = collateral branch to left lower lobe; p = pulmonary artery to left upper lobe and lingula.

ninth week of gestation (Boydon, 1970). Around the time of birth, these bronchial arteries communicate with the intraacinar arteries. These communications may persist abnormally postnatally or may proliferate when there is decreased forward pulmonary blood flow.

Throughout fetal life, as the airways are forming, true intrapulmonary arteries de-velop from the plexus within the lung buds. By the 16th week, all pre-acinar arteries are present (both the conventional arteries that run alongside the airways and many super-numerary arteries). After the 16th week, the intra-acinar arteries begin to form along the newly developing acini, which include the respiratory bronchioli and the saccules (primitive alveoli).

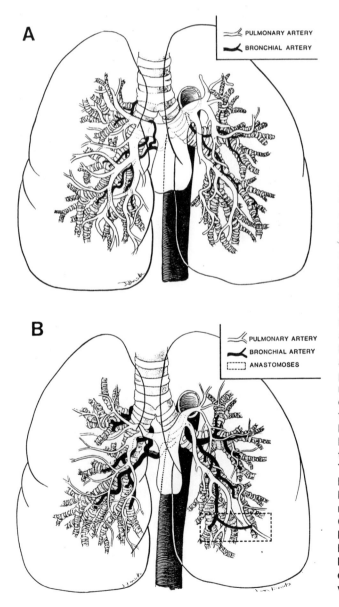

Figure 4. *A:* Normal relationship of the normal pulmonary arteries to air-ways and bronchial arteries. In the left lung, the arteries are in front of the bronchi so as not to obscure their structural features. *B:* Some of the features dissected in a patient who had tetralogy of Fallot and pulmo-nary atresia. The bronchial arteries to both lungs are enlarged. In the right lung and the left upper lobe, the axial pulmonary arteries are severely hypoplastic, but in the left lower lobe and lingula the diameters of the axial pulmonary arteries are nearly nor-mal. Large anastomoses with bron-chial arteries were seen. *C:* Dissec-tion of the vessels in the left lower lobe shows large anastomoses (a) between branches of a bronchial ar-tery (b) and a pulmonary artery (p). *D:* The postmortem arteriogram shows large anastomosis (a) between a bronchial arterial branch and a pul-monary artery in the left lower lobe. On the right, the axial arteries are hypoplastic. The dense background haze results from filling of the en-larged bronchial arteries. (Repro-duced with permission from Rabino-vitch et al., 1981.)

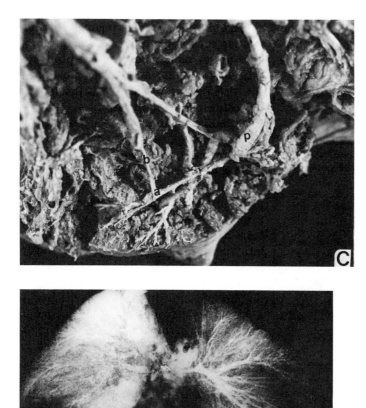

Figure 4. *Continued.*

Aortopulmonary Collaterals: A Classification Based on Morphology and Embryology

Based on these embryologic considerations, together with our dissections of lungs obtained at postmortem from patients with tetralogy of Fallot and pulmonary atresia, we devised the following simplified classification of aortopulmonary connections (Rabinovitch et al., 1981) (Fig. 2): There are essentially three types of collateral arteries based upon site of origin. The first type are the direct aortopulmonary collateral arteries which arise directly from the descending aorta. They are probably derived from primitive intersegmental arteries. The second type of indirect aortopulmonary collateral arteries are those vessels that arise from branches of the aorta, such as the subclavian, internal thoracic, coronary, or intercostal arteries. They develop only at some later point in gestation. The third type are the bronchial artery collateral vessels, which arise from the bronchial arteries. They therefore will appear only after the ninth week of gestation.

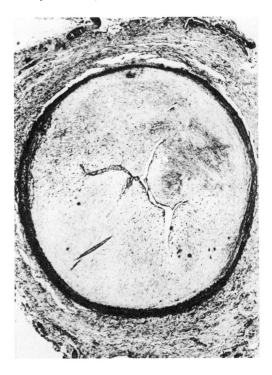

Figure 5A. The site of anastomosis between a direct aortopulmonary collateral artery and a pulmonary artery at the hilum. There is marked occlusive intimal hyperplasia. Movat Stain. Original magnification ×50.

There are three types of anastomoses that collateral arteries will form with pulmonary arteries. These are based on location and may be at the *hilar* margin of the lung, may be *intrapulmonary* (or inside the lung), or they may be *extrapulmonary* (or outside the lung). Moreover, each type of systemic collateral artery has a preferential means of anastomosing with a pulmonary artery.

Direct aortopulmonary collateral arteries are usually replaced at the hilum or in the intrapulmonary perihilar region by a vessel that is "pulmonary" in both its histology and its distribution and which follows the airways. The region of anastomosis is characterized by "intimal hyperplasia" and probably represents an incomplete attempt of the primitive intersegmental artery to involute. The stenosis caused by the intimal hyperplasia prevents the transmission of

high flow and pressure from the aorta to the intrapulmonary arteries and thus protects the vascular bed from vascular disease. The "poststenotic" pulmonary arteries are frequently tortuous and dilated. Usually, but not always, there are additional anastomoses between these pulmonary arteries and those in adjoining lobes or segments of lobes that can be traced back to a central (true) pulmonary artery. It is only in the presence of such anastomoses that the direct aortopulmonary collateral arteries can be safely ligated at surgery at the time that flow is established from the right ventricular outflow tract to the pulmonary arteries. If there are no anastomoses to vessels that can be traced back to a central pulmonary artery, then the direct aortopulmonary collaterals must be considered as providing the main blood supply to a lung lobe or segment. In these circumstances, they may not safely be ligated at surgery without running the risk of pulmonary infarction (Fig. 3).

Indirect aortopulmonary collateral arteries frequently anastomose with the extrapulmonary components of the right or left central pulmonary arteries. They are also observed to fan out over the pleural surface of the lung and join the most distal intra-acinar pulmonary arteries. Bronchial arterial collaterals always form intrapulmonary anastomoses with relatively peripheral pre-acinar or intra-acinar pulmonary arteries (Fig. 4).

The Aortopulmonary Anastomosis

Because the anastomosis between a collateral artery and a pulmonary artery is usually stenotic, only rarely is pulmonary vascular disease manifest (Haworth 1980; Haworth and Macartney 1980; Thiene et al., 1979). Although it has not been determined what governs progressive stenosis at the site of an anastomosis, we had the opportunity to study such a segment when it was surgi-

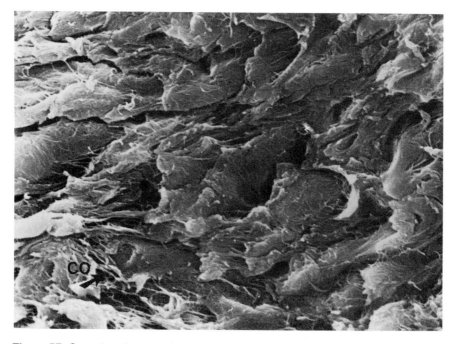

Figure 5B. Scanning electron microscopy of the endothelial surface (see arrow on light photomicrograph) reveals jagged cells with underlying exposed collagen (CO). Original magnification ×200.

cally removed. Scanning electron microscopy revealed a jagged endothelial surface. Endothelial cells were lifted and the subendothelium was exposed (Fig. 5). This area appears to be a site of turbulance and the resulting endothelial injury may predispose to thrombus formation.

The Arterial Duct as a Collateral Artery

The arterial duct can serve as a special type of "direct" aortopulmonary collateral artery. It usually supplies the entire lung by anastomosing at the hilum with a vessel that is "pulmonary" in terms of its histology and in its branching pattern in the lung (Freedom et al., 1984). If the duct closes after birth, then the sequels will be as might be expected with an "absent pulmonary artery," namely, there will be generalized hypoplasia of the intrapulmonary arteries. If

the duct constricts, then the lung will be protected from pulmonary vascular disease (Heath and Edwards, 1958). If it remains patent, this complication will likely develop (Figs. 6 and 7).

At our institution, we have successfully banded an arterial duct supplying a left pulmonary artery in a two-year-old child with tetralogy of Fallot and pulmonary atresia. This allowed regression of early pulmonary vascular changes and permitted subsequent repair into that lung (Fig. 7).

Growth of the Central Arteries

The key questions related to surgical repair of tetralogy of Fallot with pulmonary atresia revolve around whether the central pulmonary arteries will supply most of the lung parenchyma and/or whether they can be made to grow after surgical palliation, particularly palliative procedures such as

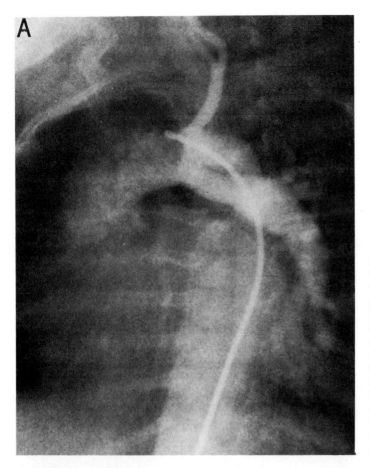

Figure 6. *A:* Cineangiogram taken from a two-year-old patient with tetralogy of Fallot and pulmonary atresia and left-sided arterial duct to the left lung. *B:* Photomicrograph of the vascular bed shows evidence of medial hypertrophy of the pulmonary arteries (arrows denote medial muscular coat). *C:* regression of medial hypertrophy is observed following banding of the duct. Movat stain. Original magnification ×320.

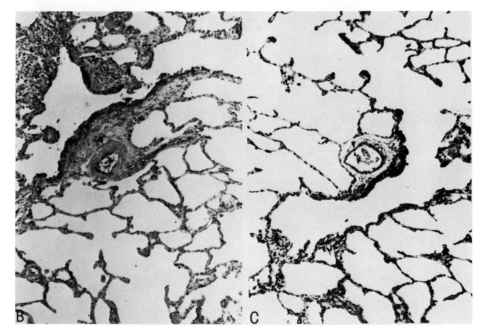

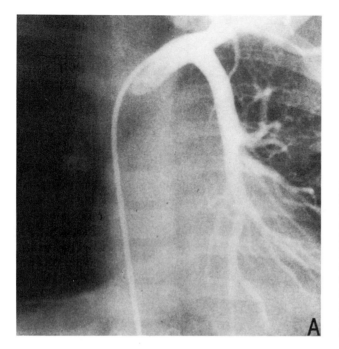

Figure 7. Cineangiogram showing left ductal supply to the left lung in a four-year-old patient with tetralogy of Fallot and pulmonary atresia and left pulmonary venous stenosis. Photomicrograph of the lung in *B* shows advanced vascular changes of intimal fibrosis (arrows). Left pneumonectomy was subsequently performed owing to recurrent hemoptysis and infection. Movat stain. Original magnification ×320.

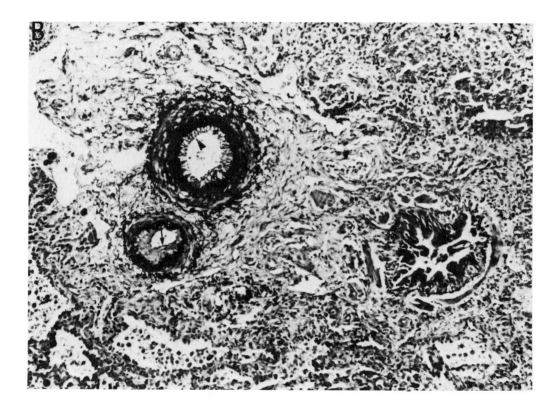

unifocalization of the aortopulmonary collateral arteries. Adequate flow is certainly an essential determinant of growth of the central pulmonary arteries (Gill et al., 1977; Kirklin et al., 1977). Since in some patients with technically adequate shunts, growth of the pulmonary arteries is not achieved, it has been my impression that "intrinsic" factors might also be important. It had been previously observed that the pulmonary arteries in patients with tetralogy of Fallot had decreased elastin (Farrar et al., 1965). It is therefore possible that a critical proportion of elastin in the subendothelium and media is necessary for growth.

We recently carried out a study in patients with cyanotic congenital heart defects (Rosenberg et al., 1986), in which we obtained a minute full-thickness section of the pulmonary artery at the time of placement of a systemic-to-pulmonary arterial shunt.

We applied quantitative techniques in analysis of electron photomicrographs of the artery so as to determine the relative proportions of elastin, collagen, smooth muscle, and ground substance in the media. We also measured the size of the central pulmonary arteries before and 7 to 27 months after surgical placement of the shunt. We were able to show a direct correlation between the density of elastin in the subendothelium and media and growth of the pulmonary arteries (Fig. 8).

Growth of the Peripheral Pulmonary Vascular Bed

It is essential in patients with tetralogy of Fallot and pulmonary atresia to consider

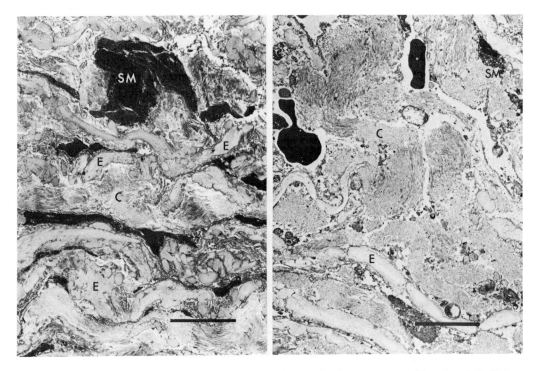

Figure 8. Electron photomicrographs of the medial layer of pulmonary artery biopsies. *Left:* Taken from a patient with good growth of the pulmonary artery, a high proportion of elastin (E) is seen at the time of placement of the shunt. *Right:* Taken from a patient who subsequently had poor pulmonary arterial growth, little elastin is evident and smooth muscle (SM) and collagen (C) predominate. (Reproduced with permission from Rosenberg et al., 1986.)

the extreme variability in the nature of aortopulmonary collateral arterial supply, particularly in the pattern of anastomosis with pulmonary arteries which may affect growth and development of the distal pulmonary vascular bed. Blood supply may be inadequate either because of deficient branching or because of multiple and severe stenoses not just at the hilum but distally as well. Further obstruction to flow may result from thromboses, particularly if polycythemia is severe. Moreover, occlusive vascular disease will ensue after surgical placement of a systemic-to-pulmonary arterial shunt (Newfeld et al., 1977), particularly if the shunt supplies only a limited area of a lung. Morphometric studies have been carried out on lungs obtained at postmortem from patients with tetralogy of Fallot and pulmonary atresia in order to assess peripheral pulmonary arterial size, number, and muscularity (Rabinovitch et al., 1981). There was much variability in the cases examined

in the nature of aortopulmonary collateral blood supply to different regions, but in all cases, the arterial size was small as judged relative to the accompanying airway (Fig. 9). Such an arrangement is also found in patients with tetralogy of Fallot (Hislop and Reid, 1973). There was normal muscularity judged both by arterial wall thickness and by the degree of extension of muscle into peripheral vessels. The number of arteries was normal or slightly increased relative to total alveoli (Fig. 10A). Since, however, the total number of alveoli was reduced, the absolute number of arteries was also decreased. The lung was not as small in volume as might be expected. This was because the decreased alveolar number was compensated by an increase in alveolar size (Fig. 10B). This, however, results in "relative emphysema" and explains the abnormal diffusing capacity with exercise seen in patients with tetralogy of Fallot even after repair (Strieder et al., 1977).

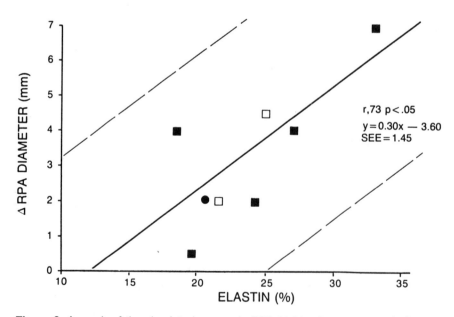

Figure 9. A graph of the absolute increase in RPA (right pulmonary artery) diameter and volume proportion of elastin. A significant correlation is seen between the two parameters. Squares represent tetralogy of Fallot with pulmonary atresia; the circle represents pulmonary atresia with intact ventricular septum; open squares represent tetralogy of Fallot. (Reproduced with permission from Rosenberg et al., 1986.)

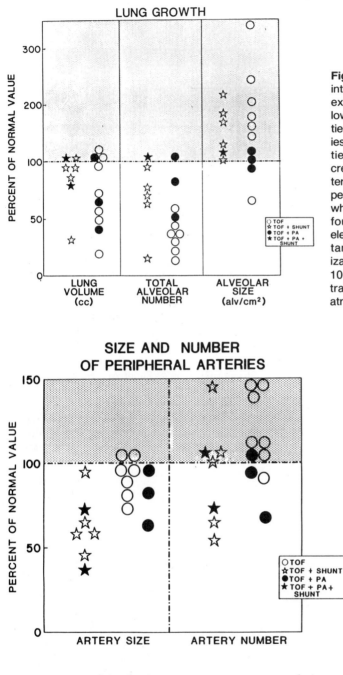

Figure 10A. The size and number of intra-acinar arteries per 100 alveoli expressed as a percentage of the lower normal. More than half the patients have small intra-acinar arteries; the most severely affected patients were those with surgically created systemic-to-pulmonary artery shunts. The number of arteries per 100 alveoli was normal or somewhat increased in most patients; in four patients, three of whom had elevated pulmonary vascular resistance documented at catheterization, the number of arteries per 100 alveoli was reduced. TOF = tetralogy of Fallot; PA = pulmonary atresia.

Figure 10B. Lung volume and number and size of alveoli as a percentage of the lowest normal value for age. Not all patients with a reduced number of alveoli have reduced lung volume, owing to a compensatory increase in alveolar size. TOF = tetralogy of Fallot; PA = pulmonary atresia. (Reproduced with permission from Rabinovitch et al., 1981.)

Conclusion

In patients with tetralogy of Fallot and pulmonary atresia, early and careful delineation of all sources of pulmonary blood supply is essential for planning optimal surgical palliation and, ultimately, correction. Palliation should be undertaken at a young age to ensure the best opportunity for growth of both the pulmonary arteries and the lungs.

References

Boyden EA. The time lag in the development of the bronchial arteries. *Anat Rec* 1970;166:611–614.

Congdon ED. Transformation of the aortic arch system during development of the human embryo. *Contrib Embryol* 1922;14:47–110.

Farrar JF, Bloomfield J, Reye RDK. The structure and composition of the pulmonary circulation in congenital heart disease. *J Pathol Bacteriol* 1965;90:97–105.

Freedom RM, Moes CAF, Pelech A, et al. Bilateral ductus arteriosus (or remnant): An analysis of 27 patients. *Am J Cardiol* 1984;53:884–891.

Gill CC, Moodie DS, McGoon DC. Staged surgical management of pulmonary atresia with diminitive pulmonary arteries. *J Thorac Cardiovasc Surg* 1977;73:436–442.

Goldstein JD, Rabinovitch M, Van Praagh R, Reid L. Unusual vascular anomalies causing persistent pulmonary hypertension in a newborn. *Am J Cardiol* 1979;43:962–968.

Haworth SG. Collateral arteries in pulmonary atresia with ventricular septal defect. *Br Heart J* 1980;44:5–13.

Haworth SG, Macartney FJ. Growth and development of the pulmonary circulation in pulmonary atresia with ventricular septal defect and major aortopulmonary collateral arteries. *Br Heart J* 1980;44:14–23.

Heath D, Edwards JE. The pathology of hypertensive pulmonary vascular disease. A description of six grades of structural changes in the pulmonary arteries with special reference to congenital cardiac septal defects. *Circulation* 1958;18:533–547.

Hislop A, Reid L. Structural changes in the pulmonary arteries and veins in tetralogy of Fallot. *Br Heart J* 1973;35:1178–1183.

Kirklin JW, Bargeron LMJ, Pacifico AD. The enlargement of small pulmonary arteries by preliminary palliative operations. *Circulation* 1977;56:612–617.

Newfeld EA, Waldman JD, Paul MH, et al. Pulmonary vascular disease after systemic-pulmonary arterial shunt operations. *Am J Cardiol* 1977;39:715–720.

Rabinovitch M, Herrera-de-Leon V, Castaneda AR, Reid L. Growth and development of the pulmonary vascular bed in patients with tetralogy of Fallot with or without pulmonary atresia. *Circulation* 1981;64:1234–1249.

Rosenberg HC, Williams WG, Trusler GA, et al. Structural composition of central pulmonary arteries: Growth potential following surgical shunts. *J Thorac and Cardiovasc Surg* 1986 (in press).

Strieder DJ, Aziz K, Zaver AG, Fellows K. Exercise tolerance after repair of tetralogy of Fallot. *Ann Thorac Surg* 1977;19:397–405.

Thiene G, Frescura C, Bini RM, et al. Histology of pulmonary arterial supply in pulmonary atresia with ventricular septal defect. *Circulation* 1979;60:1066–1074.

Shunts and Outflow Reconstruction

Ralph D. Siewers

Children with tetralogy of Fallot and pulmonary atresia, in the majority of cases, are ultimately "repairable." The intracardiac anatomy rarely presents as an obstacle to effective closure of the interventricular communication and relief of right ventricular infundibular stenosis or atresia. The pulmonary circulation, on the other hand, frequently is underdeveloped and of multifocal origin. It is these features which preclude primary correction in a majority of cases because of the resulting maldistribution of the pulmonary blood flow and unacceptably elevated pulmonary flow resistance. The need to foster growth and development of the pulmonary vascular bed provides the greatest challenge to cardiologists and surgeons alike in this subset of patients with tetralogy of Fallot.

Pulmonary Vascular Anatomy

The problem of diminutive confluent or nonconfluent pulmonary arteries and the rare lack of intrapericardial pulmonary arteries associated with various types of systemic-to-pulmonary collateral circulation has been studied and reported by Rabinovitch et al. (1981) (see Chap. 3.3), Haworth et al. (1980, 1981), Liao et al. (1985), and others. Patterns emerge that indicate a somewhat predictable range of possibilities for supply of the pulmonary circulation. When the arterial duct (patent or ligamentous) communicates with the pulmonary artery to one lung or both lungs, the pulmonary arteries to that lung (or both lungs) will nearly completely supply the pulmonary vascular bed. In this case, additional collateral vessels will usually be smaller but true bronchial collateral arteries and will communicate intraparenchymally with the pulmonary arterial distribution. In almost all cases where there is lack of an arterial duct communicating with the pulmonary artery to a lung (or lungs), large direct collaterals (usually from the descending aorta) will enter the pulmonary hilum and distribute via the normal intrasegmental or intralobar pulmonary arteries. They rarely communi-

From: Anderson, RH, Neches, WH, Park, SC, Zuberbuhler, JR, eds: *Perspectives in Pediatric Cardiology*: Mount Kisco, New York, Futura Publishing Co., © 1988.

cate with the central intrapericardial pulmonary arterial distribution. Various degrees of stenosis usually occur within these vessels. Collateral circulation from systemic arteries can also be derived from the subclavian or internal mammary vessels, the collateral arteries communicating with intrapericardial portions of the pulmonary arteries. Although these vessels may be segmentally stenotic, their distribution is via the normal intraparenchymal pulmonary arteries. In all cases, when there is less than normal blood flow to a portion of the lung, alveolar and intra-acinar pulmonary vessel growth is retarded. Since this growth is normally progressive during the first two years of life, it is reasonable to speculate that early measures to improve pulmonary blood flow to as normal a distribution as possible may most optimally achieve intraparenchymal vascular and alveolar development.

Clinical Presentation

The clinical presentation of patients with tetralogy of Fallot and pulmonary atresia depends on the adequacy of pulmonary blood flow. With duct-dependent pulmonary blood flow, impending ductal closure in the neonate often demands surgical intervention early in life, frequently during the first week. Because ductal flow to confluent pulmonary arteries is associated with the most normal pulmonary artery distribution, palliation that produces the most optimal distribution of flow will offer the best chance for pulmonary arterial growth and development. When there are nonconfluent pulmonary arteries or major areas of pulmonary artery stenosis precluding bilateral flow derived from the arterial duct, major systemic-collateral arteries will usually be present. Total pulmonary blood flow may be more "adequate" and cyanosis will be less intense. These cases may not present for evaluation until well beyond the neonatal period, often beyond infancy. It is this second group that may offer the greatest challenge to the ultimate correction of the multifocal vascular supply. This is usually in the form of small pulmonary vessels with numerous varieties of branch stenosis; major segments of the lungs may be supplied solely by the systemic-to-pulmonary collaterals.

Palliative Procedures

Systemic-pulmonary arterial shunt procedures have been, for many years, the standard for augmentation of pulmonary blood flow in patients with tetralogy of Fallot and severe pulmonary stenosis or atresia thought not suitable for primary repair. Alfieri et al. (1978), in reporting 80 patients undergoing repair of tetralogy of Fallot with pulmonary atresia at the University of Alabama between 1967 and 1968, listed 26 patients whose sole source of pulmonary blood flow was from a surgical shunt, and an additional 15 patients with prior surgical shunts and major additional collateral pulmonary blood flow. The majority of these patients came to correction over four years of age. Clearly, the shunts, most of which were standard Blalock shunts, had been variably important in relieving hypoxia and promoting pulmonary artery growth. Gale et al. (1979) have demonstrated that the Blalock-Taussig shunt can produce effective growth in right and left pulmonary arteries with no difference in the growth, either ipsilateral or contralateral to the shunt. Similar uniform experience has been less often seen in the subset of patients with pulmonary atresia, perhaps because of the generally smaller pulmonary arteries and frequency of stenosis or nonconfluence between the right and left pulmonary arteries in this group. Piehler et al. (1980) expressed dissatisfaction with conventional systemic-to-pulmonary artery shunts in the Mayo Clinic experience. They described 6 of 13 patients with anastomotic stenosis or pulmonary arterial distortion. Kirklin et al. (1977) recognized early the value of staged right ventricle-to-pulmonary artery reconstruction by patch technique for pulmonary blood flow augmentation in patients with tetralogy of Fallot and pulmonary atresia. This technique, first adopted by them in October 1973, was used in four of seven patients reported with diminutive pulmonary arteries. Their endorsement of the outflow reconstruction over conventional shunts was reserved, but based on technical and acquired problems encountered with side-to-side aortopulmonary anastomoses and Blalock-Taussig shunts in patients with very small (less than 3 mm) right or left pulmonary arteries. Support for the establishment of right ventricle-to-pulmonary arterial continuity as a palliative procedure was then offered by Gill et al. (1977), who reported the initial Mayo Clinic experience with these patients. Tucker et al. (1979) then reported on 9 of 30 infants operated upon for tetralogy of Fallot in whom complete repair was abandoned because of diminutive pulmonary arteries. In the report of the San Francisco group, 2 of those 9 patients had single right pulmonary arteries, and 4 of the 8 survivors demonstrated symmetrical pulmonary arterial growth on follow-up catheterization.

The largest reported experience with patch or conduit reconstruction of the subpulmonary outflow tract for patients with tetralogy of Fallot and pulmonary atresia has been from the Mayo Clinic. By 1980, Piehler et al. had documented 38 patients, all over two years of age, 12 of whom had prior conventional shunts. Twenty-seven of the 38 had only systemic-to-pulmonary collateral flow, 10 from collateral flow plus a shunt and one with a Waterston shunt as the only source of pulmonary blood flow. Catheterization data on 12 patients, 10 to 26 months postoperatively, demonstrated a 2.2 times increase in normalized pulmonary artery size (expressed as the sum of the diameters of the right and left pulmonary arteries divided by the diameter of the descending

thoracic aorta just above the diaphragm). Patients with previous shunts had less optimal growth and patients with pulmonary arteries of smaller size had greater growth. The improvement in systemic oxygen saturation was better than with the previous experience with conventional shunts. The most current update on the Mayo Clinic experience, reported by Millikan et al. (1986), indicates a total of 105 patients, 8 of whom underwent complete repair but because of ventricular pressure ratios of over 1.0 had the septal defect reopened. The hospital mortality was 11%. Sixty-two patients have had follow-up catheterization and 24 of the 28 judged acceptable for repair have been repaired. Seventeen of the 105 patients have had a "closed" conduit placed between the right ventricle and the pulmonary trunk using the technique described by Puga and Uretzky (1982). Patch reconstruction was used in 23% of the cases but, because of aneurysmal dilation of the patch, most of the more recent operations were done with conduits, two-thirds of which were nonvalved. All of the patients operated upon had confluent pulmonary arteries. An important benefit of this procedure, cited by Millikan and his colleagues (1986), is the improved catheter access to the central pulmonary arteries following the ventriculoarterial reconstruction. The ability to define the pulmonary arterial anatomy carefully and in detail on subsequent studies is an important advantage.

Right ventricle-pulmonary arterial reconstruction has not been without its problems. Thirty-four of the 62 patients studied postoperatively in the Mayo Clinic series were judged unacceptable for repair, largely due to inadequate distribution of pulmonary arterial flow. In addition, Freedom et al. (1983) have found a high incidence of proximal pulmonary artery stenosis, especially on the left. In their series of 15 patients reported from Toronto, 13 of the 14 survivors have been restudied and none found suitable for a second-stage repair. Two have required additional shunts and two of three have not survived attempts to relieve severe stenosis in the pulmonary arteries.

This discussion of palliative procedures designed to improve pulmonary artery growth and distribution of blood flow would not be complete without mention of balloon dilation angioplasty for branch stenosis of the pulmonary arteries. Ring et al. (1985) have reported a series of 24 children, ranging in age from 4 months to 16 years, who underwent balloon dilation angioplasty between July 1981 and April 1984, of the hypoplastic or stenotic branch pulmonary arteries. Most of these patients had tetralogy of Fallot with or without pulmonary atresia. A total of 52 dilations were done, 44 in the catheterization laboratory and 8 intraoperatively. Twenty-six of the procedures were deemed successful in producing a persistent enlargement of the pulmonary artery by over 1 mm. There was one death in their series secondary to a ruptured balloon which caused rupture of the pulmonary artery and exsanguination. In retrospect, the authors believe that this could have been managed differently to avoid death. Eight of the patients have been restudied beyond six months after the dilation procedure and show permanence of the improvement documented at the time of dilation. The authors noted an improved success rate in patients in whom the procedure was used at less than two years of age. It is quite possible that in patients following right ventricle-to-pulmonary arterial reconstruction, balloon angioplasty might offer an important role in achieving more symmetrical distribution of pulmonary arterial flow.

Management of Systemic-Pulmonary Collateral Vessels

The management of collateral blood flow in the lung at the time of palliation is controversial. Clearly, large systemic-to-pulmonary arterial vessels that are the sole source of blood flow to a segment or a lobe should be left alone. Piehler et al. (1980) emphasized that, in situations of extreme pulmonary hypoplasia, ventriculoarterial reconstruction may not alone provide enough flow. The contribution of collateral vessels to effective pulmonary blood flow may be assessed by temporary occlusion of selected competing collaterals to see if systemic oxygenation will tolerate permanent closure. There is theoretical evidence to support ligation of significant sized collateral arteries in infants since this collateral flow, if it communicates with true pulmonary arteries with central connections, may retard symmetrical pulmonary arterial development and lead to intraparenchymal pulmonary artery stenosis or aneurysm formation and hypertrophic pulmonary vascular disease. There is no current evidence to support this speculation.

Experience at Children's Hospital of Pittsburgh

Forty-four patients with tetralogy of Fallot and pulmonary atresia were operated upon at Children's Hospital of Pittsburgh between January 1970 and April 1986. Thirty-nine received conventional shunts, 31 of which were end-to-side shunts from a subclavian to a pulmonary artery. One patient came to primary repair without prior palliation and four patients have received palliation by means of nonvalved conduits placed between the right ventricle and the pulmonary trunk. Twenty of the 44 patients on initial study were found to have confluent and small, but not diminutive, pulmonary arteries. In 18, the confluent pulmonary arteries were judged diminutive, usually less than 4 mm. There were five patients in whom no pulmonary arterial confluence could be demonstrated and one patient had no identifiable intrapericardial pulmonary artery. Twelve of the 20 patients with satisfactory confluent pulmonary arteries have come to complete repair; only five of the patients judged to have diminutive confluent pulmonary arteries have progressed to repair. Of the five patients with nonconfluent pulmonary arteries, two have been repaired. Analysis of the 42 shunt procedures done in 39 patients revealed a very high complication rate with aortopulmonary shunts (Waterston and Potts) with only one of the 11 being effective without complication. Of the 31 end-to-side subclavian shunts, two produced only unilateral growth of a pulmonary artery, nine caused shunt-related pulmonary artery stenosis, and four failed. The 16 shunts deemed effective and without complication were largely in patients who, on initial study, were found to have confluent pulmonary arteries of small, but not diminutive, size. Of interest to us is that the patients presenting at less than one month of age for diagnosis and who required palliation within a month of diagnosis, had much better results, as judged by eventual repair, than did patients who had a less urgent need for palliation in the neonatal diagnosis group or who presented beyond one month of age for diagnosis. The group requiring early diagnosis and surgical palliation most frequently were found to have ductal-dependent confluent pulmonary blood flow with impending ductal closure as the prime indication of intervention. The four patients who had palliation by means of a ventriculoarterial conduit all had small confluent pulmonary arteries. Each had major systemic-pulmonary arterial collateral vessels supplying from one- to two-thirds of the pulmonary vascular bed. One patient came to us after two failed conventional shunt procedures done at another institution. The age range was 21 months to 5 years. There were no hospital or late deaths and one patient has recently come to successful total repair 11 months after his palliation. All conduits were nonvalved and all but one were made of polytetrafluorethylene (PTFE). The Dacron conduit was 8 mm in diameter, developed a muscular obstruction at the ventricu-

lar anastomosis and a thick obstructive peel within three years. It was replaced with a 10 mm PTFE conduit. A small, 6 mm PTFE conduit was found to be restrictive and was replaced within six months with a 10 mm conduit of the same material. Palliation in terms of improvement in oxygen saturation has been excellent. In no case has there been excessive pulmonary blood flow, although a fenestrated patch across the ventricular septal defect was placed in one patient because of fear of excessive flow. This patient is the one who came to repair and is the only patient in whom we have closed major collateral arteries at repair. Pulmonary arterial growth and flow distribution have not been uniform, partially, we believe, because of proximal right or left pulmonary arterial stenosis induced by the conduit and partially because of intrinsic arborization abnormalities of the pulmonary arteries.

Review of these 44 patients confirms a general dissatisfaction with conventional shunt procedures as palliation to improve pulmonary arterial growth and distribution. We are cautiously optimistic about ventriculoarterial reconstructive palliation on the basis of our brief experience and the much larger experiences of other institutions.

Conclusions

Palliative procedures for infants and children with tetralogy of Fallot and pulmonary atresia must relieve hypoxia and promote pulmonary arterial growth and development. The great majority of these patients will have at least one, and usually two, intrapericardial pulmonary arteries, most of which are confluent. Systemic-to-pulmonary shunts in neonates with small, but not diminutive, pulmonary arteries may provide good palliation and promote symmetrical growth and development of the pulmonary arteries. These shunts in the neonates, however, often cause right or left pulmonary arterial distortion or stenosis which may be challenging to repair and which may retard symmetrical pulmonary arterial growth. Right ventricle-to-pulmonary arterial reconstruction appears to be the palliative procedure of choice in patients with diminutive confluent pulmonary arteries and may well be the best palliative procedure in all patients with tetralogy of Fallot, pulmonary atresia, and confluent pulmonary arteries. Major systemic-pulmonary artery collaterals should probably be left undisturbed at the time of initial palliation unless they communicate with the central pulmonary arteries such that excessive pulmonary blood flow is likely to result following palliation. Since the majority of pulmonary artery growth occurs early following effective palliation, early and careful assessment of the pulmonary blood flow and distribution is essential. Ventriculoarterial reconstruction provides optimal access for subsequent study of pulmonary arterial anatomy.

References

Alfieri O, Blackstone EH, Kirklin JW, et al. Surgical treatment of tetralogy of Fallot with pulmonary atresia. *J Thorac Cardiovasc Surg* 1978;76:321–335.

Freedom RM, Pongiglione G, Williams WG, et al. Palliative right ventricular outflow tract construction for patients with pulmonary atresia, ventricular septal defect and hypoplastic pulmonary arteries. *J Thorac Cardiovasc Surg* 1983;86:24–36.

Gale AW, Arciniegas E, Green EW, et al. Growth of the pulmonary annulus and pulmonary arteries after Blalock-Taussig shunt. *J Thorac Cardiovasc Surg* 1979;77:459–465.

Gill CC, Moodie DS, McGoon DC. Staged surgical management of pulmonary atresia with diminutive pulmonary arteries. *J Thorac Cardiovasc Surg* 1977;73:436–442.

Haworth SG, MaCartney FJ. Growth and development of pulmonary circulation in pulmonary atresia with ventricular septal defect and major aortopulmonary collateral arteries. *Br Heart J* 1980;44:14–24.

Haworth SG, Rees PG, Taylor JFN, et al. Pulmonary atresia with ventricular septal defect and major aortopulmonary collateral arteries. Effect of systemic pulmonary anastomosis. *Br Heart J* 1981;45:133–141.

Kirklin JW, Bageron LM, Pacifico AD. The enlargement of small pulmonary arteries by preliminary palliative operations. *Circulation* 1977;56:612–617.

Liao PK, Edwards WD, Julsrud PR, et al. Pulmonary blood supply in patients with pulmonary atresia and ventricular septal defect. *J Am Coll Cardiol* 1985;6:1343–1350.

Millikan JS, Puga FJ, Danielson GK, et al. Staged surgical repair of pulmonary atresia, ventricular septal defect and hypoplastic confluent pulmonary arteries. *J Thorac Cardiovasc Surg* 1986;91:818–825.

Piehler JM, Danielson GK, McGoon DC, et al. Management of pulmonary atresia with ventricular septal defect and hypoplastic pulmonary arteries by right ventricular outflow construction. *J Thorac Cardiovasc Surg* 1980;80:552–567.

Puga FJ, Uretzky G. Establishment of right ventricle-hypoplastic pulmonary artery continuity without the use of extracorporeal circulation. *J Thorac Cardiovasc Surg* 1982;83:74–80.

Rabinovitch M, Herrera-de Leon V, Casteneda AR, Reid L. Growth and development of the pulmonary vascular bed in patients with tetralogy of Fallot with or without pulmonary atresia. *Circulation* 1981;64:1234–1249.

Ring JC, Bass JL, Marvin M, et al. Management of congenital stenosis of a branch pulmonary artery with balloon dilation angioplasty. Report of 52 procedures. *J Thorac Cardiovasc Surg* 1985;90:35–44.

Tucker WY, Turley K, Ullyot DJ, Ebert PA. Management of symptomatic tetralogy of Fallot in the first year of life. *J Thorac Cardiovasc Surg* 1979;78:494–501.

3.5

Homograft Reconstruction of the Right Ventricular Outflow Tract: Late Results of Homograft Function

Jane Somerville and Susan Stone

The concept of using a homograft aortic valve and length of aorta as a conduit to reconstruct the right ventricular outflow tract was introduced in 1966 by Ross (Ross and Somerville, 1966) at the National Heart Hospital in London. The patient was a nine-year-old with complex pulmonary atresia who now, 21 years later, works as a garage mechanic and is the father of three healthy children. The technique has been used, with modifications, to repair other congenital cyanotic congenital anomalies and various methods of sterilization have been tried. Unfortunately, use of the homograft was soon discouraged by certain centers in the United States, because of rapid calcific degeneration of the valve. The difference in our better late results is related to the methods of sterilization (Somerville,

1984; Somerville and Ross, 1972). Since there is now a renaissance in use of the commercially prepared homografts in America, it seems appropriate to re-examine our long-term results, paying particular attention to the fate of the homograft rather than the patient.

Material

Between 1966 and 1984, 58 patients left hospital after reconstruction of the right ventricular outflow tract using a cadaver aortic homograft with various extensions (Table 1). The anatomical diagnosis was pulmonary atresia with subaortic ventricular septal defect (33), extreme tetralogy of

From: Anderson, RH, Neches, WH, Park, SC, Zuberbuhler, JR, eds: *Perspectives in Pediatric Cardiology*: Mount Kisco, New York, Futura Publishing Co., © 1988.

Table 1
Homograft Reconstruction of the Right Ventricular Outflow Tract in 58 Patients:
RV Extension of Homograft

		Reop. obstr.	Reop. homo.	Reop. other	Deaths
Dacron tube	20	3	2	6	8
Teflon tube	2	0	0	0	0
Gusset	33				
Dacron or Teflon (13)		1	1	1	1
Pericardium (10)		0	0	1	1
Mitral leaflet (7)		0	1	1	1
Mitral leaflet + Dacron (1)		0	0	0	0
Mitral leaflet + pericardium (2)		0	1	0	0
Nothing	3	0	0	0	1
Total	58	4	5	9	12

Fallot with patent subpulmonary outflow tract (23), and tetralogy of Fallot with absent pulmonary valve (2). The age at operation was 4 to 35 years, distributed as shown in Figure 1. Homografts were sterilized as shown in Figure 2. All patients were fol-

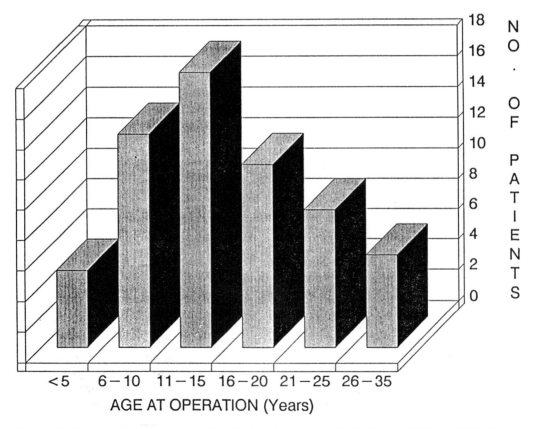

Figure 1. The age at operation of 58 patients who left hospital between 1966 and 1984 having undergone reconstruction of the right ventricular outflow tract using an aortic homograft.

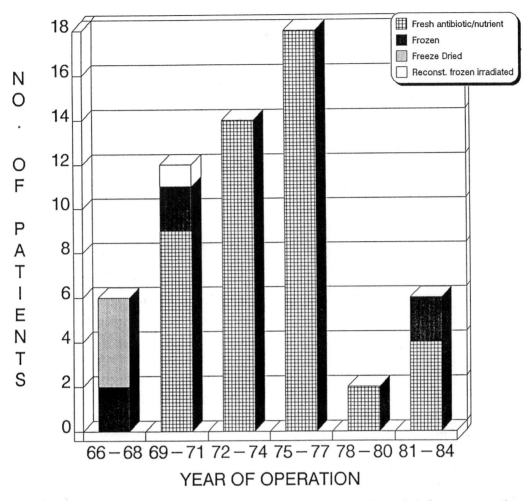

Figure 2. Diagram to show the year of operation of 58 patients who left hospital after reconstruction of the right ventricular outflow tract using an aortic homograft. The method of valve sterilization is also shown.

lowed with annual phonocardiography, radiography, electrocardiography, recently echocardiography, and clinical examination, with specific attention paid to closure of the pulmonary valve. Catheterization and angiography was performed in the majority of patients. Two or more serial studies were usually performed, determining the sites of gradients and movements of the leaflets of the homograft.

Necropsy examination was performed in 11 of the 12 deaths. The specimen was inspected by one of the authors (J.S.) when not discarded by the coroner's pathologists.

Results

Deaths

Twelve patients died (21%) at 2 months to 19 years after the procedure. The causes of death and state of the homograft are summarized in Tables 2 and 3. Two patients died from coronary arterial disease at the age of 29 and 55 years. These events occurred 8 and 19 years after homograft implantation, respectively. The leaflets of these homografts remained pliable. Only

Table 2

Homograft Reconstruction of the Right Ventricular Outflow Tract in 58 Patients:
Late Deaths

Cause of death	Number of patients	Time postop.
"Sudden" (1, VT, 1 LVF)	5	2 months–19 years
Reoperation	4	1–14 years
Ventricular failure	2	5–9 years
Reoperation: infected homograft	1*	10 years
Total	12 (21%)	2 months–19 years

LVF = left ventricular failure; Postop. = postoperatively; VT = ventricular tachycardia.
* Only one death related to homograft.

one died from a complication directly related to the homograft. In this patient, the original aortic homograft was replaced 10 years later with a pulmonary homograft and she died from uncontrolled infection from *Staphylococcus aureus*, probably present since the operation six months earlier. No patient died at reoperation for a degenerated homograft.

Reoperation

Four patients died in relation to the second or subsequent reoperation (Table 4): two with severe obstruction in Dacron conduits, one with aortic regurgitation, and one hypoxic from ligation of major systemic to pulmonary collateral arteries. The reasons for reoperation are indicated in the table. Reoperations in the 14 survivors were for

closure of a residual ventricular septal defect (3), for obstruction in a Dacron conduit (2), for obstruction of the homograft valve (5), for ligation of large systemic to pulmonary collateral arteries (1), and for aortic regurgitation (3). The state of the homografts is shown in Table 3.

Other Complications

Infective endocarditis occurred in four patients (7%), introduced in one (see Deaths), in 650 patient-years. The incidence, excluding the one case where it was introduced at the time of valve replacement, is low (5%). In two cases, the infection was on the patient's own aortic valve, occurring nine months and six years, respectively, after the insertion of the homograft, which was not involved in the infection. One epi-

Table 3

Homograft Right Ventricular Outflow Tract Reconstruction: State of Aortic Homografts
Examined in 13 Patients

Place of examination	CA++ wall	Cusps thin	Cusps CA++	Time postop.
Reoperation	7	2	5	5–16 years
Necropsy	5	6	0	2 months–19 years
Total	12	8	5	2 months–19 years

CA++ = calcified; Postop = postoperatively.

Table 4
Homograft Reconstruction of the Right Ventricular Outflow Tract in 58 Patients: Reoperations

Reason for reoperation	Time postoperatively	Number of patients	Number of deaths at reop.
Obstruction	2–13 years	4	2
Aortic regurgitation	10 months–14 years	4	1
Valve obstruction	9–16 years	5	0
Reclosure VSD	6 months–5 years	3	0
Hypoxic, shunt	1 year	1	1
Ligation collateral	1 year	1	0
Total	1–16 years	18	4

Reop. = reoperation; VSD = ventricular septal defect.

sode occurred five years later and was successfully treated with antibiotics. Ten years after operation, the patient shows progressive right ventricular dysfunction. He has gross pulmonary regurgitation with destruction of one leaflet and pulmonary hypertension.

Rhythm problems were documented in 14 patients (24%) (Table 5). Sudden death occurred in five patients aged from 18 to 55 years, one of these known to be due to ventricular tachycardia initiated by a blow on the chest. Supraventricular tachycardia was encountered in two patients (ages 17 and 33), while multiple ventricular ectopic beats occurred in two others (ages 22 and 23). Fast atrial rhythms were found in three patients (aged between 29 and 35) and nodal bradycardia complicated the course of one 22-year-old patient. One patient suffered surgically induced complete heart block and was paced, but died at the age of 20. The overall complications for the entire series are summarized in Table 6.

Pregnancy

Twenty-one pregnancies occurred in 10 patients. One woman died during the 37th

Table 5
Homograft Reconstruction of the Right Ventricular Outflow Tract: Documented Rhythm Disorders

Arrhythmia	No. of patients	Age (years)
Sudden death (1 VT)	5	18–55
SVT	2	17–33
Multiple VEs	2	22–23
Fast atrial	3	29–35
Bradycardia, Nodal	1	22
CHB Paced (died)	1	20
Total	14 (24%)	17–55

CHB = complete heart block; SVT = supraventricular tachycardia; VEs = ventricular ectopic beats; VT = ventricular tachycardia.

Table 6
Homograft Right Ventricular Outflow Tract Reconstruction: Late Complications in 28 of 58 Patients (48%) over 650 Patient-Years

Complication	No. of patients	%
Infectious endocarditis	4	7
Reop valve	5	9
Reop, other	13	22
Arrhythmias	9	15
Sudden death	5	9
Total deaths	12	21

week of pregnancy. Necropsy reported coronary thrombosis. The pathologist noted calcium in the right outflow but did not comment on any abnormality of the pulmonary valve! The patient had previously delivered a child with congenital heart disease (exact diagnosis unknown). Another died one year after her second successful delivery. A few months before, she showed evidence of deteriorating left ventricular function, which may have been related to her having had a left coronary artery supplying the pulmonary arteries. It is suspected that the blood supply to the left ventricle may have been compromised during repair at age 24 years, or perhaps before, as the result of the thieving coronary arterial fistula.

Examination of Homografts

It was possible to examine the homograft in 13 instances. Two were examined at reoperation; five were replaced at reoperation; while six were obtained at autopsy.

Calcification of the aortic wall had occurred in 12 patients, but the leaflets were thin and mobile in 8 of these. One who was examined after two months had a normal valve and normal aortic wall. Calcification of the leaflet causing obstruction and rigidity occurred in five valves, implanted 9 to 16 years previously.

In all other patients, "pulmonary" valve closure is clear, sometimes loud. In the survivors who have not required reoperation, systolic gradients greater than 25 mmHg across Dacron conduits and suture lines are present in nine. Reoperation will not be recommended until there is evidence of homograft failure, deterioration in right ventricular function, or increasing size of the heart.

Summary of Results

The results are summarized in the actuarial curves prepared by John Kirklin (Figs. 3, 4, and 5). These figures relate to

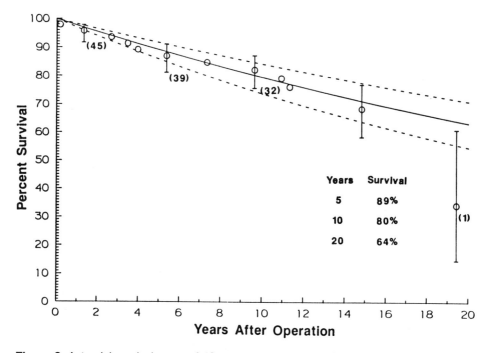

Figure 3. Actuarial survival curve of 49 patients who left hospital between 1966 and 1976 after reconstruction of the right ventricular outflow tract using an aortic homograft.

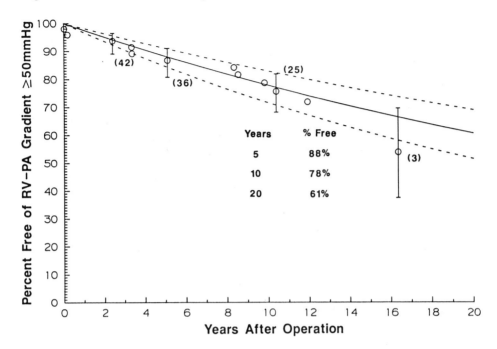

Figure 4. Actuarial estimate of freedom from right ventricular to pulmonary artery gradient > 50 mmHg of 49 patients who left hospital between 1966 and 1976 after reconstruction of the right ventricular outflow tract using an aortic homograft.

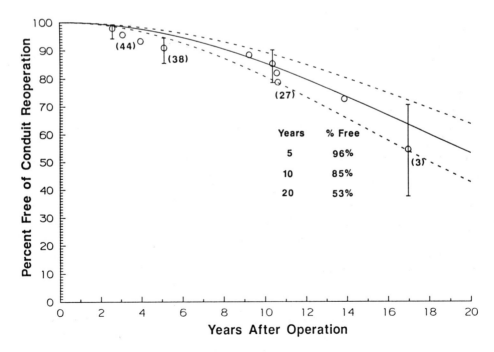

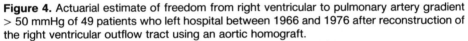

Figure 5. Actuarial estimate of freedom from reoperation on the valved conduit among 49 patients who left hospital between 1966 and 1976 after reconstruction of the right ventricular outflow tract using an aortic homograft.

only 49 of the 58 patients, namely those operated on between 1966 and 1976 in order to give at least 10 years of follow-up.

Discussion

Although 12 (21%) patients died during this long follow-up and 18 (31%) required reoperation, obstructive degeneration of the homograft valve occurred in only 5. This was not found before the ninth postoperative year, despite calcification in the aortic wall occurring routinely by the end of the first year.

In contrast, there were many more problems caused by the Dacron tubes used as extensions in 20 patients (Table 1). Obstruction was important in three and contributory to the need for reoperation in six, with eight deaths occurring in the group. Although obstruction does not occur routinely in Dacron tubes (which remained widely patent in 50%), when it did develop, particularly in the smaller-diameter tubes, reoperation was difficult, with extensive calcification in the "neointima." In particular, problems were encountered when the conduit lay to the side and obstructed the left bronchus.

The major cause of death in this group of patients was myocardial failure or "sudden," probably in relation to extensive myocardial fibrosis. Certainly the earliest postoperative death a few months after the operation occurred in a 20-year-old girl whose postoperative electrocardiogram showed a pattern suggestive of extensive infarction/necrosis. The rest of such deaths occurred 3 to 19 years after. In all but two, there was evidence of left and right ventricular myocardial disease. Whether this was related to the late age when surgery was performed, or the inadequacy of myocardial protection, is not clear. All were operated on before the era of effective myocardial protection and all had long periods of myocardial ischemia at normothermia. Arrhyth-

mias (documented) were uncommon but we cannot exclude ventricular tachycardia, either as a primary event or secondary to extensive myocardial damage, as the cause of sudden death. In one boy, lethal ventricular tachycardia was initiated by a chest blow during street fighting. At necropsy, the homograft inserted three years before was pliable and perfect and there was no macroscopic extensive fibrosis as in the other patients. We have yet to know whether in longer-term survivors, nearer to normal life expectancy will be obtained by earlier surgery and more frequent reoperation during the life span. Inevitably, even with modern techniques of graft preservation, the graft may degenerate within two decades. It is likely that the younger the patient, the more quickly this may occur in view of the differing calcium metabolism of the growing child.

We would favor not repairing with homografts too early. Repair after the age of five to six years is better when an adult-sized graft can be used together with the good techniques for myocardial protection without periods of ischemic arrest. Experience taught us early about the size of grafts. Only in the first patient was a small valve used, appropriate for a nine-year-old. Nine years later this valve was still small, particularly for a 6-foot 3-inch man, which is what he grew into. Although there was calcification, causing some obstruction in one leaflet, the real obstruction was related to the graft diameter which had not changed since implantation.

Pulmonary regurgitation, assessed at first by auscultation and now by Doppler, was common after the first one to two years but only progressive enough at the end of the eight to nine years to embarrass the right ventricle in two from residual pulmonary hypertension. Without pulmonary hypertension, progressive dysfunction of the homograft valve causing pulmonary regurgitation is unlikely to cause a problem unless the right ventricle has earlier exhibited important dysfunction. Unfortunately, pulmonary arterial hypertension from pulmonary arterial stenoses, sometimes acquired, or progressive pulmonary arteriolar disease, are not rare with pulmonary atresia, particularly in the complex with congenital systemic to pulmonary collateral arteries.

Calcification and deterioration in leaflet function is influenced by several factors, of which method of sterilization is the most important. The early reports (McGoon et al., 1982; Moodie et al., 1976; Norwood et al., 1977) damning the use of the homograft because of rapid calcific degeneration failed to mention the disastrous effects of their chosen method of sterilization, namely irradiation. Various means of sterilization were used in our series, but not irradiation (except in one patient operated on in 1969 and known to be well 15 years later). There appears to be no difference between antibiotic "fresh" valves and fresh frozen. The former technique probably carries a higher risk of infection. It is likely that, in one of the reoperations, the newly introduced pulmonary valve homograft was the source of the lethal infection with *Staphylococcus aureus.*

Pulmonary hypertension predisposes to earlier valve deterioration and failure, perhaps as systemic hypertension affects homografts in the aortic position. Surgical technique is also relevant to long-term graft behavior. Graft compression accelerates deterioration. Thus, it can be appreciated that the future of the valve, just like the future of the patient, is profoundly influenced by the underlying condition for which the operation has been performed. Even in this series, chosen deliberately for similarity of anatomy, there are differences in prognosis between those with complex pulmonary atresia (systemic-to-pulmonary collateral arteries, abnormal pulmonary arteries and branches) and those with tetralogy of Fallot or pulmonary atresia with confluent pulmonary arteries supplied by an arterial duct.

Other types of valve have been tried by choice or by need. None has the durability or number of problem-free years given by the aortic homograft. The porcine valves are disastrous, particularly in the young (Bissett et al., 1981). Valves made of fascia lata (Ross and Somerville, 1971), dura mater, and pericardium are as bad. It remains to be seen if the pulmonary valve homograft is as good or better. Whether the use of valveless conduits is viable in the long run requires evaluation. Their use predisposes to early failure with chronic and progressive right ventricular distention and damage, particularly with pulmonary hypertension from peripheral or central pulmonary arterial disease or damage. Thus, if a homograft is available, we would not consider this option. If there is no homograft, use of a valveless conduit could be better than no operation or using another biological valve in a child.

For the present, we consider our results to justify the continued use of the homograft for reconstruction of the right ventricular outflow tract. There is a low infection rate of the homograft valve, no hemolysis, no thrombosis, a reasonable guarantee of 10 or more trouble-free years from problems with the homograft, and no problems for pregnancy. For those who wish to adopt the technique, good surgery, good laws (to allow harvesting), and good sterilization are required for a successful outcome and long maintained result.

Acknowledgments: We acknowledge with admiration and appreciation the work of Mr. Donald Ross. We thank Drs. John Kirklin, Eugene Blackstone, and Nitu Mandke for their help and interest in the preparation of statistics which authenticate the results. We thank the anonymous donor who supports Susan Stone, Research Assistant, enabling us to maintain up-to-date data and statistics.

References

Bissett GS, Schwartz DC, Benzing G, et al. Late results of reconstruction of the right ventricular outflow tract with porcine xenografts in children. *Ann Thorac Surg* 1981;31:437–443.

McGoon DC, Danielson GK, Puga FJ, et al. Late results after extracardiac conduit repair for congenital cardiac defects. *Am J Cardiol* 1982;49:1741–1749.

Moodie DS, Mair DD, Fulton RE, et al. Aortic homograft obstruction. *J Thorac Cardiovasc Surg* 1976;72:553–561.

Norwood WI, Freed MD, Rocchini AP, et al. Experience with valved conduits for repair of congenital cardiac lesions. *Ann Thorac Surg* 1977;24:223–232.

Ross DN, Somerville J. Correction of pulmonary atresia with a homograft aortic valve. *Lancet* 1966;2:1446–1447.

Ross DN, Somerville J. Fascia lata reconstruction of the right ventricular outflow tract. *Lancet* 1971;1:941–943.

Somerville J. Fate of the aortic homograft used for reconstruction of the right ventricular outflow tract in pulmonary atresia and extreme tetralogy of Fallot. In Tucker BL, Lindesmith GG, Takahashi M (Eds): *Obstructive lesions of the right heart. Third Clinical Conference on Congenital Heart Disease.* Baltimore: University Park Press, 1984:275–286.

Somerville J, Ross DN. Long-term results of complete correction with homograft reconstruction in pulmonary outflow tract atresia. *Br Heart J* 1972;34:29–36.

3.6

Tetralogy of Fallot with and without Pulmonary Atresia

John W. Kirklin, Eugene H. Blackstone,
Albert D. Pacifico, James K. Kirklin,
and Lionel M. Bargeron, Jr.

Although tetralogy of Fallot with pulmonary atresia is often viewed as simply an extreme form of the cardiac anomaly called tetralogy of Fallot, patients with tetralogy and pulmonary atresia as a group have a different prevalence of coexisting morphological anomalies than do patients with tetralogy of Fallot and pulmonary stenosis (Table 1). The prevalence of the various surgical procedures also differs between the two groups of patients (Table 2).

The presence of pulmonary atresia is, in and of itself, not a risk factor for death early or late after the repair of tetralogy of Fallot (Kirklin et al., 1983). The frequent coexistence, however, in patients with tetralogy of Fallot with pulmonary atresia or pulmonary arterial problems (such as diffuse hypoplasia, incomplete distribution within the lungs, segmental absences, or peripheral stenoses) and large aortopulmonary collateral arteries, and the frequent need in the

repair for placement of a conduit between the right ventricle and the pulmonary trunk, impose a greater risk of death early or late after repair. Further, patients with tetralogy of Fallot and pulmonary atresia as a group are older at the time of repair and therefore have more advanced ventricular hypertrophy and secondary cardiomyopathy than do younger patients undergoing repair of tetralogy of Fallot and pulmonary stenosis.

Postrepair $P_{RV/LV}$

After the surgical correction of the tetralogy of Fallot with pulmonary stenosis or pulmonary atresia, the postrepair $P_{RV/LV}$ reflects the magnitude of residual obstruction to pulmonary blood flow. ($P_{RV/LV}$ is a widely accepted and well-understood abbreviation for the ratio between the peak pressure in

From: Anderson, RH, Neches, WH, Park, SC, Zuberbuhler, JR, eds: *Perspectives in Pediatric Cardiology*: Mount Kisco, New York, Futura Publishing Co., © 1988.

Table 1
Usual Morphological Characteristics in Tetralogy of Fallot with Pulmonary Stenosis and Tetralogy of Fallot with Pulmonary Atresia

Characteristic	Tetralogy of fallot with	
	Pulmonary stenosis	Pulmonary atresia
Variability of right ventricular outflow morphology	Marked	Mild
Pulmonary trunk bifurcation stenoses*	Uncommon	Uncommon
Hypoplasia of pulmonary arteries*	Variable	Variable, but often severe
Intrapulmonary distribution of unbranched hilar pulmonary arteries*	Usually Complete	Often incomplete
Segmental absences of pulmonary arteries*	Rare	Common
Peripheral pulmonary artery stenoses*	Rare	Common
Obstructive Microvasculature Disease*	Rare	Occasional
Large aortopulmonary collateral arteries	Rare	Common

Note: The generalizations in this and Table 2 are based on an experience with 337 patients (Mayo Clinic, 1955–1967) and 1,022 patients (UAB, 1967–1986) with tetralogy of Fallot, including those with pulmonary atresia.
Abnormalities marked by an asterisk are included in the phrase pulmonary arterial problems.

the right ventricle and that in the left ventricle.) The residual obstruction may result from residual infundibular, valvular, and/or annular narrowing (or an imperfect conduit between the right ventricle and the pulmonary trunk), unrelieved stenosis of the bifurcation of the pulmonary trunk, diffuse hypoplasia of the right and/or left pulmonary arteries, peripheral stenosis of the segmental pulmonary arteries, incomplete intrapulmonary distribution of the right and left pulmonary arteries, or increased pulmonary microvascular resistance. The postrepair $P_{RV/LV}$ (or $P_{RV/aorta}$) is used for reflecting these effects because it is convenient, not because it is ideal. A more precise measure of the effects of residual obstruction could be obtained by measuring right ventricular and pulmonary arterial pressure and pulmonary blood flow (or cardiac output, if it is known that there is no residual shunting), as well as left ventricular and aortic pressure.

Table 2
Procedures Used in the Repair of Tetralogy of Fallot With Pulmonary Stenosis and Tetralogy of Fallot With Pulmonary Atresia

Procedures	Tetralogy of fallot with	
	Pulmonary stenosis	Pulmonary atresia
Preliminary AP shunt	Infrequent	Nearly Routine
Infundibular dissection	Frequent	—
Pulmonary valvotomy	Frequent	—
Infundibular patch graft enlargement	Occasional	—
Transannular patch graft enlargement	Occasional	Infrequent
Valved conduit, RV to PA	Infrequent	Frequent

AP = aortopulmonary; PA = pulmonary arteries; RV = right ventricle.

Table 3
Classic Shunting Operations for Tetralogy of Fallot, University of Alabama, Birmingham, 1967–July 1982

Tetralogy of Fallot with	n	Hospital deaths		
		No.	%	CL
Pulmonary Stenosis	53	0	0%	0%–4%
Pulmonary Atresia	51	6	12%	7%–18%
Total	104	6	6%	3%–9%
p (Fisher)			.01	

Note: Classic AP shunting operation includes Blalock-Taussig shunt and Gore-Tex interposition shunt. Four of the six deaths were in neonates less than three days of age at operation.
CL = Confidence Limit.

Severe residual obstruction to pulmonary blood flow, as reflected in a high postrepair $P_{RV/LV}$, unfavorably affects the chances for survival early or late after repair of tetralogy of Fallot of all types (Kirklin et al., 1984). To some extent, postrepair $P_{RV/LV}$ is determined by the details of the operative procedure and, therefore, is a strategically important element in surgical decision making for patients with the tetralogy of Fallot.

Determinants of Early and Intermediate Results after Repair of Tetralogy of Fallot

Although the presence of pulmonary atresia rather than pulmonary stenosis is not in itself a risk factor for death early or intermediately after repair of tetralogy of Fallot, patients with tetralogy of Fallot and pulmonary atresia fare less well as a group than do those with pulmonary stenosis (Table 3, Figs. 1 and 2). The lower 10-year survival in the patients with pulmonary atresia is related not only to the somewhat higher early risks imposed by the complexities of their pulmonary circulation, but also to the considerably higher constant phase of hazard. This higher hazard extends as far as the patients have been followed (Fig. 3).

The coexisting anomalies and conditions that increase the risk of failure in the surgical treatment of patients with tetralogy of Fallot of all types are best determined by a multivariate analysis of death and other events which takes into account their time-relatedness. This analysis is currently being made at the University of Alabama in Birmingham. At this moment, only an informal determination of this kind can be made (Table 4). Knowledge of these risk factors (and comparisons of the risks and imponderables of reacting to their presence in various ways) is useful when a serious attempt is made to minimize absolutely the risks of death and disability early or late after repair.

Indications and Techniques of Surgical Treatment

In all patients with the tetralogy of Fallot, the proper treatment at some time is repair. The only exception is in those rare situations where the patient is inoperable. Patients with tetralogy of Fallot and pulmonary atresia are not managed differently in themselves from patients with pulmonary stenosis, but the coexisting demographic, morphological, and functional features are frequently such that the patients in the two subgroups should be treated differently.

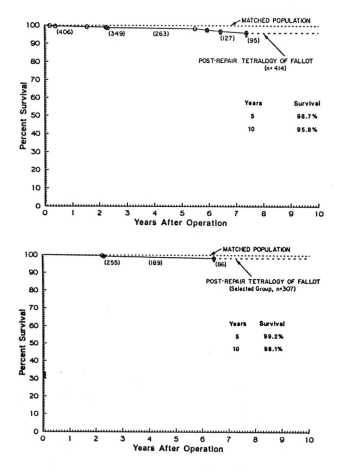

Figure 1. Percent survival after hospital dismissal of patients undergoing repair of tetralogy of Fallot with pulmonary stenosis. Each circle represents an individual death. The vertical bars represent the 70% confidence intervals. The large dashed line depicts the length of follow-up after the last death. The numbers in parentheses indicate the patients at risk at that postrepair interval. The small dashed lines represent the survival of an age-sex-race matched population (U.S. Life Tables, 1976). *Top:* All patients (UAB, 1967–1977; n = 414 hospital survivors; deaths = 9); *Bottom:* Survival of patients who were younger than 20 years of age at repair, and had either no previous operation or only a single aortopulmonary shunt (UAB, 1967–1977, selected groups; n = 307 hospital survivors, deaths = 3).

Age

When repair of *uncomplicated tetralogy of Fallot* can be accomplished by simple patch closure of the ventricular septal defect together with infundibular dissection and/ or patching but *without* a transannular patch, a primary reparative operation is advised during infancy at the age of three to six months or older. (It should be noted that,

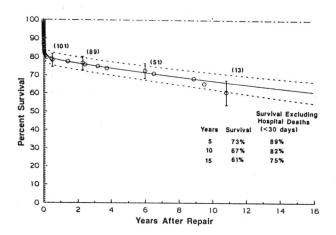

Figure 2. Percent survival, including hospital deaths, after the repair of patients with tetralogy of Fallot and pulmonary atresia (UAB; 1967–July 1983; n = 129; deaths = 38). Median age of the patients at repair was 8 years, and the range from 18 months to 51 years; mean age was 11 ± 8.7 (SD) years. The depiction is as in Figure 1. Note the 10-year survival (excluding hospital deaths) of 82% is considerably less than that of 95.8% for unselected patients with tetralogy of Fallot and 98% for the selected group (see Fig. 1).

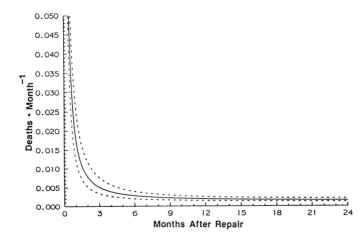

Figure 3. Hazard function for death after the repair of tetralogy of Fallot with pulmonary atresia (same data set as in Fig. 2). The dashed lines enclose the 70% confidence intervals. The hazard function has two phases, and the value for the constant phase is 0.0014. The constant phase of the hazard function for the data set in Figure 1B is 0.0001 deaths · month − 1 (informal estimate).

in this discussion, the phrase "uncomplicated tetralogy of Fallot with either pulmonary stenosis or atresia" implies absence of pulmonary arterial problems, large aorto-pulmonary collateral arteries, or major associated cardiac anomalies. It does not include tetralogy of Fallot with absence of the leaflets of the pulmonary valve.) Arguably,

Table 4

Informal Estimate of Incremental Risk Factors for Death After Repair of Tetralogy of Fallot With Pulmonary Stenosis or Atresia in the Current Era, Based Upon Previously Published Analyses*

Incremental risk factors for death	Time of death after repair		
	Early (hospital and <0.5 years)	Intermediate term (0.5–20 years)	Late (>20 years)
Demographic			
Young age (<3–12 months)	·		
Older age (>5 years)		●	●
Morphological			
Pulmonary arterial problems	●	●	
Absent pulmonary valve	●		
Major associated cardiac anomaly	●	●	
Functional			
High hematocrit	·		
More than one preliminary shunt, or a Potts or Waterston shunt	●	●	
Surgical			
High postrepair $P_{RV/LV}$ in OR	●	●	
Transannular patch	·		●
Valved extracardiac conduit	·	·	·

OR = operating room; $P_{RV/LV}$: right ventricular systolic pressure/left ventricular systolic pressure.
* Kirklin et al., 1983; Katz et al., 1982; Kirklin et al., 1984. The small dots depict a small and arguable effect, the large dots a near certain and strong effect.

a preliminary aortopulmonary shunting procedure is advisable for those in whom operation is required before the age of three months.

The management of the neonate and young infant with uncomplicated tetralogy of Fallot and either pulmonary stenosis or atresia of such morphology that it can be repaired by patch closure of the ventricular septal defect and *placement of a transannular patch* with or without infundibular dissection (but not without a transannular patch), is controversial. The available information supports the use of a preliminary GoreTex interposition shunt, rather than primary repair, up to the age of 6 to 12 months, but after that age, primary repair. When a shunt has been performed, the repair is accomplished at two to three years of age, or sooner if important cyanosis reappears.

When the repair of tetralogy of Fallot of any type requires the *placement of a valved conduit* between the right ventricle and the pulmonary trunk and the patient is younger than three to five years of age, a preliminary shunting operation is usually advisable (see below for further discussion). The intracardiac repair and placement of the conduit are best deferred until about three to five years of age when a near-adult-sized homograft valve can be used. The operation can be done earlier when and if the situation requires it.

Delay of the repair of the tetralogy of Fallot beyond three to five years of age invites the development of a secondary left ventricular (Borow et al., 1980) and right ventricular cardiomyopathy. These are truly irreversible phenomena that impose a considerable risk of premature late death. Further, such undue delay does not reduce the risk of death early after operation.

Pulmonary Arterial Problems

Patients with tetralogy of Fallot and pulmonary stenosis rarely have pulmonary arterial problems. In contrast, patients with the tetralogy and pulmonary atresia have them frequently.

A severe but fortunately uncommon form of these pulmonary arterial problems is absence of the central and unbranched hilar portions of both the right and left pulmonary arteries. In such cases, large aortopulmonary collateral arteries supply blood to the pulmonary microvasculature through the distal portions of the intrapulmonary arteries (Fig. 4). Either multiple stenoses are present in the collateral arteries or pulmonary microvascular resistance is high in patients who survive more than a short period of time. This situation, together with the undoubted technical problems, makes anything less than heart-lung transplantation impossible currently.

In between the normal complete accessibility of the pulmonary microvasculature to blood flow from the right ventricle and pulmonary trunk, and the total lack of accessibility just described, are varying degrees of incompleteness of accessibility caused by atresia (absence) of the central and unbranched hilar portion of the right or left pulmonary artery, atresia (absence) of a branched portion of one or both hilar pulmonary arteries, or by segmental absence of portions of the intrapulmonary arteries. These anomalies are usually associated with large aortopulmonary collateral arteries that supply blood to areas of the lung that are inaccessible to blood flow from the pulmonary trunk. The operative procedure of unifocalization, discussed elsewhere in this volume, represents an attempt to improve accessibility.

In any event, the amount of the pulmonary microvasculature that must be accessible to blood flow from the right ventricle and pulmonary trunk (or the central or unbranched hilar portions of the right and left pulmonary arteries) for complete repair to be successful is currently under investigation at our center (unpublished data). Tentatively, however, the likelihood of early and intermediate success from a complete repair is considered small when the micro-

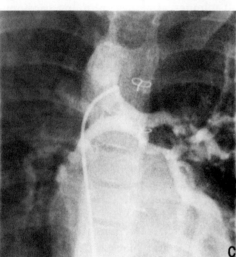

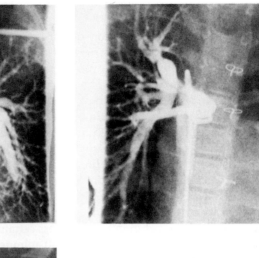

Figure 4. Cineangiograms from two patients (one in *a*, the other in *b* and *c*) with tetralogy of Fallot and pulmonary atresia. These and other films demonstrated no pulmonary trunk and no central and unbranched hilar portion of the right and left pulmonary arteries, and large aortopulmonary collateral arteries merging end-to-end with branched hilar and intrapulmonary pulmonary arteries.

vasculature of less than 10 pulmonary segments is available to blood flow from the right ventricle and pulmonary trunk. The management of patients with more than this amount of accessibility but which is still incomplete, is variable and not yet determined with precision. It is dependent in part at least upon the other characteristics of the pulmonary circulation.

In general, when a palliative connection from the right ventricle to the pulmonary trunk or a complete repair is made, aortopulmonary collateral arteries that connect end-to-side to pulmonary arteries, or are part of a dual supply to the pulmonary microvasculature, should be closed surgically or by catheter techniques. Those that merge end-to-end with intrapulmonary pulmonary arteries and are their only source of blood flow must not be ligated, although, uncommonly, banding them may be useful.

Surgical Decisions

In patients with pulmonary arterial problems of any sort, a pulmonary arteriogram with injection directly into the appropriate pulmonary artery is necessary. Only in this way can the entire pulmonary arterial tree be visualized free from the confusing effect of associated opacification of the collateral circulation to the pulmonary microvasculature. When there is only pulmonary stenosis, this can be accomplished by right heart cardiac catheterization. In patients with tetralogy of Fallot and pulmonary atresia, a GoreTex interposition shunt may be required shortly after birth because of severe cyanosis. In any event, in those with pulmonary arterial problems a shunt is needed at some time before repair in order to provide catheter access to the pulmonary arterial tree as well as for relief of cyanosis.

A complete repair should probably not be undertaken in patients with any type of tetralogy of Fallot when the predicted *late* postrepair $P_{RV/LV}$, after the most complete possible operation, is greater than 0.90 at rest. The exact limits, however, are still under investigation, since methods for making this prediction preoperatively have not yet been perfected.

In the operating room, in patients with tetralogy of Fallot with pulmonary stenosis, the decision is made to perform the repair without a transannular patch whenever the resultant predicted late postrepair $P_{RV/LV}$ is less than 0.7. In practice, about 30 minutes after the repair, the postrepair $P_{RV/LV}$ is measured and the absence of a transannular patch accepted if the $P_{RV/LV}$ at that time is less than 0.85 (if the patient is 12–24 months of age) or 1.0 (if 6 months of age) (Tables 5 and 6). Otherwise, cardiopulmonary bypass is reestablished and a transannular patch placed. If a transannular patch is not placed, and the postrepair $P_{RV/LV}$ the next morning is not less than 0.7, the patient is returned to the operating room and a transannular patch is placed (an easy and safe secondary procedure).

After repair of tetralogy of Fallot with pulmonary atresia with a valved extracardiac conduit, the limits of acceptability are less certain, but when the $P_{RV/LV}$ is 1.1 or 1.2 30 minutes after discontinuing cardiopulmonary bypass, cardiopulmonary bypass should be reinstituted and a large slit made in the patch used to close the ventricular septal defect. This is a very short procedure that can readily be accomplished through the right atrium. This procedure may also be used intentionally for palliation when too high a postrepair $P_{RV/LV}$ is predicted preoperatively.

There has been speculation as to whether there is a greater fall in postrepair $P_{RV/LV}$ between the immediate and later postrepair period when the repair is performed through the right atrium (Fig. 5). A study by Coles, Blackstone, Pacifico, and Kirklin (unpublished data, 1985) indicates

Table 5

The Correlates of the Late Postrepair $P_{RV/LV}$ after Repair of Tetralogy of Fallot, UAB, 1978–1982; $n = 100$*

Variable	Coefficient $\pm$ SD	p value
Postrepair $P_{RV/LV}$ (OR)	0.45 ± 0.068	<0.0001
Body surface area (m²)	-0.07 ± 0.028	0.01
Presence of pulmonary atresia (0, 1)	0.10 ± 0.034	0.03
Presence of pulmonary arterial problems (0, 1)	0.06 ± 0.032	0.05
Intercept	0.27	

Note: The late postrepair $P_{RV/LV}$ in an individual patient may be determined by adding to the intercept the specific product of the coefficient times the quantity of each variable. Zero and one indicate no or yes, respectively.
* The value for the late postrepair $P_{RV/LV}$ is similar 24 hours after repair and many months or years later.
Revised from Kirklin and Barratt-Boyes: *Cardiac Surgery.* New York, Wiley, 1986, Tables 23–26.

Table 6

Examples of the Prediction of the Late Postrepair
$P_{RV/LV}$ *by Measuring the Postrepair* $P_{RV/LV}$,
30 Minutes or More After Discontinuing
Cardiopulmonary Bypass (A Solution of
the Regression Equation in Table 5)

Postrepair (OR) $P_{RV/LV}$	Late postrepair $P_{RV/LV}$ (Age) months		
	6	12	24
Uncomplicated TF			
0.7	0.56	0.55	0.55
0.85	0.63	0.62	0.61
1.0	0.69	0.69	0.68
TF with PA problems			
0.7	0.62	0.62	0.61
0.85	0.69	0.68	0.68
1.0	0.76	0.75	0.75
TF with pulmonary atresia			
0.7	0.66	0.66	0.65
0.85	0.73	0.73	0.72
1.0	0.80	0.79	0.79
TF with pulmonary atresia and PA problems			
0.7	0.73	0.72	0.72
0.85	0.79	0.79	0.78
1.0	0.86	0.86	0.85

PA = pulmonary arterial; TF = tetralogy of Fallot.

that the fall is the same for the two techniques (Table 7).

Valved or Valveless Repair for the Tetralogy of Fallot

The value subsequent to repair of placing a valve between the right ventricle and the pulmonary arteries has also been controversial. Patients born with isolated absence of the leaflets of the pulmonary valve generally become symptomatic after about 40 years (Shimazaki et al., 1984). This is compatible with the finding that a transannular patch, which results in absence of a valve between the right ventricle and pulmonary trunk and pulmonary incompetence, is not a risk factor for death during the first 10 to 20 years after repair of the tetralogy of Fallot (Fuster et al., 1980; Katz et al., 1982). A transannular patch is, however, a risk factor for impaired exercise capacity within 5 to 12 years of operation (Wessel et al., 1980). Furthermore, an important secondary right ventricular cardiomyopathy will have been found to develop

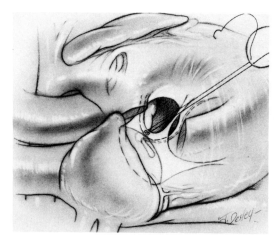

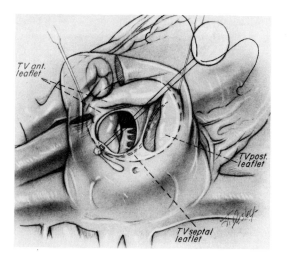

Figure 5. Depiction of the repair of the ventricular septal defect in patients with tetralogy of Fallot through the right ventricular approach (top) and the right atrial approach (bottom). Note that the morphological relations are different, but that the steps of the patch closure of the ventricular septal defect are the same. (Reproduced with permission from Kirklin and Barratt-Boyes: *Cardiac Surgery.* New York, Wiley, 1986.)

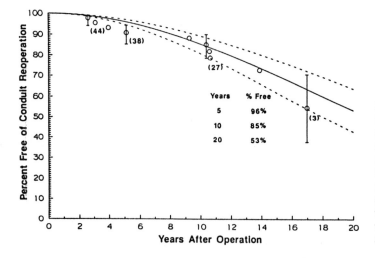

Figure 6. Percent of patients free of conduit reoperation after the repair of a ventricular septal defect and placement of a homograft valved conduit between right ventricle and pulmonary trunk (1966–1977; n = 49; events = 10). This information was very kindly provided by Dr. D. Ross and Dr. J. Somerville (1986).

Table 7

$P_{RV/LV}$ *After Repair of Tetralogy of Fallot (RV Approach 1967–1982; RA Approach 1978–1984)**

	$P_{RV/LV}$ *(mean ± SD)*		
Postrepair $P_{RV/LV}$	*RV approach (n = 391)*	*RA approach (n = 39)*	*p*
30 minutes after repair	0.56 ± 0.195	0.59 ± 0.190	0.4
20 hours or more after repair	0.47 ± 0.188	0.50 ± 0.145	0.3
Change	−0.09 ± 0.176	−0.09 ± 0.142	0.9

$P_{RV/LV}$ = ratio between systolic right ventricular and systolic left ventricular pressures; RA = right atrium; RV = right ventricle.
Note: Some patients with an RA approach had part of the procedure performed through the pulmonary artery. Transannular patch yes/no was not a correlate of the change in $P_{RV/LV}$.
* Unpublished data of Coles, Blackstone, Kirklin, and Pacifico, 1985. These data correspond in all ways to the data presented in Tables 5 and 6.

in some patients. A transannular patch may, therefore, become a risk factor for premature death after 20 years. For these reasons, it is prudent to avoid the use of a transannular patch unless it is near certain that the postrepair $P_{RV/LV}$ will be too high without it.

Should a conduit placed between the right ventricle and pulmonary artery contain a valve? The argument against a nonvalved conduit is the same as that against an unnecessary transannular patch: namely, the risk of the slow development of a progressing secondary right ventricular cardio-

myopathy secondary to the volume overload. This argument may be particularly valid in patients with the tetralogy of Fallot and pulmonary atresia. Pulmonary arterial problems in these patients may result in high pulmonary arterial and right ventricular systolic pressures and the additive effect of a right ventricular pressure overload.

The argument in favor of a valve in the conduit was difficult to sustain when the heterograft valve was used. This was because all patients receiving these prostheses in our center required reoperation within 15

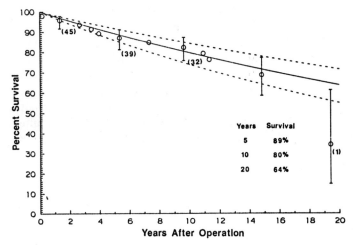

Figure 7. Percent survival after the repair of tetralogy of Fallot with pulmonary atresia using a homograft valved conduit (1966–1967; n = 49; deaths = 12). This information was very kindly provided by Dr. D. Ross and Dr. J. Somerville (1986).

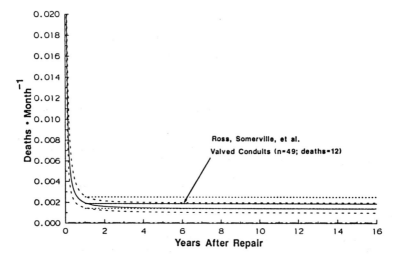

Figure 8. The constant phase of hazard function in the experience of Ross, Somerville (personal communication, 1986) shown against the background of the UAB experience (see Fig. 3). Note that the 70% confidence limits of the two experiences are overlapping.

years of their insertion (Shimazaki et al., 1984). Ross and Somerville have shown that only about 20% of homograft valved conduits require replacement within that time period, although slightly over 50% have required replacement within 20 years after insertion (Fig. 6). In 1982 therefore, a homograft bank was reestablished at the University of Birmingham in Alabama using cryopreservation techniques (Kirklin and Barratt-Boyes, 1986). Even at that time, the unsatisfactory results of the use of the heterograft valved conduits were apparent.

Nonetheless, the survival of the patients of Ross and Somerville has not been rendered optimal by the use of a homograft valved extracardiac conduit, the 10-year survival being 80% and 20-year survival 64% (Fig. 7). Interestingly, the survival of similar patients in our experience has been almost identical (see Fig. 2), even though at that time we used, for the most part, heterograft valved conduits. The hazard function during the constant phase is similar in both the National Heart Hospital and our experiences (Fig. 8). This similarity in all probability reflects the presence in both experiences of two important risk factors, older age at

operation (indicating a more advanced secondary cardiomyopathy) and inadequate myocardial protection.

Summary

Coexisting cardiac and pulmonary arterial anomalies, and a secondary cardiomyopathy from delay in repair, not the atresia itself, decrease the probability of early and late survival in patients with tetralogy of Fallot and pulmonary atresia. Application of current detailed knowledge, proper management of the details of the operation including the myocardial protection, and (when conduits are necessary) use of a homograft valved conduit, can improve results in tetralogy of Fallot of all types. Continuing studies of unsolved problems are indicated.

References

Borow KM, Green LH, Castaneda AR, Keane JF. Left ventricular function after repair of tetralogy of Fallot and its relationship to age at surgery. *Circulation* 1980;61:1150–1158.

Fuster V, McGoon DC, Kennedy MA, et al. Long-term evaluation (12 to 22 years) of open heart surgery for tetralogy of Fallot. *Am J Cardiol* 1980;46:635–642.

Katz NM, Blackstone EH, Kirklin JW, et al. Late survival and symptoms after repair of tetralogy of Fallot. *Circulation* 1982;65:403–410.

Kirklin JW, Barratt-Boyes BG. *Cardiac Surgery.* New York: John Wiley and Sons, 1986; Chapter 23.

Kirklin JW, Barratt-Boyes BG. *Cardiac Surgery.* New York: John Wiley and Sons, 1986; p. 421.

Kirklin JW, Blackstone EH, Kirklin JK, et al. Sur-

gical results and protocols in the spectrum of tetralogy of Fallot. *Ann Surg* 1983;198:251–265.

Kirklin JW, Blackstone EH, Pacifico AD, et al. Risk factors for early and late failure after repair of tetralogy of Fallot, and their neutralization. *Thorac Cardiovasc Surgeon* 1984;32:208–214.

Ross DN, Somerville J. Personal communication, 1986.

Shimazaki Y, Blackstone EH, Kirklin JW. The natural history of isolated congenital pulmonary valve incompetence: Surgical implications. *Thorac Cardiovasc Surgeon* 1984;32:257–259.

Wessel HU, Cunningham WJ, Paul MH, et al. Exercise performance in tetralogy of Fallot after intracardiac repair. *J Thorac Cardiovasc Surg* 1980;80:582–593.

IV

Complete Transposition: Optimal Treatment

4.1

Introduction

James R. Zuberbuhler

Complete transposition (the combination of concordant atrioventricular and discordant ventriculoarterial connections) was once of the most lethal of congenital cardiac malformations. If the anomaly was "uncomplicated", the presence of two parallel circulations resulted in severe hypoxemia and death as soon as the arterial duct closed. Only when an atrial or ventricular septal defect was present was there enough mixing between the two circuits to permit survival beyond the neonatal period. Pulmonary vascular disease then appeared in most of the survivors unless there was associated pulmonary stenosis.

The transition from a nearly hopeless prognosis to the present expectation of survival beyond childhood has required a great measure of therapeutic ingenuity. Rashkind's balloon septostomy (Rashkind and Miller, 1966) provided a practical means of obtaining better mixing. It quickly supplanted surgical septectomy as the palliative procedure of choice in the hypoxemic newborn. The direct surgical attack on the anomaly of correcting the basic problem of the discordant ventriculoarterial connection by "switching" the great arteries was at first

impossible (Mustard et al., 1954). The difficulties were both technical and physiological. There were no techniques for transplanting the coronary arteries from the "old" to the "new" aorta in a newborn, and this was a necessary part of the operative procedure. Since the left ventricle rapidly becomes "deconditioned" by the usual fall in pressure in the pulmonary circuit, any switch procedure could not be delayed until the infant grew larger. Because of the difficulties inherent in any arterial switch procedure, atrial redirection techniques were pursued. First the Senning (1959), then the Mustard (1964), and then again the Senning operations have found favor. At first used only beyond infancy, these techniques are now routinely performed in the first year of life, using profound hypothermia and circulatory arrest. The surgical mortality of the Mustard and Senning operations are now acceptably low in patients with uncomplicated complete transposition. (The presence of a large ventricular septal defect or of severe pulmonary stenosis complicates repair and makes surgical mortality much higher.) The long-term results of atrial redirection operations are less sanguine. Although most

From: Anderson, RH, Neches, WH, Park, SC, Zuberbuhler, JR, eds: *Perspectives in Pediatric Cardiology*: Mount Kisco, New York, Futura Publishing Co., © 1988.

survivors are without symptoms and can lead productive, as well as reproductive, lives, there is a distressing incidence of arrhythmias and sudden death. There continues to be doubt as to the ability of the right ventricle and tricuspid valve to withstand systemic pressure over a normal lifetime. Because of these concerns, the possibility of switching the great arteries was reconsidered and techniques were developed for transferring coronary arteries to the new aorta (Jatene et al., 1975). At first the operative mortality was much higher than with atrial redirection operations, but now there are reports of very low operative mortality with the switch procedure. In truth, the long-term results of the switch operation are no more known than the long-term results of the Mustard operation were 15 years ago. There is concern about the fate of the transplanted coronary arteries, but the left ventricle and mitral valve are now part of the systemic circuit. The long-term advantages of the switch over atrial redirection techniques are theoretical at present, but it is hoped that they will be proven to be real over the years.

We have designed this section to highlight the advantages and disadvantages of the two approaches. The first two chapters deal with morphological and physiological considerations. The next two chapters consider septostomy techniques and mortality and morbidity between the septostomy and surgical repair. The next three chapters address the long-term results of atrial redirection procedures, exploring abnormalities of cardiac rhythm, exercise capacity, and the incidence and cause of late death. The final chapter compares the operative mortality of the two basic surgical approaches to repair.

References

Jatene AD, Fontes VF, Paulista PP, et al. Successful anatomic correction of transposition of the great vessels. A preliminary report. *Arq Bras Cardiol* 1975;28:461–464.

Mustard WT, Chute AL, Keith JD, et al. A surgical approach to transposition of the great vessels with extracorporeal circuit. *Surgery* 1954;36:39–51.

Mustard WT. Successful two-stage correction of transposition of the great vessels. *Pediatr Surg* 1964;55:469–472.

Rashkind WJ, Miller WM. Creation of an atrial septal defect without thoracotomy: A palliative approach to complete transposition of the great arteries. *JAMA* 1966;196:991–992.

Senning A. Surgical correction of transposition of the great arteries. *Surgery* 1959;45:966–980.

Morphology of Complete Transposition

Robert H. Anderson and Siew Yen Ho

The condition to be described and discussed in this section is characterized by a concordant connection at the atrioventricular level in association with a discordant ventriculoarterial connection. As such, it can exist with usual or mirror-image atrial arrangements (Fig. 1), but cannot be found in the presence of atrial isomerism or with a univentricular atrioventricular connection. Similarly, a discordant ventriculoarterial connection in this setting is to be distinguished from the same connection found at the ventriculoarterial level together with a discordant atrioventricular connection. How, then, is it best to describe this particular morphological combination? There has been a vogue for describing the arrangement as "D-transposition," or D-loop transposition. Indeed, some continue to use this convention (Vetter et al., 1987), but we consider it far too nonspecific to be of real value. Many lesions fulfilling the required segmental combination have either a left-sided aorta or left-hand ventricular topology (L-loop), making the very terminology

meaningless (Becker and Anderson, 1983). Furthermore, many other hearts exhibiting an anterior and right-sided aorta do *not* fulfill the required morphological criteria. In our opinion, therefore, the "D" convention has little to recommend it unless it is used in the full segmental notation ("transposition {S, D, D}," and so on). Many would opt instead simply for "transposition" or "TGA." Again, in our opinion, this usage is far too nonspecific while retaining a controversial aspect. There has still been no consensus as to whether "transposition" in isolation should describe an anterior aorta or a discordant ventriculoarterial connection. Although the trend is certainly toward its use for description of the discordant connection, this remains imprecise because of the variability described above to be found at the atrioventricular junction. Our preference, therefore, is to describe the combination of concordant atrioventricular and discordant ventriculoarterial connections as *complete transposition*. This then differentiates the lesion well from congenitally cor-

From: Anderson, RH, Neches, WH, Park, SC, Zuberbuhler, JR, eds: *Perspectives in Pediatric Cardiology*: Mount Kisco, New York, Futura Publishing Co., © 1988.

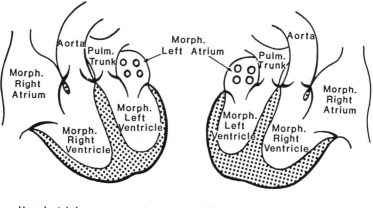

Usual atrial arrangement   Mirror-image arrangement

COMPLETE TRANSPOSITION

Concordant atrioventricular connection and discordant ventriculo-arterial connection

Figure 1. A diagram showing the chamber combinations producing the lesion we prefer to describe as complete transposition.

rected transposition (found with a discordant atrioventricular connection) and from transposition (considered as a discordant ventriculoarterial connection) coexisting with atrial isomerism, double inlet ventricle, or atrioventricular valve atresia. It could be argued that the adjective "complete" was initially used to differentiate this type of transposition from double outlet right ventricle, considered by some in the past to be a *partial transposition* because only the aorta was placed across the septum to arise from the right ventricle. If this is the case, the counterargument can then be made that this strengthens rather than weakens the use of "complete" to describe the arrangement in which both great arteries are placed across the septum, although this would then clearly apply to all forms of discordant ventriculoarterial connection rather than simply the variant found with a concordant atrioventricular connection. None of the alternatives is perfect. We must, therefore, search for the least degree of imperfection. That, to our eyes, is provided by using the combination *complete transposition* (Tynan and Anderson, 1979).

Basic Morphology

The unifying morphology is provided by the concordant atrioventricular and discordant ventriculoarterial connections. Always, therefore, the morphologically right atrium will be connected to the morphologically right ventricle which in turn will support the aorta while the morphologically left atrium will be connected to the morphologically left ventricle and thence to the pulmonary trunk (Fig. 1). These connections can be found in the usual (Fig. 2) or mirror-image (Fig. 3) variants. They can be found with overriding of either the atrioventricular or arterial orifices, providing that the degree of override is not such as to produce a univentricular atrioventricular or double outlet connection. The segmental combinations can also be found with

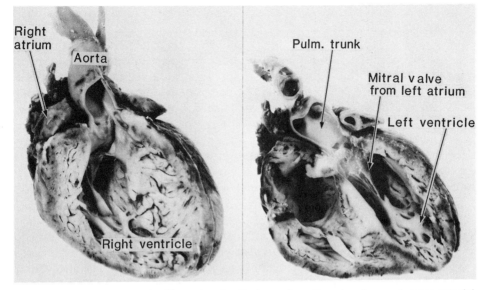

Figure 2. These sections in "four-chamber" plane show the chamber and great arterial connections of complete transposition with usual atrial arrangement.

marked variability in either arterial relationships or infundibular morphology. Within the convention we have espoused, it is the connections of the segments which determine the definition of the lesion, rather than either the position of the aorta or the presence of a complete subaortic infundibulum (conus). Thus, most often the aorta will be positioned anteriorly and to the right of the pulmonary trunk. The diagnosis of

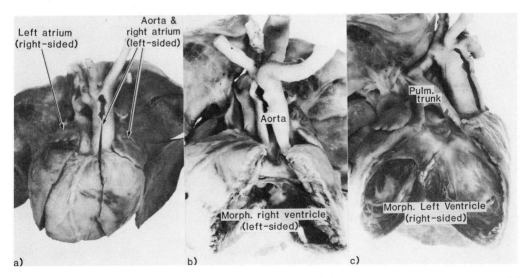

Figure 3. This montage shows the morphology of complete transposition with mirror-image atrial arrangement. The frontal view (a) shows the typical left-sided aortic position. The aorta is connected to the left-sided morphologically right ventricle (b), which is in turn connected to the left-sided right atrium. The right-sided left atrium drains to the right-sided morphologically right ventricle (c), which then gives rise to the pulmonary trunk.

complete transposition will not change, however, should the aorta be found directly anterior, in left-sided position (be there usual or mirror-image atrial arrangement) or even posteriorly and to the right ("normal relations"; Van Praagh et al., 1971; Wilkinson et al., 1975). Similarly, although there is almost always a completely muscular sub-aortic infundibulum with pulmonary-mitral valvalar continuity (Fig. 2), the segmental combination can rarely be found with bilaterally complete infundibular structures or with a subpulmonary infundibulum and aortic-atrioventricular valvular continuity. It is the segmental combinations that determine the important anatomical features, such as the disposition of the conduction tissues and the arrangement of the coronary arteries. To an extent, nonetheless, these can be modified by the important associated malformations, particularly the presence of a ventricular septal defect or fixed obstruction to the subpulmonary outflow tract from the left ventricle.

The Conduction Tissues

Since the sinus node and atrioventricular node are atrial structures, and since atrial morphology is undisturbed in complete transposition (except with juxtaposed atrial appendages), the nodal structures are to be found in their anticipated sites for the normally structured heart. The sinus node, therefore, is almost always found as a cigar-shaped structure lying laterally to the crest of the atrial appendage in the terminal groove between appendage and venous sinus of the right atrium (Fig. 4). The exceptions are those minority of cases (one-tenth in our experience; Anderson et al., 1979) in which the node takes up a "horseshoe" position astride the crest of the appendage and those hearts with juxtaposed appendages when the site of the node is deviated anterocephalad toward the atrioventricular junction (Ho et al., 1979). The atrioventricular node and its zones of atrial transitional cells are found exclusively within the triangle of Koch (Anderson et al., 1983). The atrioventricular bundle penetrates into the subpulmonary outflow tract of the left ventricle in comparable fashion to the arrangement found in the normal heart, the only difference being that the membranous septum is often lacking in complete transposition (Smith et al., 1986). Thereafter, the disposition of the ventricular conduction tissues is as for the normal heart, and the

COMPLETE TRANSPOSITION – conduction tissues

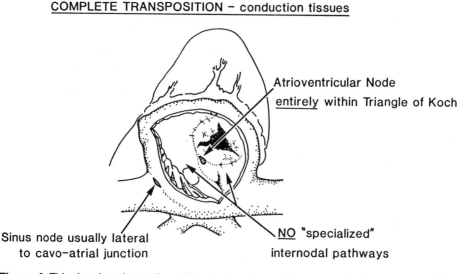

Figure 4. This drawing shows the anticipated position of the conduction tissues as might be seen by the surgeon at operation.

relationship to defects within the ventricular septum is also as expected for the normally constructed heart.

The Coronary Arteries

The disposition of the coronary arteries has become of crucial importance with the introduction and acceptance of the arterial switch procedure with coronary relocation as a means of surgical correction. It is necessary to take account of both the origin and course of the three major coronary arteries, but then to take particular note of the arrangement of the artery to the sinus node. Although there are isolated reports of coronary arteries in hearts with complete transposition which take origin from the nonfacing sinus of the aorta, in our experience, together with that of our colleagues in Liverpool (Smith et al., 1986) and Leiden (Gittenberger-de-Groot et al., 1983), the arteries always take origin from one or the other of the aortic sinuses which are adjacent to, or *face*, the pulmonary trunk (Fig. 5). There are various ways of describing these sinuses. We originally termed them "right" and "left" facing sinuses (Anderson and Becker, 1981). Our Leiden colleagues pointed to the problem with this convention when the

great arteries were side by side, since the sinuses were then anterior and posterior. They suggested a numerical approach, considering the sinuses from the stance of the surgeon standing in the nonfacing sinus and looking toward the pulmonary trunk (Fig. 6). In the Leiden convention, the sinus to the left hand is then termed "Sinus 2" while the right hand sinus is "Sinus 1." This has the problem of taxing the memory! The convention is first class, but we suggest it may be better to describe right hand and left hand facing sinuses, thereby relieving the memory banks of one small task. Since there are three major coronary arteries (anterior interventricular, circumflex, and right arteries), and since they arise from only two sinuses, there are eight possible combinations of sinusal origin (Table 1). Thus far, not all of these have been seen in practice, and some, basing their approach on clinical experience, prefer an alphanumeric system for description of the variability (Yacoub and Radley-Smith, 1978). Apart from the obvious additional toll this approach places on the memory banks, it seems likely that, in time, all possibilities will be seen. This will then entail either procrustean remedies or else expansion of the present fivefold classification. In either event, by far the greater majority of cases fall into two patterns. The most common is for the right coronary artery to arise from the left-hand facing sinus while the anterior interventricular and circumflex arteries take origin from the right-hand sinus (about two-thirds of cases). The second most common pattern is for the right coronary and the circumflex arteries to arise from the left-hand sinus, the circumflex branch taking a retropulmonary course as it passes to the left atrioventricular junction. The anterior interventricular artery arises from the right-hand sinus. This pattern accounts for up to one-quarter of cases. The other patterns make up the rest, all coronary arteries arising from the same sinus being the most troublesome arrangement for the surgeon. This, and other less usual patterns, are seen with some degree of frequency when the great arteries are positioned side

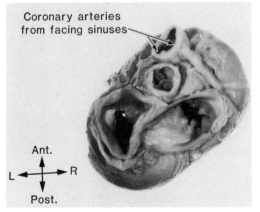

Coronary arteries from facing sinuses

Ant.

L ← → R

Post.

Figure 5. This dissection shows the base of the heart as viewed from above and reveals the typical origin of the coronary arteries from the facing sinuses of the aorta.

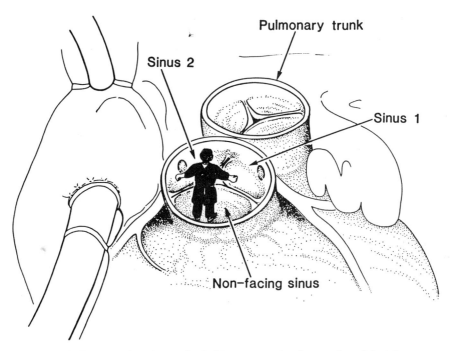

Figure 6. This drawing shows the Leiden convention for naming of the sinuses of the aorta in complete transposition. Our preference is to call sinus 1 the right-hand and sinus 2 the left-hand facing sinus.

by side. Origin of the artery to the sinus node is also of major significance. Although this is not an end-artery, and there is circumstantial evidence to suggest that its section is not a catastrophic event, it seems sensible to preserve the artery during surgery if this is possible. Usually, the artery arises from the proximal portions of either the right or circumflex coronary arteries and then courses through the anterior interatrial groove toward the superior cavoatrial junction. As it runs through the anterior interatrial area, it can burrow intramyocardially and approach close to the rim of the oval

Table 1

Possible Origins of Coronary Arteries

Right-hand sinus (Sinus 1)	Left-hand sinus (Sinus 2)
• Right coronary artery	Circumflex and anterior descending artery
• Right coronary artery and circumflex	Anterior descending artery
• Right coronary artery and anterior descending artery	Circumflex
• Right coronary artery, anterior descending artery, and circumflex	——
• ——	Right coronary artery, anterior descending artery, and circumflex
• Circumflex	Anterior descending artery and right coronary artery
• Anterior descending artery	Circumflex and right coronary artery
• Circumflex and anterior descending artery	Right coronary artery

fossa. This is of significance during surgical septectomy or atrial redirection procedures. Having reached the cavoatrial junction, the artery can pass procavally, retrocavally, or it can form an arterial circle as it supplies the node (Anderson et al., 1979). Two further variables are of surgical significance. The first, found with some frequency in our material (Rossi et al., 1986), is pertinent for all surgical procedures. It is when the artery arises from the lateral part of the right coronary artery and courses across the appendage to reach the terminal groove (Fig. 7). The second is when the artery takes a separate and unique origin from one of the aortic sinuses. Under these circumstances, it makes sense to relocate the artery to the sinus node along the other arteries during the arterial switch procedure. It would also seem prudent to limit dissection of the

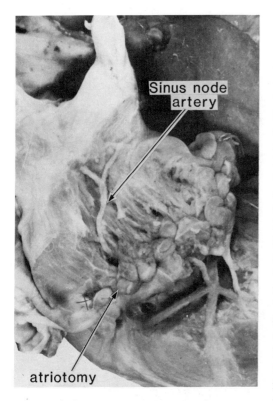

Figure 7. This dissection shows a lateral sinus node artery in complete transposition. Note that the standard atriotomy has divided the artery.

proximal artery giving rise to the sinus nodal artery should this be encountered during liberation of the arteries.

The Ventricular Septal Defect

A deficiency within the ventricular septum is the most critical of the associated malformations. It can occur with the same variability as observed in the normally connected heart, and can be categorized in similar fashion (Anderson and Becker, 1981; Soto et al., 1980). In complete transposition, however, most defects are of the malalignment type with the outlet septum parallel to the rest of the ventricular septum and inserted within the right ventricle. Such defects can extend to become perimembranous (Fig. 8a) or can have a muscular posteroinferior rim (Fig. 8b) which, when present, protects the conduction tissue axis. Of necessity, because of the septal malalignment, these defects are associated with overriding of the pulmonary trunk. Indeed, depending on the degree of overriding, a clear spectrum of malformation exists which terminates in double outlet right ventricle with subpulmonary ventricular septal defect. A strong case can be made for considering all hearts of this type, with the pulmonary trunk overriding a defect opening to the outlet of the right ventricle, as variants of the Taussig-Bing malformation, just as it is known that tetralogy of Fallot is characterized by overriding of the aorta between the extremes of concordant and double outlet ventriculoarterial connections. In this setting, two points are of surgical significance. The outlet septum can often be resected in its entirety since it contains no structures of vital significance (Fig. 9). It may, nonetheless, give rise to tension apparatus of the tricuspid valve. The second point, therefore, is that rather than being resected, the septum can be liberated and reimplanted, thereby preserving the integrity of the tension apparatus to the tricuspid valve (Le-

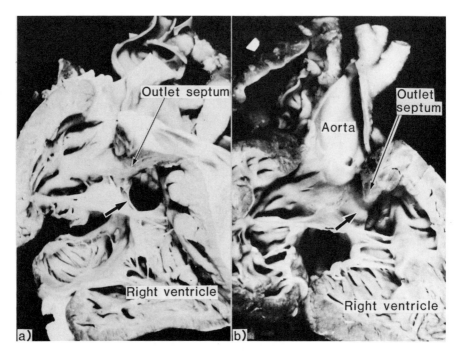

Figure 8. These views from the right ventricle show (*a*) a perimembranous and (*b*) a muscular malalignment outlet defect in complete transposition. The arrow points to the muscular posteroinferior rim in (*b*) but to tricuspid-pulmonary continuity in (*a*).

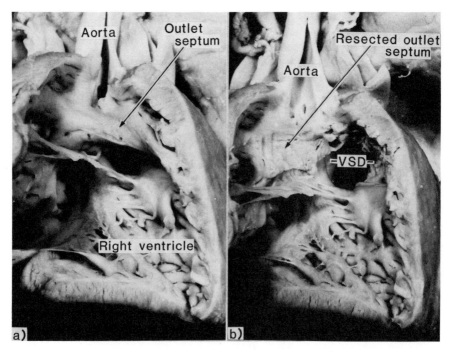

Figure 9. This dissection shows how the outlet septum can safely be resected to increase the size of a malalignment outlet defect.

compte, in press). It should not be presumed from this discussion that all defects in complete transposition are of malalignment type. Perimembranous defects can exist without malalignment (Fig. 10) and can open to inlet or outlet of the right ventricle or become confluent. Muscular defects can be found opening to inlet, apical trabecular, or outlet components of the right ventricle without septal malalignment. Juxtaarterial defects (with aortic-pulmonary valvular continuity) can be found either with muscular posteroinferior rims or extending to become perimembranous. The latter are particularly frequent when the aorta is anterior and to the left with usual atrial arrangement (Lincoln et al., 1975). As well as malalignment of the outlet septum, there may be

malalignment between the atrial and ventricular septal structures with overriding of the tricuspid valve and all the consequences of an abnormal conduction tissue axis (Milo et al., 1979). All of these variants, nonetheless, can be well described within the system outlined in Chapter 1.2.

Obstruction of the Subpulmonary Outflow Tract

Any of the structures which, in the normally structured heart, produce subaortic obstruction can produce subpulmonary obstruction in the setting of complete transposition. Thus, when the septum is intact, the obstruction may be due to a fixed subpulmonary shelf which directly overlies the left bundle branch. When severe, this type of obstruction can produce tunnel obstruction and can be combined with anomalous attachment of the tension apparatus of the mitral valve, another potential source of obstruction (Fig. 11). Bulging of the septum, with or without hypertrophy, can produce obstruction, and this too can be associated with a subpulmonary fibrous shelf. Aneurysmal tissue tags, derived from either the membranous septum, tricuspid valve (in presence of a septal defect), or mitral valve, are further substrates for stenosis. When there is a ventricular septal defect, then, in addition to the above possibilities, the most likely cause of obstruction is posterior deviation of the outlet septum. This is associated with overriding of the aortic valve and sets the scene for repair using the Rastelli procedure. In any surgical procedure, it should be remembered that the outflow tract is encircled by structures at considerable risk (Wilcox et al., 1983). Although the structures can in many cases be safely resected, the use of a conduit provides a means of bypassing the danger area.

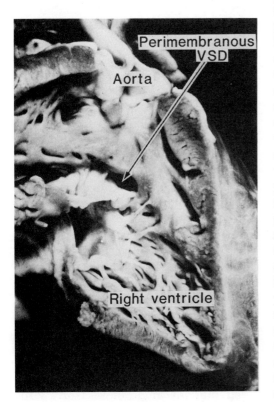

Figure 10. In this illustration, a perimembranous ventricular septal defect is seen without any malalignment of the outlet septum.

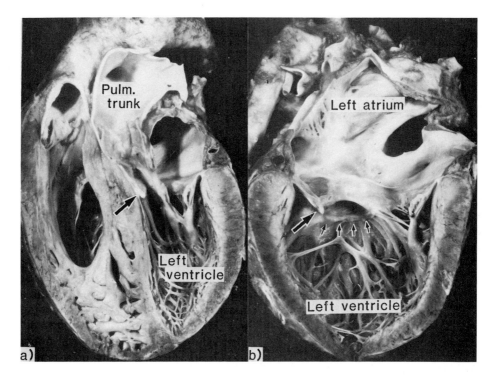

Figure 11. This "four-chamber" section (a) and view of the left heart chambers (b) show a fibrous subpulmonary shelf (arrow in a and small arrows in b) coexisting with anomalous attachment of the tension apparatus of the mitral valve (large arrow in b).

Other Associated Malformations

Any lesion that is morphologically possible should be kept in mind when diagnosing associated malformations. Juxtaposition of the atrial appendages has already been mentioned, and is particularly likely when the aorta is anterior and left-sided in a patient with usual atrial arrangement. Most patients have a deficiency of the atrial septum within the oval fossa, and it is this deficiency which is enlarged by balloon or blade septostomy (see below). Other types of interatrial communication are extremely rare, but should not be dismissed. If an atrioventricular septal defect is encountered, however, care should be taken to exclude atrial isomerism before diagnosing the case as complete transposition. Coarctation of the aorta frequently accompanies cases

with malalignment outlet defects of Taussig-Bing type in which the deviated outlet septum obstructs the subaortic infundibulum (Milanesi et al., 1982; Waldman et al., 1984). Not all cases of aortic coarctation are associated with this type of defect in complete transposition but the association is a frequent one. Certainly, if there is aortic coarctation, care should be taken to exclude subaortic obstruction, particularly if an arterial switch is contemplated as the means of surgical repair. Muscle bundles within the outflow tracts of the right ventricle are often found in complete transposition and they, too, can produce problems of subpulmonary obstruction after the arterial switch procedures. In this respect, it should be remembered that the angle of take-off of the "new" pulmonary trunk will differ markedly from that originally held by the aorta prior to an arterial switch. Anomalous muscle bundles can well exacerbate this altered geometry sufficiently to produce subpulmonary obstruction in the post-switch period. Finally, the presence of the patency of the arterial duct can be highly significant in complete transposition and must be excluded.

References

Anderson KR, Ho SY, Anderson RH. The location and vascular supply of the sinus node in the human heart. *Br Heart J* 1979;41:28–32.

Anderson RH, Becker AE. Complete transposition—Morphology. In Becker AE, Losekoot TG, Marcelletti C, Anderson RH (Eds): *Paediatric Cardiology (Vol 3)*. Edinburgh: Churchill Livingstone, 1981:167–178.

Anderson RH, Ho SY, Becker AE. The surgical anatomy of the conduction tissues. *Thorax* 1983;38:408–420.

Becker AE, Anderson RH. How should we describe hearts in which the aorta is connected to the right ventricle and the pulmonary trunk to the left ventricle? A matter for reason and logic. *Am J Cardiol* 1983;51:911–912.

Gittenberger-de-Groot AC, Sauer U, Oppenheimer-Dekker A, Quaegebeur J. Coronary arterial anatomy in transposition of the great arteries. A morphologic study. *Pediatr Cardiol* 1983;4:15–24.

Ho SY, Monro JL, Anderson RH. The disposition of the sinus node in left-sided juxtaposition of the atrial appendage. *Br Heart J* 1979;41:129–132.

Lecompte Y. Anatomic repair of complete transposition of the great arteries associated with ventricular septal defect (with or without pulmonary outflow tract obstruction). In Anderson RH, Macartney FJ, Shinebourne EA, Tynan M (eds): *Perspectives in Pediatric Cardiology (Vol 2)*. Mount Kisco, NY: Futura, (in press).

Lincoln C, Anderson RH, Shinebourne EA, et al. Double outlet right ventricle with 1-malposition of the aorta. *Br Heart J* 1975;37:453–463.

Milanesi O, Thiene G, Bini RM, Pellegrino PA. Complete transposition of great arteries with coarctation of aorta. *Br Heart J* 1982;48:566–571.

Milo S, Ho SY, Macartney FJ, et al. Straddling and overriding atrioventricular valves morphology and classification. *Am J Cardiol* 1979; 44:1122–1134.

Rossi BM, Ho SY, Anderson RH, et al. Coronary arteries in complete transposition: The significance of the sinus node artery. *Ann Thorac Surg* 1986;42:573–577.

Smith A, Arnold R, Wilkinson JL, et al. An anatomical study of the patterns of the coronary arteries and sinus nodal artery in complete transposition. *Int J Cardiol* 1986;12:295–304.

Smith A, Wilkinson JL, Anderson RH, et al. Architecture of the ventricular mass and atrioventricular valves in complete transposition with intact septum compared with the normal: I. The left ventricle, mitral valve, and the interventricular septum. *Paediatr Cardiol* 1986;6:253–257.

Soto B, Becker AE, Moulaert AJ, et al. Classification of ventricular septal defects. *Br Heart J* 1980;43:332–343.

Tynan MJ, Anderson RH. Terminology of transposition of the great arteries. In Godman MJ, Marquis RM (Eds): *Paediatric Cardiology. Vol 2. Heart Disease in the Newborn*. Edinburgh: Churchill Livingstone, 1979:341–349.

Van Praagh R, Perez-Trevino C, Lopez-Cuellar M, et al. Transposition of the great arteries with posterior aorta, anterior pulmonary artery, subpulmonary conus and fibrous continuity between aortic and atrioventricular valves. *Am J Cardiol* 1971;28:621–631.

Vetter V, Tanner C, Hardy C. Electrophysiologic studies after arterial switch repair of D-transposition of the great arteries. *J Am Coll Cardiol* 1987;9:165A.

Waldman JD, Schneeweiss A, Edwards WD, et al. The obstructive subaortic conus. *Circulation* 1984;70:339–344.

Wilcox BR, Henry GW, Anderson RH. The transmitral approach to left ventricular outflow tract obstruction. *Ann Thorac Surg* 1983;35:288–293.

Wilkinson JL, Arnold R, Anderson RH, Acerete F. "Posterior" transposition reconsidered. *Br Heart J* 1975;37:757–766.

Yacoub MH, Radley-Smith R. Anatomy of the coronary arteries in transposition of the great arteries and methods for their transfer in anatomical correction. *Thorax* 1978;33:418–424.

4.3

Complete Transposition: Physiological Considerations on the Neonatal Transition

Julien I. E. Hoffman, Michael A. Heymann, and Abraham M. Rudolph

Before birth, the fetus with complete transposition (concordant atrioventricular and discordant ventriculoarterial connections) has no known cardiovascular disability. There are, however, some differences from normal. The normal lamb fetus ejects about 65% of the combined ventricular output from the right ventricle into the pulmonary trunk which distributes a small proportion to the lungs (about 10% of the combined ventricular output at term) and delivers the rest to the descending aorta through the arterial duct (ductus arteriosus). This blood has an arterial oxygen tension of about 18 mmHg. The remaining 35% of the combined ventricular output is ejected by the left ventricle into the ascending aorta. About 23% of the combined ventricular output with an oxygen tension of about 24 mmHg is distributed to the head and upper limbs, and about 12% crosses the aortic isthmus into the descending aorta (Heymann et al., 1973; Rudolph, 1974; Rudolph and Heymann, 1970). Because there is more flow to the developing brain in the human than in the lamb fetus, proportionately more of the combined ventricular output in the human fetus is ejected by the left ventricle. On the reasonable assumption that the flow per gram of brain is similar in human and lamb fetuses, it is possible to calculate what the total flow to the brain would be in each species and hence to assess the relative outputs of right and left ventricles in the human fetus. This calculation suggests that the right ventricle in the

Supported in part by Program Project Grants HL 24056 and 25847 from the United States Public Health Service and by BRSG Grant SO7 RR05355 awarded by the Biomedical Research Support Program, Division of Research Resources, National Institutes of Health.

From: Anderson, RH, Neches, WH, Park, SC, Zuberbuhler, JR, eds: *Perspectives in Pediatric Cardiology*: Mount Kisco, New York, Futura Publishing Co., © 1988.

human fetus near term ejects about 55% of the combined ventricular output, a proportion matched by that obtained by echocardiographic-Doppler studies of human fetuses (Meijboom et al., 1985; Sahn et al., 1980).

If there is complete transposition, then the right ventricle ejects blood into the ascending aorta so that the head and upper limbs receive blood at the lower oxygen tension of 18 mmHg, whereas the left ventricle ejects blood with the higher oxygen tension of 24 mmHg into the pulmonary arteries. Because pulmonary vascular resistance is very sensitive to oxygen tension in the fetus, pulmonary blood flows may be higher in fetuses with transposition than in those with normal hearts. There is no information about the outputs of each ventricle when there is transposition. If we argue that outputs are determined primarily by afterload (Rudolph and Heymann, 1973; Thornburg and Morton, 1983), then the proportions of right and left ventricular outputs might be reversed in the setting of complete transposition. On the other hand, if outputs are determined largely by the venous return to each ventricle, then the ascending aorta will receive more than it normally does. Consequently, the residual flow across the aortic isthmus could be increased to about 20% of combined ventricular output. This may explain why the aortic isthmus is usually wide in newborn infants with complete transposition, and why associated coarctation of the aorta is so rare in them.

After birth, many of the normal neonatal transitional changes tend to take place. Pulmonary vascular resistance falls and flow into the left atrium increases. Systemic vascular resistance rises because of removal of the low-resistance placental circulation. In the normal infant these changes raise left more than right atrial pressures and so tend to close the flap valve of the foramen ovale. In the infant with complete transposition, the changes in pulmonary vascular resistance and pulmonary flow cause left atrial pressure to rise, as in normal infants, but the

rise in systemic vascular resistance causes right atrial pressure to rise as well. The similarity of atrial pressures therefore tends to keep the foramen ovale open and permits continued right-to-left atrial shunting. The disparity between aortic and pulmonary arterial pressures and resistances facilitates aortic-to-pulmonary shunting. Both of these changes result in flow of desaturated systemic venous blood into the pulmonary circuit where it can be oxygenated. In complete transposition, however, there must also be shunting of oxygenated blood into the systemic circulation. And, in the absence of a ventricular septal defect, this shunting must occur at the duct or atrial levels. When the arterial duct is widely open in the immediate newborn period, then during systole left ventricular ejection imparts enough kinetic energy to the blood that some of the left ventricular ejectate passes through the duct into the descending aorta, thus introducing oxygenated blood into the systemic circulation (Rudolph, 1986). During diastole, aortic blood enters the pulmonary circulation because of its lower vascular resistance. At this stage, the infant can get enough interchange between the two circulations to be minimally cyanotic and to avoid severe hypoxemia. Eventually, however, the arterial duct begins to close, so that bidirectional shunting through it diminishes in importance. What happens then depends on how much bidirectional shunting occurs through the foramen ovale. If the valve of the foramen ovale is incompetent and the foramen itself is large, then an adequate bidirectional shunt can occur to sustain systemic oxygenation at a safe level. During ventricular diastole, blood shunts from right into left atrium because of the lower resistance to filling of the left ventricle, whereas in ventricular systole blood shunts from left into right atrium because the left atrium is less distensible than is the right atrium and has the higher pressures at that phase of the cycle (Carr, 1971; Kjellberg et al., 1959). If, on the other hand, the foramen is small or its valve is competent, then only a small right-to-left atrial shunt can occur, left atrial pressure will rise, and the infant will become severely hypoxemic.

At the time when oxygen delivery to the tissues is beginning to decrease because of closing of the arterial duct, other major changes are taking place. Before birth, the combined cardiac output of the two ventricles in fetal lambs is about 500 ml/min/kg body weight (Rudolph and Heymann, 1970). Of this amount, about 300 ml/min/kg goes to the body. Immediately after birth the flow to the body (left ventricular output) is 300–400 ml/min/kg, so that combined ventricular output rises to about 600–800 ml/min/kg depending on ambient temperature (Klopfenstein and Rudolph, 1978; Sidi et al., 1983). Therefore, combined ventricular output (excluding flow to the placenta) almost doubles. At the same time, oxygen consumption per kilogram of body weight doubles, related to increased metabolism, the need to maintain body temperature, increased body movement (including the increased work of breathing), and beta-adrenergic receptor stimulation (Breall et al., 1984; Lister et al., 1979). (Should the infant be exposed to a low ambient temperature, then oxygen consumption may rise even more, largely in response to nonshivering thermogenesis [Adamson et al., 1965; Bruck, 1970; Dawkins and Hull, 1964; Hey, 1969; Hey and Katz 1970]. It is thus particularly important to maintain a neutral thermal environment in these infants.) Because of these changes, there is a markedly increased requirement for oxygen delivery to the tissues in the immediate postnatal period. In infants with complete transposition, this increased oxygen demand comes at a time when closure of the arterial duct may prevent the infant from being able to supply the oxygen that is needed. Furthermore, in newborn infants there is still a high proportion of fetal hemoglobin which, because of its increased avidity for oxygen, limits oxygen extraction by the tissues. For example, in the fetal lamb near term, it takes 37.5 ml of flow to the fetal body to supply 1 ml of oxygen. One week after birth, despite the high oxygen demand, it takes only 28.5 ml of flow to the body to supply 1 ml of oxygen. By six weeks after birth, the flow needed to supply 1 ml of oxygen to the body is only 19 ml (Klopfenstein and Rudolph, 1978).

Because of the low arterial oxygen tension and saturation, there will be some peripheral vasodilation in these infants. Systemic blood flow therefore tends to be raised. The increased cardiac output, however, is not sufficient to produce a severe volume overload of the right ventricle, and congestive heart failure is usually not seen with simple complete transposition. On the other hand, the arterial hypoxemia has certain important metabolic consequences. If hypoxemia becomes severe—and this frequently occurs in these infants—then metabolically active tissues like the kidneys, liver, and brain have to turn to anaerobic metabolism. They then use glycolysis to generate sufficient adenosine triphosphatase (ATP) to sustain mechanical and biochemical processes. Because glycolysis is relatively inefficient in generating the triphosphatase (one molecule of glucose yields six molecules of ATP by anaerobic glycolysis but 36 molecules of ATP by aerobic oxidation via the Krebs cycle), there is excess glucose utilization by all tissues and also excess lactate production. Consequently, the glucose that is stored in the liver as glycogen begins to be depleted rapidly. This event may be catastrophic for the brain. At rest, when skeletal muscles are not active, the brain in the newborn infant uses about 70% of the total body oxygen consumption (Holliday, 1971) and 95% or more of the total production of glucose by the liver (Bier et al., 1977). Severe hypoxemia and an increased glycolytic rate, therefore, may deplete the brain of its supply of oxygen and glucose with resultant damage to the nervous system. A second consequence of hypoxemia and accelerated glycolysis is the production of excess lactate. Normally, lactate produced in the body by metabolism is transported to the liver where it is converted back to glucose. When there is severe hypoxemia, however, this conversion may not occur. Lactate accumulates in the blood, the pH falls in blood and tissues, and impaired cellular function occurs. Given the deleterious changes that are likely to occur postnatally, it is no wonder that the natural history of untreated complete transposition is so bad, and that the introduction of balloon atrial septostomy produced such a major improvement in these infants.

References

Adamsons K Jr, Gandy GM, James LS. The influence of thermal factors upon oxygen consumption of the newborn human infant. *J Pediatr* 1965;66:495–508.

Bier DM, Leake RD, Haymond MW, et al. Measurement of "true" glucose production rates in infancy and childhood with 6,6-dideuteroglucose. *Diabetes* 1977;26:1016–1023.

Breall JA, Rudolph AM, Heymann MA. Role of thyroid hormone in postnatal circulatory and metabolic adjustments. *J Clin Invest* 1984; 73:1418–1424.

Bruck K. Heat production and temperature regulation. In Steve U (Ed): *Physiology of the Perinatal Period*. New York: Appleton-Century-Crofts, 1970.

Carr I. Timing of bidirectional atrial shunts in transposition of the great arteries and atrial septal defect. *Circulation* 1971;44 (Suppl II):70.

Dawkins MJR, Hull D. Brown adipose tissue and the response of new-born rabbits to cold. *J Physiol* 1964;172:216–238.

Hey EN. The relation between environmental temperature and oxygen consumption in the newborn baby. *J Physiol* 1969;200:589–603.

Hey EN, O'Connell B. Oxygen consumption and heat balance in the cot-nursed baby. *Arch Dis Child* 1970;45:335–343.

Heymann MA, Creasy RK, Rudolph AM. Quantitation of blood flow patterns in the foetal lamb

in utero. In Comline KS, Cross KW, Dawes GS, Nathanielsz PW (Eds): *Foetal and Neonatal Physiology: Proceedings of the Sir Joseph Barcroft Centenary Symposium*. Cambridge: Cambridge University Press, 1973:129–135.

Holliday MA. Metabolic rate and organ size during growth from infancy to maturity and during late gestation and early infancy. *Pediatrics* 1971;47:169–179.

Kjellberg SR, Mannheimer E, Rudhe U. *Diagnosis of Congenital Disease*. Chicago: Year Book Publishers, 1959.

Klopfenstein HS, Rudolph AM. Postnatal changes in the circulation and responses to volume loading in sheep. *Circ Res* 1978;42:839–845.

Lister G, Walter TK, Versmold HT, et al. Oxygen delivery in lambs: Cardiovascular and hematologic development. *Am J Physiol* 1979;237:H668–H675.

Meijboom EJ, de Smedt MCH, Visser GHA. Cross-sectional Doppler echocardiographic evaluation of the fetal cardiac output during the second and third trimesters of pregnancy: A longitudinal study. In Jones CT, Nathanielsz PW (Eds): *The Physiological Development of the Fetus and the Newborn*. London: Academic Press, 1985:749–752.

Rudolph AM. *Congenital Diseases of the Heart*. Chicago: Year Book Medical Publishers, 1974.

Rudolph AM. Aortopulmonary (complete) transposition—medical and surgical treatment during the first week of life. In Marcelletti C, Anderson RH, Becker AE, et al. (Eds): *Paediatric Cardiology*. Edinburgh: Churchill Livingstone, 1986;6:298–306.

Rudolph AM, Heymann MA. Circulatory changes during growth in fetal lamb. *Circ Res* 1970;26:289–299.

Sahn DJ, Lange LW, Allen HW, et al. Quantitative real-time cross-sectional echocardiography in the developing normal human fetus and newborn. *Circulation* 1980;62:588–597.

Sidi D Kuipers, JRG Heymann, MA, Rudolph AM. Effects of ambient temperature on oxygen consumption and the circulation in newborn lambs at rest and during hypoxemia. *Pediatr Res* 1983;17:254–258.

Thornburg KL, Morton MJ. Filling and arterial pressures as determinants of RV stroke volume in the sheep fetus. *Am J Physiol* 1983;244:H656–H663.

Techniques for Atrial Septostomy

Sang C. Park

Balloon Atrial Septostomy

Balloon atrial septostomy was enthusiastically accepted when it was introduced by Rashkind and Miller in 1966. Its development was an important historical milestone, since it was the first therapeutic intervention in the pediatric cardiac catheterization laboratory. The procedure has been widely used with great success and has been regarded as the initial procedure of choice in all patients with complete transposition (the combination of concordant atrioventricular and discordant ventriculoarterial connections).

Types of Balloon Septostomy Catheter

Early catheters had a bulky balloon section that made it difficult to introduce the catheter into the femoral vein. The first balloons frequently ruptured and, on at least one occasion, the proximal tie slipped distal to the side hole, making it impossible to deflate the balloon. With time, the construction and quality of the balloon catheters improved considerably. The latest Rashkind septostomy catheter (USCI) has a recessed balloon that can be passed through a 6 Fr sheath. Its balloon capacity is 2 ml and it attains a maximum diameter of 12 mm (Fig. 1). The Fogarty septostomy catheter (American Edwards Laboratory) has a 1.8 ml capacity but requires a 7 Fr sheath (Fig. 1). An especially large balloon septostomy catheter with a 4 ml capacity Miller septostomy catheter (American Edwards Laboratory) can be obtained on special order. It has a maximum diameter of 16 mm (Fig. 1) and can be used when it is desired to achieve a large interatrial opening. An 8 Fr sheath is required for introduction of this catheter. It is important to use a sheath with a built-in back bleeding control device to prevent excessive blood loss occurring due to the discrepancy between the sizes of the sheath lumen and the catheter.

Approach

The femoral vein has been the conventional approach, but the umbilical vein can be an alternative site of access in the new-

From: Anderson, RH, Neches, WH, Park, SC, Zuberbuhler, JR, eds: *Perspectives in Pediatric Cardiology*: Mount Kisco, New York, Futura Publishing Co., © 1988.

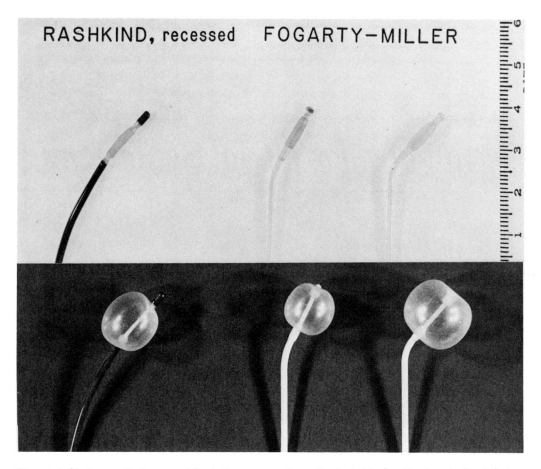

Figure 1. Various catheters used for balloon septostomy illustrated before (top) and after inflation (bottom).

born less than three to four days of age in whom there has been no anatomical closure of the venous duct. Access to the umbilical vein is not predictable and maneuvering the catheter is often difficult, since a sharp angulation between the umbilical and the inferior caval veins must be negotiated. Despite these limitations, balloon septostomy via the umbilical vein has been as effective and as safe as that through the femoral vein (Kaye et al., 1974; Newfeld et al., 1974; Rosuin et al., 1984). Some prefer the umbilical venous approach since it avoids the possibility of ileofemoral vein thrombosis, which may occur following balloon atrial septostomy (Hawker et al., 1971; Mathews et al., 1979). If a percutaneous sheath is used for

the umbilical approach, a sheath with a back bleeding control device should again be used routinely to avoid excessive blood loss or air embolism.

Guidance

In the past, fluoroscopic guidance has been the standard technique. Cross-sectional echocardiography, however, has recently been used as the sole imaging method for balloon septostomy in the newborn nursery or intensive care unit (Allan et al., 1982; Baker et al., 1984, Bullaboy et al., 1984; Steeg et al., 1985). Unfortunately, he-

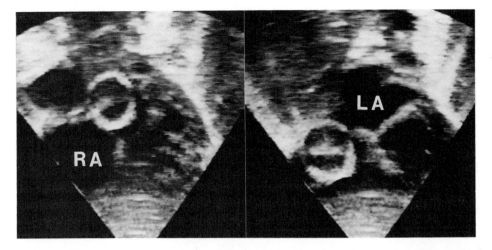

Figure 2. Cross-sectional echocardiography from the subcostal approach demonstrating the balloon portion of a septostomy catheter within the left atrium (LA) and the right atrium (RA).

modynamic evaluation and/or angiocardiography cannot be accomplished in this setting, should it unexpectedly become indicated. Some have advocated combined fluoroscopy and cross-sectional echo guidance in the cardiac catheterization laboratory (Lin et al., 1986; Perry et al., 1982). The location of the balloon catheter in the cardiovascular system can be readily confirmed by echo study (Fig. 2) and radiation exposure minimized. The availability of a cardiac catheterization laboratory and geographic limitations are the determining factors in deciding on either echocardiographic guidance alone or fluoroscopic guidance in the cardiac catheterization laboratory.

Procedure

Once the decision has been made to proceed with balloon septostomy, an appropriate-sized balloon catheter is selected. A 2 ml balloon is generally adequate in children under one year of age or less than 10 kg of body weight. A 4 ml balloon catheter is recommended in older children. Once the balloon catheter tip is placed in the left atrium, the balloon should be inflated

slowly to prevent inadvertent rupture of a pulmonary vein or the left atrial appendage. The balloon should be withdrawn to the right atrium as soon as the balloon has been fully inflated to its maximum size in order to prevent blockage of pulmonary venous return and consequent bradycardia. The essence of the balloon septostomy maneuver is not simply a steady withdrawal of the catheter into the right atrium, but more a distinctly jerky motion. To practice this maneuver, form a fist with the thumb and index fingertips together and pretend to hold the balloon catheter. Then, place the hand along a table edge with a distance of 5 cm between the ulnar surface of the fist and the table edge. Move the fist toward the table edge as quickly as possible, coming as close as possible to the table without contacting it. This type of motion results in a jerky movement of the fist. When reproduced during balloon septostomy, it will prevent the inadvertent passage of the inflated balloon into the inferior caval vein. In general, this withdrawal maneuver is performed several times to ensure an adequate tear of the atrial septum. To estimate the size of the interatrial communication before and after septostomy, a balloon catheter is inflated in the left atrium to a diameter

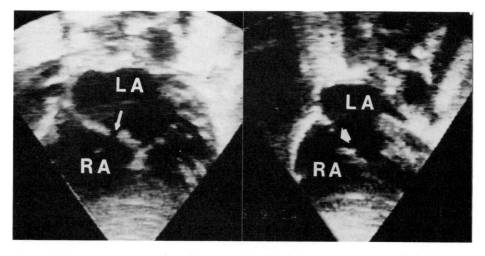

Figure 3. Cross-sectional echocardiography from the subcostal view in a patient with complete transposition prior to balloon atrial septostomy (left) and after the procedure (right), demonstrating enlargement of the interatrial communication (arrows).

larger than that of interatrial communication and is gently pulled against the atrial septum. The balloon is then gradually deflated until it passes through the defect, recording the passage on video and/or cineangiogram. A calibrated measuring grid is also recorded at the level of the right atrium to calculate the magnification factor. A measured interatrial communication greater than 12 mm is regarded as a good therapeutic result. One under 8 mm is usually inadequate. A cross-sectional echocardiographic study facilitates the measurement of interatrial opening (Fig. 3). The assessment of the opening tends to give lower values when studied by echocardiographic measurement than by balloon withdrawal. If the echocardiographic measurement of the interatrial opening is greater than 8 mm, the opening should be adequate. Less than 5 mm is inadequate. The change in arterial oxygen saturation is another important criterion of success.

62% (Hawker et al., 1974) to 89% (Neches et al., 1973) of cases. In the early years of its use, there were frequent complications (9%; Baker et al., 1971) including a mortality rate of 2% (Neches et al., 1973). Most of the complications reported in the early stage of this procedure were related to malfunction of the balloon, such as rupture or inability to deflate the balloon (Scott, 1970; Williams et al., 1970). Such complications have been reduced with improvement in quality of balloon construction but still occasionally occur (Blanchard et al., 1983).

Despite the availability of good catheters and experienced operators, we find it impossible to create an adequate interatrial communication in approximately one-fifth of patients with complete transposition. Failure to create an adequate interatrial communication is largely related to a thickened atrial septum which cannot be torn. Repeat balloon septostomy has rarely been effective in our hands (Baker et al., 1971).

Complications and Results

The initial success of balloon atrial septostomy has been reported to vary from

Blade Atrial Septostomy

To overcome the limitations of balloon atrial septostomy indicated in the previous section, we developed a technique of blade atrial septostomy (Park et al., 1975). Animal studies established its efficacy and safety. Clinical use of this technique was successful initially in a limited number of patients (Park et al., 1978). Following an extensive collaborative study among multiple centers (Park et al., 1982), the procedure is now widely used both in the United States and abroad. (Lin et al., 1986; Rao 1984; Perry et al., 1986; Ward et al., 1986). The technique has also been used in an adult with primary pulmonary hypertension and right-sided heart failure (Rich et al., 1983).

Procedure and Technique

The details of the technique are well described in our previous communication (Park et al., 1982). Initially, only a catheter with a 12 mm blade was available for general use. Subsequently, 16 mm and 21 mm blade catheters (Cook, Inc.) have become available and can be used in older children in whom a larger interatrial communication is required. Excessive blood loss was an occasional problem in the early stage of development of this technique. This was a particular problem when the procedure was done using the percutaneous technique and there was mismatch between the size of the catheter and the luminal diameter of the percutaneous sheath. Development of a percutaneous sheath with a device that controls back bleeding has largely eliminated this problem. A recessed balloon catheter is also helpful, since this arrangement gives a more appropriate match with the sheath size.

The blade catheter has a long straight metal component that has a slight angulation between its tip and the catheter proper (Fig. 4). This arrangement may cause difficulty in passing the tip of the catheter into the left atrium, particularly in a patient with a small left atrium or an unusual location of the interatrial communication (Fig. 4). In this situation, a long percutaneous sheath

such as the Mullins transseptal sheath (USCI), is helpful for introduction of the catheter tip into the left atrium. Prior to introduction, the length of the sheath should be carefully measured to ensure that the balloon catheter will protrude beyond its distal end. If the sheath is too long, it can be cut off. Even with the standard 6 Fr blade catheter, a 7 Fr sheath is recommended to permit easy manipulation within the sheath. Intermittent or slow continuous infusion of intravenous fluid through the side port of the sheath is desirable. This prevents both the possibility of air embolism (due to air entrapment during catheter exchange) and thrombus formation within the sheath.

The sheath is introduced into the right atrium using a conventional guidewire and a long dilator (Fig. 5-1). The wire and dilator are then removed and a regular woven Dacron catheter is introduced into the sheath and passed into the left atrium (Fig. 5-2). The sheath is then slipped over the catheter into the left atrium and the regular catheter is withdrawn, leaving only the tip of the sheath within the left atrium (Fig. 5-3). The blade septostomy catheter is then passed through the sheath into the left atrium (Fig. 5-4). The sheath is withdrawn while the tip of the blade catheter remains in the left atrium. The blade component can now be opened and rotated in a counterclockwise direction so that the blade faces anteriorly in the lateral fluoroscopic view. Gentle but steady force is maintained until a sudden loss of resistance is felt and the catheter passes into the right atrium. If the atrial septum is unusually thick and tough, the blade may reach to the level of diaphragm before it "pops." The maneuver is safe, nonetheless, as long as resistance is met in the usual midportion of the atrium and there is no loss of resistance or sudden change of angulation during traction. We recommend several passes of the blade catheter across the atrial septum with a slightly different angulation each time to ensure multiple cuts. A balloon septostomy catheter is then introduced into the left

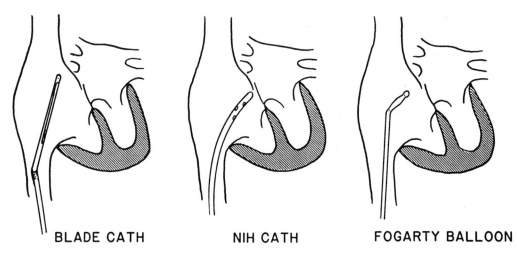

BLADE CATH   NIH CATH   FOGARTY BALLOON

Figure 4. A catheter for blade septostomy positioned in the right atrium showing a long straight metal component and minimal angulation. The woven Dacron NIH and Fogarty balloon septostomy catheters have a gentle curve at the tip.

atrium (Fig. 5-6 and 5-7) and balloon septostomy is performed in the usual fashion, this procedure further enlarging the newly created interatrial communication (Fig. 5-8). It is important to emphasize that during blade or balloon septostomy, the sheath and

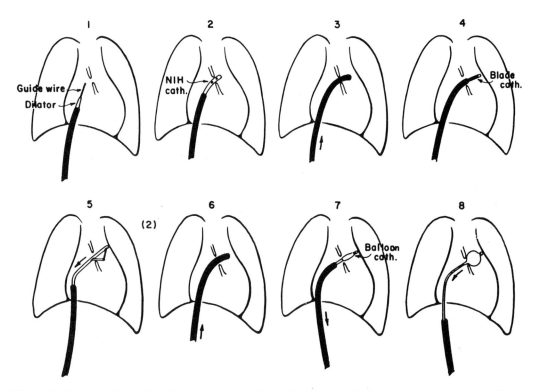

Figure 5. Diagrams illustrating the use of a long sheath for blade and balloon atrial septostomies. (See text for further discussion of insertion of catheters.)

the septostomy catheter must be pulled in unison so that the distal tip of the long sheath is not damaged during septostomy. In patients with an intact atrial septum or with an unusual location of the interatrial communication, the left atrium can be entered by transseptal puncture prior to blade septostomy.

Indications for Blade Atrial Septostomy

Balloon atrial septostomy is the procedure of choice in the majority of patients, particularly newborns, who have complete transposition. Blade atrial septostomy, however, is recommended in several conditions. It may be required subsequent to failure of an initial balloon atrial septostomy. Alternatively, it may be needed in patients over one month of age in whom the interatrial septum is anticipated as being too thick to be torn by a balloon. A further indication is presence of an unusually thickened interatrial septum as determined echocardiographically. This holds even if the patient is a neonate. Finally, blade septostomy may be indicated in patients with intact atrial septum, this indication necessitating additional use of the transseptal technique.

Complications and Results

In our early experience with blade septostomy, we conducted the procedure with the blade component facing superiorly in the first instance. Complete rotation of the catheter tip was then required after the blade was opened. This was not ideal, so we modified the design of the catheter to permit the blade to protrude toward the inferior and concave aspect of the curved catheter tip. This arrangement promoted considerably less chance of cardiac damage. Blood

loss from mismatch between the sheath size and balloon catheter was also a problem, but this complication was eliminated with use of sheaths to control back bleeding. The incidence of insult to the central nervous system following the procedure has also decreased, probably because the back bleeding control device not only controls blood loss but also prevents air embolism during catheter exchanges, particularly with a long sheath. As indicated above, the blade catheter has a straight metal component that is often difficult to pass into the left atrium, particularly in small infants or in patients with an unusual location of the interatrial communication. Prolonged manipulation of the catheter within the heart can result in perforation of either the right atrium (Ward et al., 1986) or the right ventricle (Park et al., 1982). A fatal outcome for this complication, however, is rare, and only one death was encountered in our early experience with the procedure. The introduction of a long sheath virtually eliminated the problem of prolonged catheter manipulation. Catheter malfunction has occurred occasionally. Difficulty in retracting the blade component back into the catheter lumen is probably related to opening the blade beyond the recommended level. Thus, careful inspection and trial attempts at opening the blade are essential prior to introduction of the catheter into the patient. Intermittent or slow continuous infusion of heparinized fluid through the side port of the blade catheter will prevent clot formation that might interfere with retraction of the blade component into the catheter lumen. Despite these precautions, certain limitations of blade septostomy remain. If the left atrial diameter is smaller than 2 cm, the blade cannot be opened within the left atrium. This occurs most frequently in patients with mitral and/or aortic atresia complex and is rare in the setting of complete transposition.

Blade septostomy produced clinical improvement in 79% of the patients in a recent collaborative study (Park et al., 1982) who had various cardiac malformations. A recent survey of board-certified pediatric cardiologists indicated that their overall experience with blade septostomy has been limited in both duration and number of cases treated (unpublished data, Park et al., 1986). The survey indicated, nonetheless, that the procedure was effective in the majority of cases and that complications were rare. With further experience and availability of various sizes of blade catheters and supportive accessories (such as long sheaths and back bleeding control devices), the technique should become increasingly safe and effective.

Management Following the Septostomy Procedure

Adequacy of the interatrial communication achieved can be evaluated by sizing with a withdrawal of a balloon catheter from the left atrium to the right atrium or by cross-sectional echocardiography. When either balloon and/or blade septostomy is performed, the interatrial communication can be adequately enlarged to greater than 10 mm diameter in almost all patients with complete transposition. A number (10–15%) of patients, however, experience persistent hypoxemia following the septostomy procedure despite an adequate interatrial communication. Expansion of intravascular volume using transfusion of packed cells or plasma may promote interatrial mixing, especially but not exclusively in patients who have experienced excessive blood loss. Prostaglandin E_1 has also been used (Beitzke et al., 1983; Henry et al., 1981; Weldon et al., 1983). This agent promotes atrial mixing by increasing ductal flow and by reducing pulmonary vascular resistance. If the patient responds, prostaglandin may be continued for 48 to 72 hours. If the response is unsatisfactory despite an adequate interatrial communication, definitive surgical repair should be considered.

Conclusions

Nonsurgical procedures achieving atrial septostomy have made a significant contribution to the overall survival of patients with complete transposition and with other cardiac defects where an adequate interatrial communication is essential for survival. A new experimental technique for septostomy using laser technology has been described (Bommer et al., 1983) but this has yet to be tested in clinical trials. The recent success of the "arterial switch" for neonatal surgical correction of transposition may make septostomy for this segmental combination unnecessary in the future. Until that time, nonsurgical septostomy techniques will continue to be useful, as they are in other congenital cardiac malformations in which an adequate interatrial communication is hemodynamically advantageous.

References

Allan LD, Leanage R, Wainwright R, et al. Balloon atrial septostomy under two dimensional echocardiographic control. Br Heart J 1982;4:41–43.

Baker F, Baker L, Zoltun R, Zuberbuhler JR. Effectiveness of the Rashkind procedure in transposition of the great arteries in infants. Circulation 1971;43 & 44(Suppl I):1–6.

Baker EJ, Allan LD, Tynan MJ, et al. Balloon atrial septostomy in the neonatal intensive care unit. Br Heart J 1984;51:337–338.

Beitzke A, Suppan CH. Use of prostaglandin E2 in management of transposition of great arteries before balloon atrial septostomy. Br Heart J 1983;49:341–344.

Blanchard WB, Knauf DG, Victorica BE. Interatrial groove tear: An unusual complication of balloon atrial septostomy. Pediatr Cardiol 1983;4:149–150.

Bommer WJ, Lee G, Riemenschneider TA, et al. Laser atrial septostomy. Am Heart J 1983; 106:1152–1156.

Bullaboy CA, Jennings RB Jr, Johnson DH. Bedside balloon atrial septostomy using echocardiographic monitoring. Am J Cardiol 1984;53:971.

Hawker RE, Celermajer JM, Cartmill TB, Bowdler JD. Thrombosis of the inferior vena cava following balloon septostomy in transposition of the great arteries. *Am Heart J* 1971;82:593–595.

Hawker RE, Krovetz LJ, Rowe RD. An analysis of prognostic factors in the outcome of balloon atrial septostomy for transposition of the great arteries. *Hopkins Med J* 1974;134:95–106.

Henry CG, Goldring D, Hartmann AF, et al. Treatment of d-transposition of the great arteries: Management of hypoxemia after balloon atrial septostomy. *Am J Cardiol* 1981;47:299–306.

Kaye HH, Tynan M. Balloon atrial septostomy via the umbilical vein. *Br Heart J* 1974;36:1040–1042.

Lin AE, Di Sessa TG, Williams RG. Balloon and blade atrial septostomy facilitated by two-dimensional echocardiography. *Am J Cardiol* 1986;57:273–277.

Mathews RA, Park SC, Neches WH, et al. Iliac venous thrombosis in infants and children after cardiac catheterization. *Cathet Cardiovasc Diagn* 1979;5:67–74.

Neches WH, Mullins CE, McNamara DG. Balloon atrial septostomy in congenital heart disease in infancy. *Am J Dis Child* 1973;125:371–375.

Newfeld EA, Purcell C, Paul MH, et al. Transumbilical balloon atrial septostomy in 16 infants with transposition of the great arteries. Pediatrics 1975;54:495–497.

Park SC, Zuberbuhler JR, Neches WH. A new atrial septostomy technique. *Cathet Cardiovasc Diagn* 1975;1:195–201.

Park SC, Neches WH, Zuberbuhler JR, et al. Clinical use of blade atrial septostomy. *Circulation* 1978;58:600–606.

Park SC, Neches WH, Mullins CE, et al. Blade atrial septostomy: Collaborative study. *Circulation* 1982;66:258–266.

Perry LW, Ruckman RN, Galioto FM Jr, Echocardiographically assisted balloon atrial septostomy. *Pediatrics* 1982;70:403–408.

Perry SB, Lang P, Keane JF, et al. Creation and maintenance of an adequate interatrial communication in left atrioventricular valve atresia or stenosis. *Am J Cardiol* 1986;58:622–626.

Rao PS. Transcatheter blade atrial septostomy. *Cathet Cardiovasc Diagn* 1984;10:335–342.

Rashkind WJ, Miller WW. Creation of an atrial septal defect without thoracotomy: Palliative approach to complete transposition of the great arteries. *JAMA* 1966;196:991–992.

Rich S, Lam W. Atrial septostomy as palliative therapy for refractory primary pulmonary hypertension. *Am J Cardiol* 1983;51:1560–1561.

Rosuin N, Sujov P, Montag J. Transumbilical balloon atrial septostomy for transposition of the great arteries in infants under the age of 60 hours. *Am Heart J* 1984;107:174–176.

Scott O. A new complication of Rashkind balloon septostomy. *Arch Dis Child* 1970;45:716–717.

Steeg CN, Bierman FZ, Hordof AJ, et al. Bedside balloon septostomy in infants with transposition of the great arteries: New concepts using two-dimensional echocardiographic techniques. *J Pediatr* 1985;107:944–946.

Ward KE, Mullins CE, Huhta JC, et al. Restrictive interatrial communication in total anomalous pulmonary venous connection. *Am J Cardiol* 1986;57:1131–1136.

Weldon CS, Hartmann AF Jr, Kelly JP. Current management of transposition of the great arteries: Immediate septostomy, occasional prostaglandin infusion, and early Senning operations. *Ann Thorac Surg* 1983;36:10–18.

Williams GD, Ahrend TR, Dungan WT. An unusual complication of balloon-catheter atrial septostomy.*Ann Thorac Surg* 1970;10:556–559.

Morbidity and Mortality in the First Year of Life

William H. Neches

The introduction of balloon atrial septostomy in the mid-1960s (Rashkind and Miller, 1966) was the single most important factor to influence the survival of the infant with complete transposition (the combination of concordant atrioventricular and discordant ventriculoarterial connections). Many other milestones have occurred over the last three decades that have had a major influence on the survival of these patients (Table 1). Systemic-to-pulmonary arterial anastomoses were developed in the mid-1940s (Blalock and Taussig, 1945; Potts et al., 1946), making it possible to improve pulmonary blood flow in those patients with pulmonary stenosis. Atrial septectomy became available in 1950 (Blalock and Hanlon, 1950) and this resulted in improved survival for those infants with an intact ventricular septum. Although the first atrial redirection procedure was also described toward the end of that decade (Senning, 1959), most surgeons were unable to perform this procedure successfully and it was therefore abandoned. A few years later, the

introduction of another interatrial redirection procedure (Mustard, 1964) revolutionized the approach toward the management of the patient with complete transposition. Widespread success with this procedure made it possible to repair the anomaly successfully and a much more aggressive approach to the management of the newborn and small infant with this disorder resulted.

With the development of balloon atrial septostomy, it became possible to palliate the young infant with complete transposition without an operation and with low risk. In the 1970s the development of blade septostomy (Park et al., 1975) and the arterial switch procedure (Jatene et al., 1976) modified our approach to these patients. Prostaglandin E_1 was introduced in 1977; its use improved oxygenation of newborns until palliative or definitive procedures can be performed.

It is becoming increasingly common in many centers, including our own, to attempt repair of complete transposition in the early months of life. To compare the results of

From: Anderson, RH, Neches, WH, Park, SC, Zuberbuhler, JR, eds: *Perspectives in Pediatric Cardiology*: Mount Kisco, New York, Futura Publishing Co., © 1988.

Table 1
Chronology of Management

1945: Blalock-Taussig and Potts anastomoses
1950: Blalock-Hanlon procedure
1959: Senning's operation
1964: Mustard's operation
1966: Rashkind balloon septostomy
1975: Park blade septostomy
1976: Jatene arterial switch
1977: Prostaglandin E_1

Table 2
Time Periods of Management, Children's Hospital of Pittsburgh

Period 1: 1953–1964
—Surgical atrial septectomy
—Systemic-to-pulmonary anastomosis
—Baffes procedure
—Senning's operation

Period 2: 1965–1974
—Balloon septostomy
—Mustard's operation

Period 3: 1975–1984
—Blade septostomy
—Prostaglandin E_1
—Profound hypothermia
—Senning's operation

this approach with other means of therapy, it is important to know the expected morbidity and mortality that prevail if operation is delayed until or beyond the end of the first year of life. This review describes our experience with all infants with complete transposition who were seen during their first year of life since the Pediatric Cardiology Division of Children's Hospital of Pittsburgh was founded in 1954. These three decades span three major eras in management (Table 2). The first period, from 1953 through 1964, constituted the prerepair era. Palliative surgical procedures were available as discussed above, and in addition, the Baffes procedure (Baffes, 1956) was attempted in a few patients but was largely unsuccessful. Although Senning's operation had been described, no patient under one year of age was submitted to this procedure in our center. The second period, 1965 through 1974, marked the introduction of balloon atrial septostomy and Mustard's operation; these procedures dramatically changed the survival of our patient population. In the third period, 1975 through 1984, profound hypothermia and circulatory arrest were used for the repair of all patients with complete transposition. The Senning operation again became popular in this period and was used in preference to the Mustard operation.

Although the major advances in therapy have been outlined above, it must be remembered that many improvements in other areas had a profound influence on the management, morbidity, and mortality of infants with complete transposition. During the second period, we became increasingly aware that, in addition to polycythemia, anemia or relative anemia were also important factors in the progress of the hypoxic infant. The early 1970s saw the development of intensive care units together with the specialty of critical care medicine, both of which factors improved survival of extremely ill patients before and after palliative or reparative procedures. Critical care facilities have continued to improve during the last decade and new inotropic agents have been developed. We have also seen a striking improvement in emergency transport facilities. Helicopter transport is now available in most tertiary referral centers and a team of skilled physicians and nurses can be sent to outlying areas to effect rapid and stable transport of critically ill patients.

Patient Population

Over the 32-year period of this investigation, 281 patients with complete transposition were seen at Children's Hospital of Pittsburgh (Table 3). In addition to a breakdown by time period, these patients are further divided according to the presence of

Table 3
Complete Transposition, Children's Hospital of Pittsburgh, 32 Years

Type	1953–1964	1965–1974	1975–1984	Total
IVS or small VSD	62	72	73	207 (74%)
VSD	14	20	13	47 (17%)
Complex	10	11	6	27 (9%)
Total	86	103	92	281 (100%)

IVS = intact interventricular septum; VSD = ventricular septal defect.

associated anomalies. The largest group, which contains 207 patients (74% of the total), have an intact interventricular septum or a small and hemodynamically insignificant ventricular septal defect. The next group of 47 patients (17%) had a large ventricular septal defect and pulmonary hypertension. The smallest group consisted of 27 patients (9%) with complex lesions defined as the association with ventricular septal defect and pulmonary stenosis. Two of these patients had associated stenosis of the tricuspid valve and hypoplasia of the right ventricle. Patients with double inlet ventricle, atrioventricular or arterial valve atresia, or those with atrial isomerism (heterotaxy syndromes) were not included in this study. As can be seen from the Table 3, the distribution was relatively similar among the three groups during the three periods.

Results

Complex Transposition

Our experience with patients with complex transposition (those with associated ventricular septal defect and pulmonary stenosis) parallels that of other centers (Table 4). Patients with this complex have a good balance between pulmonary and systemic blood flow and rarely exhibit either profound hypoxemia or congestive heart failure during the first year of life. In the first time period, 9 of the 10 patients required no procedure and all 10 patients survived the first year of life. Balloon atrial septostomy has been routinely performed in subsequent years at the time of the initial cardiac catheterization and, again, only a

Table 4
Complete Transposition: Complex Form (VSD + PS), Children's Hospital of Pittsburgh (n = 27)

Procedure	1953–1964	1965–1974	1975–1984
None	9 (9)	4 (4)	—
Atrial septectomy (AS)	—	1 (1)	—
Catheter septostomy (CS)	—	5 (5)	6 (6)*
CS + AS	—	—	—
Shunt	1 (1)	—	1 (1)*
AS + shunt	—	1 (0)	—
Repair	—	—	—
Total	10 (10)	11 (10)	6 (6)
	100%	91%	100%

( ) = survival to one year of age; * = one patient with CS + shunt; Shunt = systemic-to-pulmonary artery anastomosis; PS = pulmonary stenosis; VSD = ventricular septal defect.

Table 5
Complete Transposition and Ventricular Septal Defect, Children's Hospital of Pittsburgh (n = 47)

Procedure	1953–1964	1965–1974	1975–1984
None	6 (3)	—	—
Atrial septectomy (AS)	4 (2)	3 (2)	—
Catheter septostomy (CS)	—	1 (0)	2 (2)
PT banding	2 (1)	3 (2)	1 (0)
CS + PB	2 (1)	8 (5)	7 (7)
CS + AS + PB	—	3 (3)	—
PB + AS	—	2 (2)	—
CS + repair	—	—	3 (1)
Total	14 (7)	20 (14)	13 (10)
	50%	70%	77%

AS = atrial septostomy; CS = catheter septostomy; PT = pulmonary trunk; PB = banding of the pulmonary trunk.

few patients have required any additional palliative procedure. Although 26 of the 27 patients in this group survived until one year of age, the mortality in our center, as well as in others, occurred during childhood at the time of repair of this combination of lesions.

Association with Large Ventricular Septal Defect

The results in the 47 patients with ventricular septal defect are shown in Table 5. During the first time period, one-half of the patients did not survive to one year of age. In the second period (from 1965 to 1974), survival to one year of age increased to 70%. All patients had some form of palliative procedure, usually including banding of the pulmonary trunk. In the most recent period, survival improved further to 77%. Surgical atrial septectomy was largely abandoned in this small group but a few patients underwent catheter septostomy and subsequently had complete repair during the first year of life.

Patients with Intact Ventricular Septum

The third, and by far the largest group in this series was made up by the 207 patients with an intact ventricular septum (or a small ventricular septal defect) (Table 6). The outlook for these patients was dismal in the first time period, overall survival being only 35% (22 of the 62 patients). Twenty-four patients had no palliative procedures and most died. It is perhaps surprising that four of the patients in this group did survive until one year of age without any palliative procedures being performed. More than half of the patients had atrial septectomy but less than 50% of these survived. In the second time period, 10% of the patients had palliation alone by atrial septectomy. All procedures were performed during the early years of this time period prior to the availability of balloon septostomy. Again, a significant percentage of those patients treated did not survive. The remaining 65 patients in that group had balloon atrial septostomy. In 45 of these 65, this was the only palliative treatment required during the first year of life. Forty-two of these 45 patients survived.

Table 6

Complete Transposition with Intact Septum or Small VSD, Children's Hospital of Pittsburgh (n = 207)

Procedure	1953–1964	1965–1974	1975–1984
None	24 (4)	—	1 (0)
Atrial septectomy (AS)	37 (17)	7 (3)	—
Catheter septostomy (CS)	—	45 (42)	39 (32)
CS + AS	—	20 (18)	5 (5)
CS + shunt	1 (1)[+]	—	3 (3)
CS + repair	—	—	25 (24)
Total	62 (22)	72 (63)	73 (64)
	35%	88%	88%

( ) = survival to one year of age; + = shunt only during this period; Shunt = systemic-to-pulmonary arterial anastomosis; VSD = ventricular septal defect.

The remaining patients also had a surgical atrial septectomy during the first year of life. In contrast to the high mortality in patients with a primary atrial septectomy, 90% of these patients who had an atrial septectomy as a secondary procedure survived. It is likely that improved preoperative and postoperative care greatly enhanced survival but, in addition, these procedures were performed on older infants.

In the last time period, 72 of 73 patients underwent balloon atrial septostomy. In 39 of these (54%), a catheter septostomy (balloon and in some cases a subsequent blade septostomy) was the only palliation that was required in the first year of life. A few additional patients required either atrial septectomy or a systemic-to-pulmonary arterial anastomosis with no mortality in either group. With the advent in this period of profound hypothermia and circulatory arrest, 25 of the patients (35%) who had an initial catheter septostomy subsequently underwent complete repair during the first year of life. A Mustard operation was performed during the 1970s and, since the early 1980s, a Senning procedure. In the first half of this time period, the age for elective repair at our institution was between 12 and 15 months of age. Patients who required a secondary procedure during

the first year of life, however, usually underwent repair rather than a second attempt at palliation. In the second half of this time period we began electively to repair patients between 8 and 15 months of age. As a result, most of these patients had their repair electively under the age of one year rather than because of increasing cyanosis. Twenty-four of the 25 patients (96%) undergoing repair during this time period survived to one year of age. In the overall group of 73 patients, 64 (88%) survived. Although this seems to be no change from the survival rate in the previous time period, it must be remembered that 24 of these survivors (39%) had undergone complete repair.

In this latter time period, 7 of the 39 patients who underwent catheter septostomy as their only palliative procedure died some time during the first year of life. At first glance this seems to be excessive, especially when one considers the survival rate in patients who underwent other procedures during the same period. A number of additional factors must be considered. Although there has been considerable improvement in the care of the critically ill newborn infant, this very improvement has resulted in more referrals of such neonates, often with multiple anomalies, who previously would have died either at the referring institution or during transport. This is supported by the fact that, during the second period, balloon atrial septostomy was performed at a mean age of 13.7 days and that only two-thirds of the patients were less than one week of age at the time of the procedure. In contrast, during the third period, balloon atrial septostomy was performed at a mean age of 3.4 days and 96% of the procedures were performed on patients less than one week of age. Indeed, four-fifths were performed on the first day of life. Three of the deaths occurred during the early newborn period. One was a result of complications during balloon atrial septostomy, while the other two occurred in critically ill and extremely hypoxic newborns who were on mechanical ventilation prior to cardiac catheterization. Three additional patients had other major congenital anomalies which probably contributed to death during the first few months of life. The last patient who died did so suddenly at four months of age. Thus, there was a 12% mortality in this time period. Now, however, with the early recognition of the lesion, the ever-increasing abilities of critical care and the use of prostaglandin, mortality related to hypoxemia can be minimized and well over 90% survival should be expected.

Morbidity

The incidence of nonfatal complications is summarized in Table 7. Surprisingly, there were no serious nonfatal complications during the first time period. Despite this, only 39 of the 86 patients (45%) survived until one year of age. It is likely that most patients who suffered any serious complications during this interval died as a result of the complication. In the second time period, 87 of the 103 patients (84%) survived until one year of age. Three of these 87 patients had cerebrovascular acci-

Table 7
Complete Transposition: Morbidity,
1st Year of Life

Period 1: 1953–1964: 39/86 (45%) survivors
  None
Period 2: 1965–1974: 87/103 (84%)
  survivors
  CVA = 3 (2 Cath-related)
  Other vascular = 2 (1 Cath-related)
  Other CNS = 2
                7/87 (8%)
Period 3: 1975–1984: 80/92 (87%) survivors
  CVA = 8 (5 Cath-related)
  Other CNS = 1
                9/80 (11%)

CNS = central nervous system abnormality; CVA = cerebrovascular accident.

dents, two of these being related temporally to cardiac catheterization. Two additional patients had major vascular complications. Renal venous thrombosis occurred in one following cardiac catheterization and, in the other, a spontaneous thrombosis occurred at the bifurcation of the abdominal aorta. Two additional patients developed seizure disorders during the first year of life. Thus, of the 87 who survived during the second time period, 7 patients (8%) had significant morbidity. In the third time period, 80 of 92 patients (87%) survived until a year of age. Eight patients had a cerebrovascular accident during the first year of life; five of these were temporally related to cardiac catheterization, and two of these five patients were extremely ill and hypoxic neonates who suffered a major insult to their central nervous system subsequent to their initial cardiac catheterization. One additional patient had a cerebrovascular accident following a blade septostomy. This was prior to the availability of the side port sheath. Use of this sheath permits flushing with heparinized solution while the catheter is inserted. Prior to its use, it is likely that a thrombus formed in the sheath and embolized. Thus, nine of 80 patients surviving to one year of age (11%) had significant morbidity, all related to the central nervous system.

Summary

The outlook for patients with complete transposition has improved markedly over the last three decades. At present, survival until one year of age should be anticipated for well over 90% of the infants born with this disorder, achieved either subsequent to balloon septostomy alone or some combination of other palliative or reparative procedures. There is, however, a continued 10% incidence of serious complications, mostly neurological, during the first year of life. Thus, early operation either with balloon atrial septostomy followed by an atrial baffle procedure or an arterial switch operation is advisable in the neonatal period. If procedures are performed on hypoxemic patients, careful attention must be paid to even the smallest of details during cardiac catheterization in order to minimize hazards related to the procedure.

References

Baffes TG: A method for surgical correction of transposition of the aorta and pulmonary artery. *Surg Gynecol Obstetr* 1956;102:227–233.

Blalock A, Hanlon CR. The surgical treatment of complete transposition of the aorta and the pulmonary artery. *Surg Gyn Obst* 1950;90:1–15.

Blalock A, Taussig HB. The surgical treatment of malformations of the heart in which there is pulmonary stenosis or pulmonary atresia. *JAMA* 1945;128:189–198.

Jatene AD, Fontes VF, Paulista PP, et al. Anatomic correction of transposition of the great vessels. *J Thorac Cardiovasc Surg* 1976;72:364–370.

Mustard WT. Successful two-stage correction of transposition of the great vessels. *Surgery* 1964;55:469–472.

Park SC, Zuberbuhler JR, Neches WH, et al. A new atrial septostomy technique. *Cath Cardiovasc Diag* 1975;1:195–201.

Potts WJ, Smith S, Gibson S. Anastomosis of the aorta to a pulmonary artery. Certain types in congenital heart disease. *JAMA* 1946;132:627–631.

Rashkind WJ, Miller WW. Creation of an atrial septal defect without thoracotomy. A palliative approach to complete transposition of the great arteries. *JAMA* 1966;196:991–992.

Senning A. Surgical correction of transposition of the great vessels. *Surgery* 1959;45:966–980.

4.6

Assessment of Cardiac Rhythm Following Atrial Redirection Procedures

Lee B. Beerman, Robert A. Mathews,
Frederick J. Fricker, Donald R. Fischer,
William M. Gay, William H. Neches,
and James R. Zuberbuhler

The hemodynamic and functional results of the atrial redirection procedure for complete transposition (the combination of concordant atrioventricular and discordant ventriculoarterial connections) have generally been quite favorable and have resulted in good quality of life in the long-term survivors of the operation. Despite this, a major area of concern for these patients is the development of disturbances of cardiac rate and rhythm. Various studies have shown a wide range of arrhythmias in patients who have had the Mustard, or more recently the Senning, procedure with an incidence ranging between 13 and 100% (Beerman et al., 1983; Byrum et al., 1986; Clarkson et al., 1976; El-Said et al., 1972, 1976; Epstein et al., 1983; Flinn et al., 1984; Gillette et al., 1980; Hayes and Gersony, 1986; Saalouke et al., 1978; Southall et al., 1980; Vetter and Horowitz, 1982). The most commonly described abnormalities include sinus node dysfunction, supraventricular and ventricular ectopy, and atrioventricular conduction disturbances. The bradycardia-tachycardia syndrome is one of the more common arrhythmias that occurs and is illustrated by two rhythm strips from the same patient in Figure 1. This example shows a slow junctional rhythm alternating with episodes of atrial flutter. In this chapter, the results of a review of the electrophysiological function of 86 long-term survivors of the Mustard operation at our institution using surface

From: Anderson, RH, Neches, WH, Park, SC, Zuberbuhler, JR, eds: *Perspectives in Pediatric Cardiology*: Mount Kisco, New York, Futura Publishing Co., © 1988.

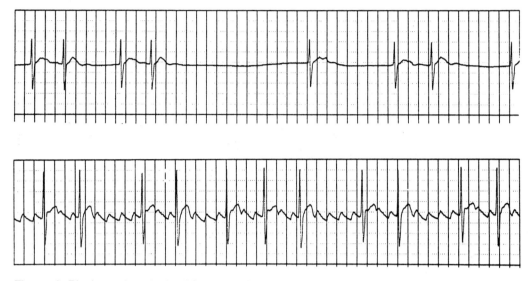

Figure 1. Rhythm strips obtained from a patient with complete transposition and the bradycardia-tachycardia syndrome. Top tracing demonstrates a slow junction rhythm with occasional atrial activity. Bottom tracing shows atrial flutter.

electrocardiography, Holter monitoring, exercise electrocardiograms, and intracardiac electrophysiological studies are presented. Data from a review of the short-term results of 30 survivors of the Senning operation are also presented.

Mustard Operation

Methods

The data from 86 long-term survivors of the Mustard operation performed at the Children's Hospital of Pittsburgh between 1965 and 1981 were analyzed. The current and all preceding surface electrocardiograms were reviewed in each patient and pertinent information regarding rhythm and conduction was tabulated. The mean duration of follow-up was 10.2 years with a range of 2 to 20.7 years. Twenty-four-hour ambulatory Holter monitors were obtained in 46 patients. A total of 78 studies were performed, including 20 patients with serial assessments of cardiac rhythm. The mean age at the time of the study was 13.6 years

with a range between 5.3 and 28.2 years. The interval from the time of operation until the study ranged between 4 and 20.7 years with a mean of 10 years. This group included 9 patients who were over the age of 18 years and 7 individuals who had been followed for more than 15 years since the Mustard operation.

Several criteria were used to detect abnormalities during the analysis of the surface electrocardiograms and Holter monitoring data. Sinus node dysfunction was defined as excessive sinus bradycardia for age, prolonged sinus pauses, or a non-sinus-node pacemaker occurring by default due to a slow sinus rate (Table 1). This latter category included junctional and ectopic atrial rhythms in addition to isorhythmic dissociation. Ventricular and supraventricular ectopy were characterized as either simple or complex. Simple ectopy was used to describe isolated premature beats occurring with a frequency of less than 30 per hour. Complex ectopy was defined as isolated premature beats occurring more frequently than 30 per hour, two or more consecutive ectopic beats, and, in the case of ventricular arrhythmias, ectopic beats of multiform

Table 1
Criteria for Sinus Node Dysfunction

1. Sinus Bradycardia

| | Heart rate (beats/min) | |
Age	Day	Night
>11 years	<50	<40
7 to 11 years	<55	<45
<7 years	<60	<50

2. Sinus Pauses
   Duration >3.0 seconds

3. Non-Sinus Pacemaker by Default
   Junctional rhythm
   Isorhythmic dissociation
   Ectopic atrial rhythm

configuration. The arrhythmia was categorized as simple if only rare couplets were noted in conjunction with infrequent isolated ectopy.

Intracardiac electrophysiological studies were performed in a total of 61 patients, either pre- or postoperatively or both. Standard procedures using one or two intracardiac electrode catheters were used for the atrial pacing studies and His-bundle recordings. The upper limits of normal in our laboratory for the A-H and H-V intervals are 120 and 55 msec, respectively. The development of atrioventricular block at an atrial pacing rate of 160 beats/min or less was considered abnormal. Sinus node function was assessed by the determination of corrected sinus node recovery time following rapid atrial pacing (absolute sinus node recovery time minus resting sinus cycle length). A value of greater than 275 msec or a non-sinus recovery time were defined as abnormal responses. Atrial extrastimulus studies were performed in a smaller number of patients (3 pre- and 10 postoperatively) in order to assess refractory periods of the atrium and atrioventricular node.

A total of 71 exercise tests were performed on 46 patients and the data from the exercise electrocardiography obtained were also analyzed.

Results

Surface Electrocardiogram

All patients had normal rate, rhythm, and conduction prior to the operation except for two individuals who had ectopic atrial rhythm and one with first-degree atrioventricular block. The results obtained from the review of the most recent electrocardiogram of these 86 patients are shown in Table 2. Normal sinus rhythm was present in only 39 of the patients (45%). By far the most common abnormality seen was sinus node dysfunction, which occurred in 29 patients (34%). Although atrioventricular block was noted in 10 (12%), it was usually of the first-degree pattern. A few patients had combinations of sinus node dysfunction, atrioventricular block, or ectopy, but either supraventricular or ventricular ectopic beats were very infrequent. The review of all previous electrocardiograms indicated there were 10 patients who had evidence of the bradycardia-tachycardia syndrome. In these patients, supraventricular tachycardia, usually atrial flutter, intermittently occurred in patients who had a slow junctional pacemaker as their dominant rhythm. The time of onset of sinus node dysfunction could be determined in 34 patients. There was a de-

Table 2
Arrhythmias Following Mustard Operation, Current Electrocardiogram

Normal sinus rhythm		39 (45%)
Sinus node dysfunction		29 (34%)
Atrioventricular block		10 (12%)
First-degree	8*	
Third-degree	2**	
SND + 1°AVB		2 (2%)
SND + PVC		1 (1%)
3° AVB + PVC		1 (1%)
PVC		2 (2%)
Supraventricular ectopy		1 (1%)
Atrial flutter		1 (1%)
Total		86 (100%)

* Includes two patients who currently have AAI pacemaker.
** One patient has VVI pacemaker.
AVB = atrioventricular block; SND = sinus node dysfunction; PVC = premature ventricular contractions.

layed onset beyond one year postoperatively in 46% of the patients and, in 9 of these patients (26%), rhythm abnormalities were not found until 5 years after the Mustard procedure.

Holter Monitor

The results of the 24-hour ambulatory recordings of an unselected subgroup of 46 patients are shown in Table 3. The same spectrum of abnormalities noted on the surface electrocardiograms are seen, although the incidence of these findings was considerably higher using Holter monitoring. Once again, sinus node dysfunction proved to be the most prevalent abnormality, being found in 27 patients (59%). Most of these patients had periods of sinus rhythm alternating with episodes of sinus node dysfunction. Only five of the 27 individuals had marked suppression of sinus node function throughout the 24-hour period with rare sinus activity. The incidence of ectopy, particularly ventricular, was strikingly more common during 24-hour recordings than would be expected from its infrequent presence on surface electrocardiograms. Over half (57%) of the patients had ventricular ectopy, ranging in severity from rare to complex. Although in 10 of these 26 patients it occurred only rarely

Table 3
Arrhythmias Following Mustard Operation, Holter Monitor (n = 46)

A. Sinus node dysfunction		27 (59%)
B. Atrioventricular block		8 (17%)
First-degree	3	
Second-degree	3	
Mobitz I	1	
Mobitz II	2	
Third-degree	2*	
C. Ventricular ectopy**		26 (57%)
Rare	10	
Simple	6	
Complex	10	
D. Supraventricular ectopy**		20 (43%)
Rare	6	
Simple	4	
Complex	10	
E. Normal***		8 (17%)

* VVI pacemaker in one patient.
** 17 patients had both ventricular and supraventricular ectopy.
*** Includes patients with only rare ectopy (<1/hour).

Table 4
Intracardiac Electrophysiology Following Mustard Operation, His-Bundle and Rapid Atrial Pacing

	AH interval >120 msec	HV interval >55 msec	RAP AVB ≤ 160/min
Preop	2 (6%) (n = 32)	1 (3%) (n = 32)	1 (3%) (n = 31)
Postop	1 (3%) (n = 32)	3 (9%) (n = 32)	8 (18%) (n = 45)

RAP = rapid atrial pacing.

(less than one isolated ectopic beat per hour), another 10 patients had complex ventricular ectopy. These rhythm disturbances were rarely, if ever, associated with symptoms. Supraventricular ectopy was present in 20 patients (43%) and was classified as complex in half of this group. Atrioventricular block occurred in 8 patients (17%) and was first-degree in 3, second-degree in 3, and third-degree in 2 patients. A combination of abnormalities was found in many patients and only 8 (17%) had completely normal 24-hour recordings.

Intracardiac Electrophysiology

Intracardiac electrophysiological studies were performed in 61 patients. The results of the His-bundle recordings and rapid atrial pacing are shown in Table 4. Abnormalities of A-H or H-V intervals were uncommon both before and after surgery. With rapid atrial pacing, atrioventricular block at an abnormally low rate occurred in only one patient (3%) preoperatively compared to 8 patients (18%) postoperatively. The results of sinus node function studies are depicted in Table 5. Only 2 of 29 (7%) preoperative patients had abnormal results, while 12 of 45 (27%) postoperative patients had either an abnormally prolonged corrected sinus node recovery time or an abnormal recovery site following cessation of rapid atrial pacing. An abnormality of the corrected sinus node recovery time was found in 67% of the patients who had evidence of sinus node dysfunction on either the surface electrocardiogram or Holter

Table 5
Intracardiac Electrophysiology Following Mustard Operation, Sinus Node Function

Normal CSNRT		33 (73%)
Abnormal CSNRT		12 (27%)
Prolonged CSNRT		6
275–500 msec	4	
>500 msec	2	
Abnormal recovery site		6
Junctional	3	
Ectopic atrial focus	3	
Total		45 (100%)

CSNRT = corrected sinus node recovery time.

Table 6
Intracardiac Electrophysiology Following Mustard Operation, Extrastimulus Studies

	Normal	Prolonged	Total
Refractory periods			
AERP or AFRP	9*	1 (10%)	10
AVNERP or AVNFRP	10	0 (0%)	
Intraatrial conduction			6
HRA-LSRA	4	2 (33%)	

* Three of these patients had values > 1 standard deviation above the mean.
AERP = atrial effective refractory period; AFRP = atrial functional refractory period; AVNERP = atrioventricular node effective refractory period; AVNFRP = atrioventricular node functional refractory period; HRA = high right atrium; LSRA = low septal right atrium.

monitor. However, there was imperfect correlation between intracardiac electrophysiology and these clinical studies. An abnormal electrophysiological result was found in 13% of patients with no evidence of abnormal sinus node function by electrocardiogram or Holter monitor studies, while 21% of those who had a normal corrected sinus node recovery time had sinus node dysfunction by clinical criteria. Atrial extrastimulus studies were performed in a relatively small number of patients; these results are shown in Table 6. Only one of 10 postoperative patients had prolongation of the atrial effective or functional refractory period greater than two standard deviations beyond the mean values for normal children as determined by Dubrow et al. (1975). The refractory periods of the atrioventricular node were within normal limits in all patients. There was prolongation of the intraatrial conduction time between the high right atrium and low septal right atrium in two of six patients (33%) after the operation.

Exercise Electrocardiography

The results of exercise electrocardiography of 46 patients are reported in an accompanying paper (Mathews et al., 1987). abnormal rhythms were found in 40% of the patients during exercise. Ventricular ec-

topy occurred in 11 patients (24%), including three who had Holter records that did not show ventricular arrhythmias.

Summary

When the results of all of the testing modalities were combined, the incidence of abnormalities was high. Sinus node dysfunction occurred in 45 patients (52%), supraventricular ectopy in 29 patients (34%), ventricular ectopy in 24 patients (28%), and atrioventricular block in 19 patients (22%). Only 25 (29%) of the long-term survivors of the Mustard operation had no demonstrable abnormalities of their rate, rhythm, or conduction. The bradycardia-tachycardia syndrome occurred in 10 of the 45 patients who had sinus node dysfunction. Atrioventricular block, when present, was greater than first-degree in only 5 of the 19 patients with conduction disturbance.

Senning Operation

Methods

From 1981 until the present the Senning procedure has been the preferred technique at our institution for atrial redirection

Table 7
Arrhythmias Following Senning Procedure,
Current Electrocardiogram (n = 30)

Mean follow-up = 2.2 years		
(Range: 0.2–5.1 years)		
Normal sinus rhythm		25 (85%)
Sinus node dysfunction		4 (13%)
Brady-tachycardia	1	
Junctional rhythm	1	
Ectopic atrial pacemaker	1	
Sinus bradycardia	1	
Supraventricular ectopy		1 (3%)

repair of patients with complete transposition (Gay et al., 1986). The most recent surface electrocardiograms were reviewed in 30 of these patients, with a mean follow-up of 2.2 years and a range from 0.7 to 5.1 years. The mean age at operation of patients who had the Senning procedure was 10.7 months with a range of 5 days to 24 months.

Results

The review of the surface electrocardiograms shown in Table 7 indicates that normal sinus rhythm was present in 25 patients (83%). Sinus node dysfunction was found in 4 patients (13%), and one child had supraventricular ectopy. Intracardiac electrophysiological studies were performed in 14 postoperative patients; these results are shown in Table 8. Sinus node function was abnormal in 8 patients (57%) while atrioventricular conduction was intact in all patients tested by the response to rapid atrial pacing. Atrial functional and effective refractory periods were normal in all 9 patients in whom these parameters were evaluated.

Discussion

There have been a large number of studies that clearly document a high frequency of arrhythmias in patients who have survived the Mustard operation for complete transposition (Beerman et al., 1983; El-Said et al., 1972; Epstein et al., 1983; Gillette et al., 1980; Saalouke et al., 1978; Southall et al., 1980). These studies have consistently shown that the most prevalent abnormality is sinus node dysfunction. This is manifested either by an abnormally slow sinus rate for the patient's age or by a junctional rhythm. An important subset of these patients have a slow baseline rhythm alter-

Table 8
Senning Procedure, Postoperative
Electrophysiological Studies

A. Sinus node function			
Normal CSNRT			6 (43%)
Abnormal CSNRT			8 (57%)
Prolonged CSNRT		6	
275–500 msec	5		
>500 msec	1		
Abnormal recovery site		2	
Junctional	2		
Total			14 (100%)
B. Atrioventricular conduction			
Intact AV conduction			
≥ 180 beats/min with RAP			12 (100%)

AV = atrioventricular; CSNRT = corrected sinus node recovery time;
RAP = rapid atrial pacing.

nating with episodes of supraventricular tachycardia, usually atrial flutter (in other words, the bradycardia-tachycardia syndrome). All of the long-term studies have shown that the incidence of sinus node dysfunction increases with duration of follow-up. Atrioventricular block occurs much less frequently and the prevalence of supraventricular or ventricular ectopy has received relatively little attention (Saalouke et al., 1978).

There have been two recent reviews of this group of patients that highlight the problem well. Flinn et al. (1984) reviewed the surface electrocardiograms alone in 372 patients from multiple centers who were followed between 0.4 and 15.9 years with a mean of 4.5 years. There was a progressive increase in the incidence of sinus node dysfunction with time, and it occurred in 70% of patients who had been followed for 14 years after surgery. Although 40% of all patients had supraventricular ectopy noted on at least one occasion, the prevalence was low until after the 10th postoperative year. Second- or third-degree atrioventricular block occurred very infrequently and its incidence did not vary during the period of follow-up. Sudden death was found in 2.5% of their patient population. Its occurrence was not related statistically to the degree of bradycardia or to whether or not a pacemaker had been implanted. There was a statistically significant association between the presence of persistent supraventricular tachycardia, usually atrial flutter, and sudden death. Hayes and Gersony (1986) studied 95 patients for a follow-up period ranging from 0.3 to 13 years by analyzing Holter monitors in addition to surface electrocardiograms. Arrhythmias eventually developed in 79% of patients and there was an incidence of sudden death of 3.3% in their series. They recommended pacemaker insertion for the following indications: heart rates less than 30 beats/min, Stokes-Adams episodes, tachycardia requiring treatment other than digoxin, and bradycardia associated with poor ventricular function or ventricular ectopy.

Table 9
Arrhythmias Following Mustard Operation, Symptomatic Status (n = 73)

No treatment		65 (89%)
Asymptomatic	59	
Mild palpitations	6	
Treatment required		8 (11%)
Brady-Tachycardia*	5	
SVT	1	
Ventricular ectopy	1	
3° AVB**	1	

* Two patients with AAI pacemaker.
** VVI pacemaker.
AAI = atrial demand pacemaker; AVB = atrioventricular block; SVT = supraventricular tachycardia; VVI = ventricular demand pacemaker.

The results of our study demonstrate a similarly high incidence of sinus node dysfunction with a low incidence of second- or third-degree atrioventricular block. Furthermore, supraventricular ectopy, either associated with underlying bradycardia or in isolation, was rather common. Surprisingly, we also found a high incidence of ventricular ectopy that has not been stressed in most previous studies. Hayes et al. (1986) did find multiple premature ventricular contractions in 12% of their patients, while Saalouke et al. (1978) detected complex ventricular arrhythmias in 40% of those patients undergoing Holter monitoring. We found an overall incidence of ventricular ectopy of 28%, with 12 patients (14%) having complex forms of ventricular arrhythmias.

Despite the very high prevalence of rhythm disturbances in this group of patients, they are usually asymptomatic (Table 9). In the 73 patients whose status could be accurately determined, the great majority (89%) required no treatment and are either asymptomatic or having only mild transient palpitations. Treatment for a rhythm disorder has been necessary in only eight (11%) of these patients, including two with atrial demand pacemakers and one with a ventricular demand pacemaker. Conversely, sudden unexplained late deaths (most likely related to arrhythmias) occurred in four patients, making up 5% of the total group. The rhythm abnormalities detected in these four patients include bradycardia-tachycardia syndrome along with first-degree and intermittent second-degree atrioventricular block in one, only first-degree atrioventricular block in another, complex ventricular ectopy on exercise testing in one, and sinus node dysfunction unassociated with tachyarrhythmias in one patient.

Although patients undergoing the Senning procedure have not been studied as extensively or as long postoperatively as those with the Mustard operation, there are data to suggest that rhythm disturbances have not been eliminated by using this alternative technique for atrial redirection (Byrum et al., 1986; Epstein et al., 1983). Byrum et al. (1986) found that sinus node dysfunction occurred in 25% of their patients, being particularly prevalent in those operated upon younger than five months of age. Although our study showed that 83% of the total were in normal sinus rhythm on their surface electrocardiogram at a mean follow-up of 2.2 years, there was a 57% occurrence of an abnormal sinus node response during intracardiac electrophysiological studies.

Conclusions

Sinus node dysfunction is very common and occurs in more than half of all patients following the Mustard procedure. This abnormality is often associated with the bradycardia-tachycardia syndrome and its incidence progressively increases with duration of follow-up. Ventricular ectopy is more common than has previously been emphasized, but requires Holter monitoring and exercise testing in order to detect its presence. The great majority of patients with rhythm disturbances are asymptomatic and may not require treatment. There is, however, a disturbing incidence of sudden late death that is most likely related to arrhythmia. The specific etiology for this tragic occurrence may involve ventricular ectopy as well as sinus node dysfunction, persistent atrial flutter, or the bradycardia-tachycardia syndrome. Although less likely than the other abnormalities, atrioventricular block may be important in certain patients. Pacemakers are clearly indicated in some patients but have not been shown to prevent sudden death. Short-term follow-up of the Senning procedure would suggest that it will confer no benefit over the Mustard procedure in preventing the occurrence of arrhythmias in patients with complete transposition who undergo an atrial redirection procedure.

Acknowledgment: We thank Susan Gainor for her assistance in the preparation of this manuscript.

References

Beerman LB, Neches WH, Fricker FJ, Arrhythmias in transposition of the great arteries after the Mustard operation. *Am J Cardiol* 1983;51:1530–1534.

Byrum CJ, Bove EL, Sondheimer HM, Hemodynamic and electrophysiologic results of the Senning procedure for transposition of the great arteries. *Am J Cardiol* 1986;58:138–142.

Clarkson PM, Barratt-Boyes BG, Neutze JM. Late dysrhythmias and disturbances of conduction following Mustard operation for complete transposition of the great arteries. *Circulation* 1976;53:519–524.

Dubrow IW, Fisher EA, Amat-y-Leon F, Comparison of cardiac refractory periods in children and adults. *Circulation* 1975;51:485–491.

El-Said GM, Rosenberg HS, Mullins CE, et al. Dysrhythmias after Mustard's operation for transposition of the great arteries. *Am J Cardiol* 1972;30:526–532.

El-Said GM, Gillette PC, Mullins CE, et al. Significant of pacemaker recovery time after the Mustard operation for transposition of the great arteries. *Am J Cardiol* 1976;38:448–451.

Epstein ML, Riemenschneider TA, Mathewson JW, Hurley EJ. Postoperative hemodynamic and electrophysiological evaluation of the Senning procedure. *Cardiology* 1983;70:247–254.

Flinn CJ, Wolfe GS, Dick M, et al. Cardiac rhythm after the Mustard operation for complete transposition of the great arteries. *N Engl J Med* 1984;310:1635–1638.

Gay W, Neches WH, Park SC, et al. Dysrhythmias following Senning operation. Abstract presented at World Congress of Cardiology, Washington, D.C., 1986.

Gillette PC, Kugler JD, Garson A, et al. Mechanisms of cardiac arrhythmias after the Mustard operation for transposition of the great arteries. *Am J Card* 1980;45:1225–1230.

Hayes CJ, Gersony WM. Arrhythmias after the Mustard operation for transposition of the great arteries: A long-term study. *J Am Coll Cardiol* 1986;7:133–137.

Mathews RA, Fricker FJ, Beerman LB, et al. Exercise performance after the Mustard operation for complete transposition, 1987 (in preparation).

Saalouke MG, Rios J, Perry LW, et al. Electrophysiologic studies after Mustard's operation for d-transposition of the great vessels. *Am J Cardiol* 1978;41:1104–1109.

Southall DP, Keeton BR, Leanage R, Cardiac rhythm and conduction before and after Mustard's operation for complete transposition of the great arteries. *Br Heart J* 1980;43:21–30.

Vetter VL, Horowitz LN. Electrophysiologic residua and sequelae of surgery for congenital heart defects. *Am J Cardiol* 1982;50:588–604.

Exercise Performance After the Mustard Operation for Complete Transposition

Robert A. Mathews, Frederick J. Fricker,
Lee B. Beerman, Donald R. Fischer,
and Mary Kay Yurchak

Functional impairment has been frequently observed in patients with congenital heart disease even after successful operation. Patients who have had a Mustard procedure for repair of complete transposition are in a unique anatomical situation since the morphologically right ventricle must continue to function as the systemic ventricle. The operation may be complicated by a ventricular septal defect and/or subpulmonic stenosis that requires repair. Postoperatively, systemic venous and/or pulmonary venous drainage may become restrictive. Right ventricular dysfunction, atrial and/or ventricular arrhythmias (Beerman et al., 1983; Duster et al., 1985; Flinn et al., 1984; Graham et al., 1982; Hayes et al., 1986; Park et al., 1983; Scagliotti et al., 1984) and arterial de-saturation because of baffle leaks have also been reported. Because of these persistent postoperative problems, exercise performance may also be abnormal. Even patients with excellent postoperative hemodynamic results may develop significant arrhythmias during exercise that may limit overall performance. In our previous study of 21 patients with complete transposition (Mathews et al., 1983), we noted a variety of abnormalities during exercise. This group has been followed longitudinally and 16 of these original patients and four others have undergone serial exercise testing.

This study is a review of the exercise performance data of 71 tests on 46 patients following the Mustard operation. In addition, longitudinal data from our other 20

From: Anderson, RH, Neches, WH, Park, SC, Zuberbuhler, JR, eds: *Perspectives in Pediatric Cardiology*: Mount Kisco, New York, Futura Publishing Co., © 1988.

patients will be used to determine whether any improvement or deterioration occurs with increasing time after operation.

Material and Method

Forty-six patients (31 male, 15 female) who had Mustard operation performed between 1960 and 1980 for complete transposition at Children's Hospital of Pittsburgh underwent exercise testing. The patients have been followed since operation from 6 to 21 years (mean = 9.8 years). The mean age at the time of initial Mustard operation was 8 years (range 1–15 years). Only six of the patients in this series had operation at less than 3 years of age.

Eighteen patients had uncomplicated transposition; 15 had an associated ventricular septal defect that required surgical closure; 15 had pulmonary stenosis that was relieved at operation; 12 had a prior operative atrial septectomy; four had had banding of the pulmonary trunk prior to Mustard operation. Two patients required reoperation for baffle leak and one had valve replacement because of severe tricuspid insufficiency. Complete heart block necessitating permanent pacemaker insertion occurred in two patients. All patients considered themselves to be normally active and most were students. One had a successful pregnancy and delivered a normal child. Five patients were taking medications. Two received digitalis; one each was taking propranolol, quinidine, or procainamide.

The results of the exercise studies of 227 patients without heart disease served as control data. All patients in this study had at least one postoperative cardiac catheterization, including an electrophysiological study. All have had at least one treadmill exercise test, a cross-sectional echocardiogram and a 24-hour ambulatory electrocardiogram. None has been lost to follow-up. Longitudinal evaluations of exercise perfor-

mance were available in 20 patients who had either two or three exercise tests. A determination of any change in status was thus possible in this smaller subset. This included 16 of the 21 patients previously reported (Mathews et al., 1983) and four others. Fifteen patients had two tests and five more had three exercise studies. The time interval between the first and second test was 1.5 to 6 years (mean = 4.5 years).

All patients underwent maximal graded treadmill exercise testing in the Cardio-Pulmonary Exercise Laboratory at Children's Hospital of Pittsburgh. Four limb and six precordial electrodes were placed after adequate cleansing of the skin. All patients and control subjects underwent progressive exercise testing on a treadmill (International Medical Corporation Model 200) using a modified Balke protocol. Most patients walked 3.4 miles per hour and a 4% increment in treadmill elevation was made every three minutes. Resting blood pressure, heart rate, and a 12-lead electrocardiogram were obtained in sitting, standing, and supine position, and after hyperventilation. One precordial lead was continuously monitored during each test and a 12-lead strip was recorded every minute. Blood pressure was obtained every three minutes by auscultation with an appropriate-sized arm cuff. Oxygen consumption was measured in the standing position at rest and continuously throughout the exercise test using the Waters MRM-1 Oxygen Consumption computer and/or Medical Graphics Corporation System 2001. Arterial oxygen saturations were measured noninvasively at rest and during exercise with a pulse oximeter (Nellcor). All cardiac patients and control subjects were similarly encouraged to proceed with exercise to exhaustion. Monitoring was continued for at least six minutes after exercise or until the patient's vital signs returned to baseline values.

Test results from all cardiac patients were first analyzed by individual ages comparing anthropometric and dynamic exer-

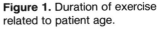

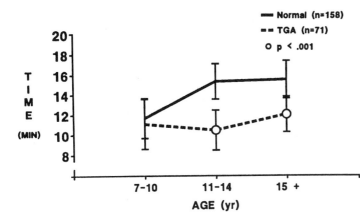

Figure 1. Duration of exercise related to patient age.

cise performance data to controls. The patients were then divided into three nearly equal subgroups by age. This produced a group of young patients less than 11 years of age (24 tests); a second intermediate group of children between 11 through 14 years of age (21 tests); and a final group of those 15 years of age and older (26 tests).

Values for each of the three age groups were compared between controls and cardiac patients. Statistical analysis with computer assistance was done using the two-sample Student t test for comparison, with a probability of less than 0.01 as the lowest level of significance accepted.

Results

Body height, weight, and surface area were similar to controls in the younger and intermediate age groups. All three parameters were statistically lower than controls in the older age group.

In terms of duration of the exercise test (Fig. 1), younger patients performed nearly as well as controls (mean times: 12.0 minutes versus 13.5 minutes). The patients in the group older than 15 years consistently fell below the mean value for duration of treadmill exercise when compared by height or age to controls ($p < 0.001$). Longitudinal data in 20 patients showed slight improvement in 12 (mean increase = 4.6 minutes), while eight patients had a shorter time or no change (mean decrease = 3.2 minutes).

Maximal level of oxygen consumption (L/min) (Fig. 2) and indexed for body weight (ml/kg/min) (Fig. 3) was normal in the younger group. Decreased utilization of oxygen was particularly evident in older children, adolescents, and young adults

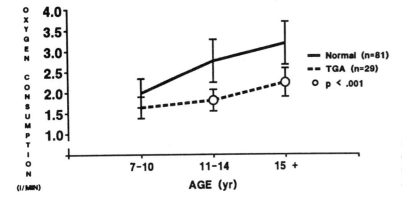

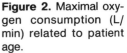

Figure 2. Maximal oxygen consumption (L/min) related to patient age.

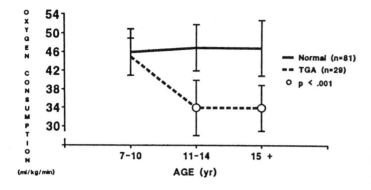
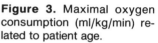

Figure 3. Maximal oxygen consumption (ml/kg/min) related to patient age.

($p < 0.001$), indicating a lower fitness level. Serial evaluation of this parameter demonstrated a rise in total oxygen consumption (L/min) with advancing age in five of seven patients (Fig. 4). There was a decrease in oxygen utilization indexed for body weight in three of these five (Fig. 5).

Maximal heart rate responses of patients were lower than most older normal individuals (Fig. 6). This decreased chronotropic response became more apparent ($p < 0.001$) in patients older than 14 years of age. Some older patients occasionally had coexistent atrial or ventricular arrhythmias. Two patients with a fixed-rate permanent pacemaker were excluded from analysis of this parameter. In longitudinal evaluation of maximal heart rate, 7 of 20 patients showed

a decreased heart rate on subsequent tests while 2 of 20 had maximal heart rate similar to that at the initial test.

Systolic blood pressure response to exercise was normal in the younger and intermediate groups. A statistically lower than normal maximal blood pressure was evident in the older patients (Fig. 7).

Arterial oxygen saturation was measured noninvasively during 41 tests in 33 patients (Table 1). Resting values were normal (greater than 92%) in 20 patients who had no change with exercise. Fourteen patients who had a normal oxygen saturation at rest had a decline in oxygen saturation to less than 92% (58–91%) during exercise. Seven patients were desaturated at rest (61–85%). No significant change in resting

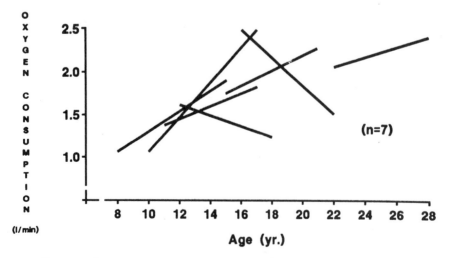

Figure 4. Serial measurements of maximal oxygen consumption (L/min).

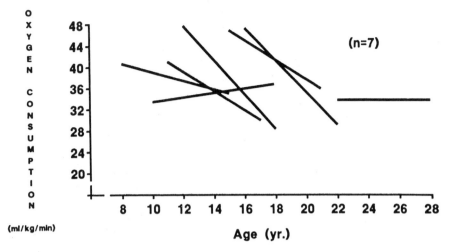

Figure 5. Serial measurements of maximal oxygen consumption (ml/kg/min).

or exercise values for oxygen saturation were seen in those patients who had serial evaluations.

Abnormal cardiac rhythms were present in 19 tests at rest and became apparent in 21 more during exercise (Table 2). Fifty-two tests had sinus rhythm at rest, but sinus rhythm was present in only 31 tests (60%) during exercise. Premature atrial systoles were seen during three studies, atrial tachycardia and/or atrial flutter was precipitated during exercise in one. Premature ventricular contractions were seen during 11 tests. Longitudinal study of 45 tests in 20 patients demonstrated the development of a variety of arrhythmias in those who were in normal sinus rhythm during their initial study (Table 3).

Three patients in the total series (6.5%) have died during the follow-up period. Two of these patients were represented in our earlier report and had right ventricular dysfunction and a history of multiform premature ventricular contractions. A third patient with sinus node dysfunction and progressive conduction abnormalities died suddenly. No deaths were associated with exercise.

Discussion

The exercise capability of patients who had Mustard operation for complete transposition may be subnormal or abnormal in

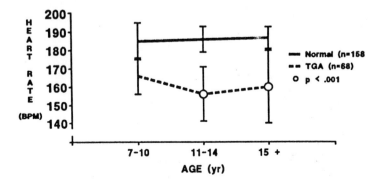

Figure 6. Maximal heart rate response to exercise.

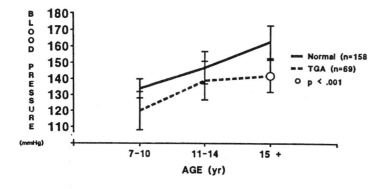

Figure 7. Maximal systolic blood pressure response to exercise.

one or several parameters. Some of these patients may have underlying abnormal hemodynamics that predispose them to abnormal exercise performance. A few patients, however, appear to have excellent postoperative results but manifest subnormal capability or exercise-induced abnormalities. Most patients have adapted well to their limitations and report few, if any, symptoms. Even significant arrhythmias are not apparent to most patients. Despite this subjectively normal functional state, a number of parameters objectively measured during maximal exercise testing may be abnormal or in the lower range of normal.

Chronotropic response to exercise is typically gradual, reaching a value near 200 beats/min in most normal pediatric subjects. Pediatric and young adult patients with complete transposition as a group, however, are generally unable to reach the usual maximal level. Several patients with evidence of sinus or atrioventricular node dysfunction would be expected to have a blunted chronotropic response to exercise. Some patients in this study showed intermittent junctional rhythm alternating with

sinus rhythm. The progressive decremental change in maximal heart rate seen with increasing age is worrisome. This trend suggests that an increased incidence of sinus node dysfunction may become more evident as more patients reach adulthood.

Blood pressure response to exercise is also blunted, but to a lesser degree. This dynamic response does not appear to be significantly less than normal until after 14 years of age. This subnormal response may be secondary to the decreased ability of the right ventricle to generate the same level of blood pressure as a normal left ventricle during stress.

Maximal oxygen consumption, expressed as total body uptake or indexed for body weight, differed significantly from normal. The normal trend of increasing uptake (in L/min) with advancing age until late adolescence was seen, but at a significantly lower level ($p < 0.001$) in patients over ten years of age (54% increase versus a 100% increase in controls). When maximal oxygen consumption index was compared to controls, a precipitous decline was evident from a normal value of 49 ml/kg/min

Table 1
Arterial Oxygen Saturation (41 Tests in 36 Patients)

Number	Rest	Exercise
19	Normal (more than 92%)	Normal
15	Normal	Desaturation (58–91%)
7	Desaturation (84–90%)	Further desaturation (61–85%)

Table 2
Cardiac Rhythms and Arrhythmias during Resting and Exercise (71 Tests)

Resting	Exercise	
Normal sinus rhythm (52)	Sinus rhythm	31
	Junctional	6
	Atrioventricular block	3
	Supraventricular tachycardia	1
	Atrial premature	3
	Ventricular premature:	
	unifocal	5
	multifocal	3
Sinus rhythm, ventricular premature, multifocal (1)	Sinus rhythm, ventricular premature, multifocal	1
Junctional rhythm (9)	Sinus rhythm	5
	Junctional	2
	Junctional with ventricular premature	2
Atrioventricular dissociation (6)	Atrioventricular dissociation	4
	Sinus rhythm	1
	Ventricular premature, unifocal	1
Atrioventricular block (3)	Atrioventricular block	3

seen in younger children to 33 ml/kg/min in both older groups.

Arrhythmias induced by exercise may account for decreased duration of exercise and subnormal maximal responses of heart rate and blood pressure. Although abnormal rhythm was occasionally provoked, most patients were in sinus or junctional rhythm during exercise. Premature ventricular contractions were precipitated during 11 of 52 tests (21%) in patients with normal sinus rhythm.

Table 3
Longitudinal Exercise Study: Rhythms and Arrhythmias (45 Tests in 20 Patients)

First exercise study	Last exercise study	
Normal sinus rhythm (14)	Junctional rhythm	5
	Sinus rhythm	3
	Supraventricular tachycardia	1
	Atrial premature beats	1
	First-degree heart block	1
	Ventricular premature beats, unifocal	3
Sinus rhythm and ventricular premature beats, unifocal (1)	Junctional rhythm and atrial premature beats	1
Junctional rhythm (2)	Junctional rhythm	1
	Sinus rhythm	1
Atrioventricular block or dissociation (3)	Atrioventricular block or dissociation	3

Desaturation at rest and provoked during exercise may theoretically cause myocardial ischemia. No patient, however, complained of chest pain during or after exercise. It was impossible to determine electrocardiographic evidence of ischemia conclusively because of the presence of right ventricular hypertrophy in all patients. Nonetheless, no patient had a change in T wave morphology or developed new Q waves on electrocardiogram during exercise.

Right and even left ventricular dysfunction secondary to tricuspid insufficiency or myocardial disease has previously been well documented in numerous postoperative studies using echocardiographic and radionuclide techniques in this patient population (Murphy et al., 1983; Parrish et al., 1983; Ramsey et al., 1984). Since exercise may provoke borderline cardiopulmonary dysfunction, its presence may be suspected if subnormal maximal heart rate and blood pressure responses are found during exercise.

Comprehensive exercise rehabilitation programs can improve cardiopulmonary endurance in adults as well as in children with various cardiac abnormalities (Bradley, 1985; Mathews et al., 1983). Whether significant long-term improvement in endurance to exercise would benefit postoperative patients with complete transposition remains to be determined.

Conclusion

Subnormal or abnormal exercise dynamics are common in many older patients after the Mustard operation for complete transposition. With advancing age, exercise performance decreases, exemplified by decreased endurance and fitness. Longitudinal and isolated evaluations have demonstrated trends that suggest the right ventricle will eventually be unable to sustain normal function as a systemic ventricle in many pa-

tients, especially during exercise. Arrhythmias and abnormal basic cardiac rhythm may contribute to an already compromised cardiac reserve and reduce the effective overall cardiopulmonary response to exercise. As alternative surgical approaches to this malformation continue to develop, and as improved myocardial preservation techniques have appeared, allowing safer operations at a younger age, it is hoped that the long-term outlook will improve.

References

Beerman LB, Neches WH, Fricker FJ, et al. Arrhythmias in transposition of the great arteries after the Mustard operations. *Am J Cardiol* 1983;51:1530–1534.

Bradley LM, Galioto FM, Vaccaro P, et al. Effects of intense aerobic training on exercise performance in children after surgical repair of tetralogy of Fallot or complete transposition of the great arteries. *Am J Cardiol* 1985;56:816–818.

Duster MC, Bink-Boelkens M, Wampler D, et al. Long-term follow up of dysrhythmias following the Mustard procedure. *Am Heart J* 1985;110:1323–1326.

Flinn CJ, Wolff GS, Dick M, et al. Cardiac rhythm after the Mustard operation for complete transposition of the great arteries. *N Engl J Med* 1984;310:1635–1638.

Graham TP. Hemodynamic residua and sequelae following interatrial repair of transposition of the great arteries: A review. *Pediatr Cardiol* 1982;2:203–213.

Hayes CJ, Gersony WM. Arrhythmias after the Mustard operation for transposition of the great arteries: A long-term study. *J Am Coll Cardiol* 1986;7:133–137.

Mathews RA, Fricker FJ, Beerman LB, et al. Exercise studies after the Mustard operation in transposition of the great arteries. *Am J Cardiol* 1983;51:1526–1529.

Mathews RA, Nixon PA, Stephenson RJ, et al. An exercise program for pediatric patients with congenital heart disease: Organizational and physiologic aspects. *J Cardiol Rehab* 1983;3:467–475.

Murphy JH, Barlai-Kovach MM, Mathews RA, et

al. Rest and exercise right and left ventricular function late after the Mustard operation: Assessment by radionuclide angiography. *Am J Cardiol* 1983;51:1520–1526.

Parrish MD, Graham TP Jr, Bender HW, et al. Radionuclide angiographic evaluation of right and left ventricular function during exercise after repair of transposition of the great arteries. Comparison with normal subjects and patients with congenitally corrected transposition. *Circulation* 1983;67:178–183.

Park SC, Neches WH, Mathews RA, et al. Hemo-dynamic function after the Mustard operation for transposition of the great arteries. *Am J Cardiol* 1983;51:1514–1519.

Ramsey JM, Venables AW, Kelly MJ, Kalff V. Right and left ventricular function at rest and with exercise after the Mustard operation for transposition of the great arteries. *Br Heart J* 1984;51:364–370.

Scagliotti D, Strasberg B, Duffy CE, et al. Inducible polymorphous ventricular tachycardia following Mustard operation for transposition of the great arteries. *Pediatr Cardiol* 1984;5:39–44.

4.8

Late Deaths Following Mustard/Senning Procedure for Complete Transposition

Cora C. Lenox

Between January 1964 and July 1986, the Mustard or Senning procedures were used at Children's Hospital of Pittsburgh in the operative treatment of complete transposition. During that period, the total number of hospital discharges following the operation was 135. Since their discharge, 16 patients have died, which yields an incidence of 12% for late deaths. These late deaths have been reviewed to determine the particular problems associated with these operative procedures and the late consequences.

Material and Methods

Sixteen late deaths after the Mustard/Senning procedure were studied according to year of surgery, age at surgery, length of survival after surgery, and cause of death. Features evaluated included procedures and studies from the preoperative course and

details of the surgical operation. The immediate postoperative course was carefully evaluated along with the follow-up care, including any special studies. The circumstances of death were established in all cases. Autopsy reports in 11 of the 16 patients aided in determination of cause of death.

Results

The 16 late deaths after the Mustard or Senning operation could be divided into two distinct groups based on length of survival after discharge from the hospital. The first group (Table 1) was comprised of eight patients who lived for one to nine months (mean of three months) after surgery. The second group (Table 2), also of eight patients, consisted of patients who survived 5 to 15 years (mean of 10 years). In Table 3,

From: Anderson, RH, Neches, WH, Park, SC, Zuberbuhler, JR, eds: *Perspectives in Pediatric Cardiology*: Mount Kisco, New York, Futura Publishing Co., © 1988.

Table 1

Late Deaths after Mustard/Senning, Less Than One-Year Survival

Patient no.	Sex	MU/SE Age	MU/SE Year	Death Age	Death Year	Survival	Other defects	Complications Early	Complications Late	Death	Cause	Autopsy
1	M	7 y	1970	7 y	1970	3 m	VSD, PB	—	—	sudden	not known	no
2	F	16 m	1975	18 m	1975	2 m	—	—	PVO	surgical	pulmonary hypertension	no
3	F	23 m	1975	26 m	1975	3 m	PAR	ARR, CHY	SVO	cardiac arrest	uncertain	yes
4	M	18 y	1976	19 y	1976	3 m	VSD, PSV	—	CHF, AIA	CHF syncope	shock	yes
5	M	17 m	1977	26 m	1978	9 m	VSD	—	SVO seizures	sudden	sepsis	yes
6	M	19 m	1978	22 m	1978	3 m	VSD	—	PPS SVO	surgical	meningitis acidosis shock	no
7	F	2 y SE	1980	25 m	1980	1 m	VSD, PDA	—	seizures	sudden	emboli to brain	yes
8	M	1y SE	1981	15 m	1981	3 m	VSD, ANV PSI	ECMO-6 days brain damage	—	sudden	acute MYO	yes

MU = Mustard procedure; SE = Senning procedure; M = male; F = female; y = years; m = months; VSD = ventricular septal defect; PB = pulmonary band; PVO = pulmonary venous obstruction; PAR = partial anomalous pulmonary venous return; ARR = arrhythmia; CHY = chylothorax; SVO = systemic venous obstruction; CA = cardiac arrest; PSV = pulmonary valvar stenosis; CHF = congestive heart failure; AIA = acquired aortic insufficiency; PPS = postpericardiotomy syndrome; PDA = patent ductus arteriosus; ANV = aneurysm of the membranous septum; PSI = subpulmonic stenosis; ECMO = extracorporeal membrane oxygenation; MYO = myocarditis.

Table 2

Late Deaths after Mustard, 5- to 15-Year Survival

Patient no.	Sex	MU		Death		Survival	Other defects	Complications		Death	Cause	Autopsy
		Age	Year	Age	Year			Early	Late			
1	M	9 y	1969	15 y	1975	6 y	VSD, PB	—	PSS, PVO ADR, VDR	surgical	PVO, ADR	yes
2	F	8 y	1966	23 y	1981	15 y	LSC	ARR	—	sudden	ARR-prob	yes
3	F	3 y	1971	14 y	1982	11 y	—	ARR	neurological	sudden	ARR-prob	yes
4	F	3 y	1970	14 y	1982	12 y	VSD, PSI	ARR	RVD, TIA	RVD, CHF shock	same	yes
5	F	10 y	1974	20 y	1983	10 y	VSD, ANV PSI, IVC	ARR CHF	ARR-PM CHF, VDR, MIA RVD	surgical	CHF, RVD	yes
6	M	2 y	1973	13 y	1984	11 y	VSD	ARR	ARR	sudden	ARR-prob	no
7	F	5 y	1976	15 y	1986	10 y	VSD, PB	—	ARR RVD	sudden	ARR-prob RVD	yes*
8	F	15 y	1977	24 y	1986	9 y	VSD, PVD	palliative	—	sudden	PVD	no

* Coroner's case.
PSS = pulmonic supravalvar stenosis; ADR = residual atrial septal defect, baffle leak; VDR = residual ventricular septal defect; LSC = left superior vena cava to coronary sinus; Prob = probably; RVD = right ventricular dysfunction; TIA = tricuspid insufficiency, acquired; IVC = absent inferior vena cava; ARR-PM = arrhythmia-pacemaker; MIA = mitral insufficiency, acquired; PVD = pulmonary vascular disease; others as in Table 1.

Table 3
Relation of Year of Surgery and Year of Death
in Group I and Group II

Group I year of death	Year of surgery both groups	Group II year of death
	1966	1981
	1967	
	1968	
	1969	1975
1970	1970	1982
	1971	1982
	1972	
	1973	1984
	1974	1983
1975, 1975	1975	
1976	1976	1986
1978	1977	1986
1978	1978	
	1979	
1980	1980	
1981	1981	

the year of operation is in the left column and the year of death for that patient is shown in the right column corresponding to short-term or long-term survivors. There is some overlap of the two groups in the mid-1970s. The patients who died soon after the procedure had surgery mostly in the late 1970s through 1981. Those surviving longer had undergone surgery in the earlier years (1966–1977). The two patients who died soon after surgery in 1980 and 1981 had the Senning procedure. These are the only late deaths in the total experience with the Senning procedure in this center. In the patients who died early, except for two older patients, the age at time of surgery was between one and two years. In contrast, in those who died some time after the procedure were aged 2 to 15 years at the time of operation.

Following the operative procedures, there were significant residual defects that contributed to death in both groups. These were more common in those who died early. Problems with the baffle (a leak in the baffle or obstruction to caval or pulmonary venous

flow) were related to the recent surgery. Four (50%) of the patients who died early had these problems, whereas only one of those dying later was similarly afflicted. Aortic insufficiency occurred postoperatively in an older patient who died soon after surgery and two infants had evidence of thromboembolization to the brain, the timing of embolization being estimated to be about the time of surgery. In one patient who died some time later, there was both a baffle leak and evidence of pulmonary venous obstruction. The patient also had severe supravalvular pulmonary stenosis which required reoperation. Another in the group who survived for some time had a large residual ventricular septal defect.

The cause of death in each case was determined by clinical findings, surgical findings, postoperative studies, and autopsy (in 11 cases). The findings are listed in Tables 1 and 2. Two of the patients dying early (Table 1, nos. 5 and 6) died of acute infection not related directly to the surgical procedure (no. 5 with sepsis and acute purulent meningitis, and no. 6 with acute viral myocarditis, the latter also having thromboembolization to the brain). Severe congestive heart failure was the cause of death in an 18-year-old boy (no. 4). His postoperative course had been uneventful but when he returned three months postoperatively with severe failure, he was found to have aortic insufficiency. He was being treated vigorously with diuretics when he developed a syncopal episode and hypotension which persisted in spite of all treatment. He died eight hours later. No arrhythmias were recorded. At autopsy there were two fenestrations in the aortic leaflets. One appeared traumatic but, in spite of the small size, there was a jet lesion present. This, plus his injudicious use of salt, probably accounted for the degree of congestive heart failure. Two patients (nos. 2 and 6) died at the time of reoperation, although both had relief of their baffle problems. Patient no. 2 had persistence of severe pulmonary hypertension and could not be weaned from bypass. Patient no. 6 was very ill at the time of cardiac catheterization, had an arrest, but responded to resuscitation and was sent to surgery as an emergency. He died the next day, and his death was attributed to shock and metabolic problems. One of the patients treated with the Senning procedure (no. 7) did well postoperatively and was discharged on the 12th postoperative day. At home, her course appeared normal. She fell from the porch while playing, had a convulsion, and was taken to a local emergency room where she died. Her autopsy, performed at Children's Hospital, surprisingly showed old thromboembolization to the brain, with lesions which were estimated to date from the time of reparative surgery. There were two sudden deaths in those dying early. Patient no. 1 was a seven-year-old boy who had been operated upon three months previously and died at home; no autopsy was obtained. No arrhythmias had ever been noted on the electrocardiograms taken before or after surgery. The other sudden death, patient no. 3, afflicted a two-

year-old girl who had had first-degree heart block after surgery (PR interval = 0.28 sec) and on one occasion had junctional rhythm recorded. She had required reoperation for tamponade in the immediate postoperative period and later developed chylothorax. After discharge, she was found to have complete obstruction of the superior caval vein but there was good azygos drainage to the unobstructed inferior caval vein. She was doing well when she became acutely ill with vomiting and dehydration and was taken to the emergency room. There she had cardiac arrest at time of venepuncture but responded to resuscitation. A few hours later she developed apnea and bradycardia during suction which progressed to ventricular fibrillation and then cardiac arrest from which she could not be resuscitated. No special cause for this death was found on postmortem study; possibly she had profound vagal stimulation when undergoing suction.

The causes of death were different in the second group from those in the first, although two cases followed a second operation. Patient no. 1, who had had a Mustard operation six years previously, had a baffle leak and pulmonary venous obstruction. There was additional supravalvular pulmonary stenosis at the site of a band placed previously on the pulmonary trunk. The band had been removed at the time of the Mustard operation, the pulmonary trunk being considered adequate in size. The significance of the baffle problems was not realized at the time of reoperation and he died intraoperatively. A 20-year-old girl (no. 5) had a closure of a large residual ventricular septal defect together with replacement of the mitral valve because of insufficiency due to torn cords. She had had a pacemaker inserted one month previously because of third-degree heart block and died six days postoperatively because of myocardial dysfunction. Patient no. 4 died after slowly progressive right ventricular dysfunction and tricuspid insufficiency 12 years after the

Mustard procedure. Her death was due to severe congestive heart failure and terminal hepatic and renal failure. She had had problems before the Mustard operation, with a shower of thrombi, probably from the right ventricle, passing to various parts of the body. She also had a problem with atrial arrhythmias after the Mustard procedure, especially with atrial flutter.

There were five sudden, unexpected deaths. One was a 24-year-old woman (no. 8) who had had a palliative Mustard procedure performed at age 15 years. Although she obtained much relief from the operation, and was able to resume school and graduate from high school, she continued to have pulmonary vascular disease and died suddenly at home. No autopsy was performed. The only arrhythmia recorded in her long history was an occasional isolated premature ventricular beat on the electrocardiogram. The remaining four cases of patients who died suddenly were all considered to be due to arrhythmias. A 23-year-old woman (no. 2) had been very well, was married, and was planning a family. On exercise testing she had exhibited a few premature ventricular beats and developed bigeminy in the first two minutes after exercise. Two ventricular ectopic beats were noted on her last electrocardiogram. The resting right ventricular ejection fraction as measured in radionuclide studies was 0.62% and, with exercise, was 0.1%. The only abnormal finding on cardiac catheterization had been a small right-to-left shunt at the atrial level. Autopsy, except for the small atrial defect, demonstrated a heart as anticipated for complete transposition. Another patient who died suddenly (no. 3) had had a cerebrovascular accident at four months of age, leaving a number of neurological defects requiring medications for seizures and hyperactivity. After the Mustard procedure at the age of three years, he had had various degrees of atrioventricular block together with atrial flutter. He and his sibling were ill with a respiratory infection when he died quietly in the living room. No special cause was found on postmortem study. The surgical repair was judged good. The third sudden death (no. 6) occurred in a 13-year-old boy who had had a significant atrial arrhythmia and varying degrees of heart block after the Mustard procedure. He was followed up elsewhere, but it was reported that he had had seizures one month and again two days before death. He died suddenly at home and no postmortem examination was performed. Because of the marked sinus node dysfunction and heart block, the most likely diagnosis was an arrhythmic death. The two episodes of seizures could have been Stokes-Adams attacks. The fourth sudden death (no. 7) occurred in a 15-year-old girl who had atrioventricular rhythm problems after a Blalock-Hanlon procedure. She had sinus node arrhythmias subsequent to the Mustard procedure, demonstrating slow junctional rhythm on various studies. Electrophysiological studies showed an abnormal sinus node recovery time. She had also been found to have myocardial dysfunction. She had complained of palpitations and, on the morning of sudden death, she complained of shortness of breath. The coroner did not report any acute findings on the autopsy but did report "heart damage." Arrhythmias in the second group of patients were documented on electrocardiography, on the exercise test, and with Holter monitoring (Table 4). Arrhythmias were less common in those who died early, and were mostly mild in these patients. In contrast, atrial arrhythmias were more common in those who died late and were progressively more severe as the patient became older.

Since myocardial dysfunction was important, although not always the direct cause of death in patients who died late, this problem was reviewed. Assessment was done clinically (including study of the electrocardiogram and chest x-ray) and hemodynamically by echocardiography, catheterization, and cineangiography. The response

Table 4
Documented Arrhythmias, 16 Patients

Arrhythmia	Less than one year survival (no.)	Survival from 5–15 years (no.)
Sinus bradycardia	—	2
Atrial flutter	1	2
Atrial fibrillation	1	2
Junctional rhythm	3	3
Heart block (1–3rd)	3 (1st)	7 (1–3rd)
Premature ventricular beats	—	5
Premature atrial beats with aberrancy	—	1

to exercise and measurement of the ejection fraction were done by radionuclide study. Only three of the eight had not shown any abnormality of myocardium on any studies performed (Table 5).

Discussion

Late deaths after the Mustard or Senning operation can usually be related to one or more of the following factors: atrial arrhythmias or conduction disturbances, systemic and/or pulmonary venous obstruction, residual shunts, pulmonary vascular disease, ventricular dysfunction, atrioventricular valve malfunction, or subpulmonary obstruction (Park et al., 1983). The 16 late deaths reported all fit into the above categories.

Assessment of the results of surgery for congenital heart disease is a continuing process (Graham, 1982). Assessment must be made by all involved in the care of the patient and an honest and critical evaluation made individually and as a group. It is important to share these results with other centers because, even though much has already been learned elsewhere, more information is still needed. Pathological studies of the sinus node in early deaths (Edwards et al., 1978) and the conduction tissue in sudden deaths (Bharati et al., 1979) have influenced the methods of cannulation of the superior caval vein and the techniques of stitching the baffle in the area of the atrioventricular node. The possibility of damaging the tricuspid valve and its later function when a ventricular septal defect is closed through the valve (Arciniegas et al., 1981) and attention to the tailoring of the

Table 5
Myocardial Dysfunction in Patients Surviving 5 to 15 Years

(Number of Patients = 8)

Abnormal function by:	
Clinical evidence	3
Tricuspid and/or mitral regurgitation	3
Hemodynamic study catheterization	3 Abnormal = 5/8
Abnormal exercise response	4
Radionuclide study	4
Good function	3 Normal = 3/8

baffle to prevent venous obstruction (Trusler et al., 1980) have helped decrease early surgical complications. Better protection of the myocardium during surgery (Arciniegas et al., 1981) has improved the short-term survival rate. The effects of long-term survival are yet to be determined. The study of anatomy and function of the heart after atrial redirection procedures should include, where possible, preoperative and postoperative electrophysiological studies (Beerman et al., 1983; Gillette, 1980; Hayes et al., 1986; Southall et al., 1980); hemodynamic evaluations (Hagler et al., 1979; Park et al., 1983); exercise testing (Mathews et al., 1983); radionuclide and exercise studies (Benson et al., 1982; Hurwitz et al., 1985; Murphy et al., 1983) and echocardiographic and Doppler evaluation (Chin et al., 1985; Silverman et al., 1981; Thompson et al., 1981). Standardization of preoperative and postoperative data gathering should be correlated with that from other centers for final analysis.

As we search for the "whys," all the problems of myocardial function, arrhythmias, and pathological changes must be researched. It is possible that the long-term changes in structure of the heart may follow all surgical procedures. Indeed, this possibility has already been suggested by Bharati and Lev (1982) and by Vetter and Horowitz (1982). On the other hand, alterations in the function of the atria following Mustard or Senning operation (Wyse et al., 1980) may, through poorer filling of the ventricles or some other functional abnormality, secondarily affect the function of the ventricles. The role of hypoxia subsequent to damage to the coronary arteries and impairment of the blood supply to the muscle may possibly be more marked in complete transposition, tetralogy of Fallot, and other cyanotic heart disease. The dysfunction seen in the left ventricular muscle in older patients with tricuspid atresia could possibly be due to the same cause. The age at time of surgery may also be a factor.

Conclusion

It is not possible from the review of these 16 late deaths following the Mustard or Senning procedures at Children's Hospital to reach any conclusion regarding the superiority of either of these procedures. The special problems in those who died some time after the operation were not common in those who died almost immediately, but these latter patients did not survive long enough to allow us to draw any conclusions concerning long-term problems. There is likely to be a common denominator in the eight late deaths with late deaths seen in other postoperative congenital defects such as tetralogy of Fallot. Operation at an earlier age may be the crucial point, and not the type of operation. These questions need to be answered before everyone switches to "the switch."

References

Arciniegas E, Farooki ZQ, Hakimi M, et al. Results of the Mustard operation for dextro-transposition of the great arteries. *J Thorac Cardiovasc Surg* 1981;81:580–587.

Beerman LB, Neches WH, Fricker FJ, et al. Arrhythmias in transposition of the great arteries after the Mustard operation. *Am J Cardiol* 1983;15:1530–1534.

Benson LN, Bonet J, McLaughlin P, et al. Assessment of right ventricular function during supine bicycle exercise after Mustard's operation. *Circulation* 1982;65:1052–1059.

Bharati S, Molthan ME, Veasy LG, Lev M. Conduction system in two cases of sudden death two years after the Mustard operation. *J Thorac Cardiovasc Surg* 1979;77:101–108.

Bharati S, Lev M. Sequelae of atriotomy and ventriculotomy on the endocardium, conduction system and coronary arteries. *Am J Cardiol* 1982;50:580–587.

Chin AJ, Sanders SP, Williams RG, et al. Two-dimensional echocardiographic assessment of caval and pulmonary venous pathways after the Senning operation. *Am J Cardiol* 1983;52:118–126.

Edwards WD, Edwards JE. Pathology of the sinus node in d-transposition following the Mustard operation. *J Thorac Cardiovasc Surg* 1978;75:2:213–218.

Gillette PC, Kugler JD, Garson Jr A, et al. Mechanisms of cardiac arrhythmias after the Mustard operation for transposition of the great arteries. *Am J Cardiol* 1980;45:1225–1230.

Graham Jr TP. Assessing the results of surgery for congenital heart disease: a continuing process. *Circulation* 1982;65(6):1049–1051.

Hagler DJ, Ritter DG, Mair DD, et al. Right and left ventricular function after the Mustard procedure in transposition of the great arteries. *Am J Cardiol* 1979;44:276–283.

Hayes CJ, Gersony WM. Arrhythmias after the Mustard operation for transposition of the great arteries: A long-term study. *J Am Coll Cardiol* 1986;7:133–137.

Hurwitz RA, Caldwell RL, Girod DA, et al. Ventricular function in transposition of the great arteries: evaluation by radionuclide angiocardiography. *Am Heart J* 1985;110:600–605.

Mathews RA, Fricker FJ, Beerman LB, et al. Exercise studies after the Mustard operation in transposition of the great arteries. *Am J Cardiol* 1983;15:1526–1529.

Murphy JH, Barlai-Kovach MM, Mathews RA, et al. Rest and exercise right and left ventricular function late after the Mustard operation: Assessment by radionuclide ventriculography. *Am J Cardiol* 1983;15:1520–1526.

Park SC, Neches WH, Mathews RA, et al. Hemodynamic function after the Mustard operation for transposition of the great arteries. *Am J Cardiol* 1983;15:1514–1519.

Silverman NH, Snider AR, Cole J, et al. Superior vena caval obstruction after Mustard's operation: Detection by two-dimensional contrast echocardiography. *Circulation* 1981;64:392–396.

Southall DP, Keeton BR, Leanage R, et al. Cardiac rhythm and conduction before and after Mustard's operation for complete transposition of the great arteries. *Br Heart J* 1980;43:21–30.

Thompson K, Serwer GA. Echocardiographic features of patients with and without residual defects after Mustard's procedure for transposition of the great vessels. *Circulation* 1981; 64:1032–1041.

Trusler GA, Williams WG, Izukawa T, Olley PM. Current results with the Mustard operation in isolated transposition of the great arteries. *J Thorac Cardiovasc Surg* 1980;80:381–389.

Vetter VL, Horowitz LN. Electrophysiologic residua and sequelae of surgery for congenital heart defects. *Am J Cardiol* 1982;50:588–604.

Wyse RK, Macartney FJ, Kohmer J, et al. Differential atrial filling after M Mustard and Senning repairs. Detection by transcutaneous Doppler ultrasound. *Br Heart J* 1980;44:692–698.

4.9

Current Management of Patients with Complete Transposition

John W. Kirklin and Eugene H. Blackstone

Simple complete transposition (the combination of concordant atrioventricular and discordant ventriculoarterial connections) and complete transposition with moderate-sized or large (important) ventricular septal defect have generally been considered to deserve somewhat different treatment protocols, and to present somewhat different results after treatment. Yet it is not certain that this is the case. An atrial switch repair

has, for many years, been considered the appropriate operation for patients with complete transposition, but most groups have practiced deferral of the repair until 3 to 12 months after the initial balloon atrial septostomy, at times with an intervening Blalock-Hanlon atrial septostomy. Some patients treated in this manner die before repair. Both the Mustard and Senning techniques for the atrial switch repair continue

Most of the data presented in this chapter are from the 1986 analysis of a 20-institution cooperative study of The Congenital Heart Surgeons Society. The surgeons and institutions in the Society and in the study are E.A. Arciniegas (Children's Hospital of Michigan, Detroit, MI); P.G. Ashmore (British Columbia Children's Hospital, Vancouver, B.C.); D.M. Behrendt (University of Michigan Medical Center and Mott Children's Hospital, Ann Arbor, MI); F.O. Bowman and J.R. Malm (Columbia Presbyterian Medical Center, New York, NY); A.R. Castaneda (The Children's Hospital, Boston, MA); G.R. Daicoff (All Children's Hospital, St. Petersburg, FL); G. Danielson and D.C. McGoon (Mayo Clinic, Rochester, MN); A.R. Dobell (The Montreal Children's Hospital, Montreal, Canada); D.B. Doty (University of Utah Medical Center and Primary Children's Medical Center, Salt Lake City, UT); P.A. Ebert (University of California, San Francisco, CA); F.S. Idriss (Children's Memorial Hospital, Chicago, IL); G.A. Kaiser (University of Miami and Jackson Memorial Hospital, Miami, FL); H. Laks (UCLA School of Medicine, Los Angeles, CA); G.G. Lindesmith (Children's Hospital of Los Angeles, Los Angeles, CA); W.I. Norwood and L.H. Edmunds (Children's Hospital of Pennsylvania, Philadelphia, PA); A.D. Pacifico, J.W. Kirklin, and J.K. Kirklin (University of Alabama at Birmingham Medical Center, Birmingham, AL); R.L. Replogle (University of Chicago and Michael Reese Hospital and Medical Center, Chicago, IL); A. Starr (Oregon Health Sciences University, Portland, OR); S. Subramanian (State University of New York at Buffalo, Buffalo, NY); G.A. Trusler and W.G. Williams (Hospital for Sick Children, Toronto, Canada).

From: Anderson, RH, Neches, WH, Park, SC, Zuberbuhler, JR, eds: *Perspectives in Pediatric Cardiology*: Mount Kisco, New York, Futura Publishing Co., © 1988.

to have their advocates, but no one knows if one is better than the other. Recently, the arterial switch repair has been adopted by some groups. Although it is not a new operation, only a few detailed reports of the results in sizable groups of patients are available.

This report evaluates the results in the current era of the various treatment options for complete transposition and the effect of the morphological features of the heart of the patient upon these. Since discussions of this type are based to a considerable extent upon comparisons and predictions, and since these are best done using equations that not only define the answer but also the degree of uncertainty inherent in the answer, the report will be based entirely on experiences for which such equations have been developed. Each pediatric cardiology medical and surgical group will need to supplement information of this type with studies of late postoperative cardiac function and rhythm to form their own protocols and inferences concerning the management of patients with complete transposition.

The Congenital Heart Surgeons Society Study

Since a great deal of this report is based on the study of the Congenital Heart Surgeons Society, some information concerning that study is pertinent. The criteria for entry of patients into the study were very strict (Table 1). These criteria make the patients as unselected as possible (Table 2). They provide results that are generally applicable to patients born with complete transposition of all sorts. There were 245 patients enrolled in the study between January 1, 1985 and June 1, 1986 and these are the basis of the data presented in this report. Enrollment of patients into the study will continue until January 1, 1988, by which time it is reliably estimated that 519 neo-

Table 1
Criteria for Entrance into the Study of Transposition by the Congenital Heart Surgeons Society (CHSS)

- Diagnosis: TGA of any morphological subcategory, with or without associated cardiac or other anomalies
- Entrance in CHSS Hospital <15 days of age
- No reparative operation prior to entrance

Note: For this study, complete transposition (TGA) is defined as a congenital cardiac anomaly in which the atrioventricular connection is concordant and the ventriculoarterial connection is discordant (aorta arises more than 50% from the right ventricle, and the pulmonary trunk more than 50% from the left ventricle).

nates will have been enrolled. All patients will be followed for at least 10 years.

Other Data and Equations

Equations are also used in the presentation; these are derived from an update of April 1986 of the published Leiden experience with the arterial switch repair for transposition of various types (n = 90) (Quaegebeur et al., 1986). Other equations are derived from the experience of The Toronto Hospital for Sick Children with simple transposition and a protocol leading to an atrial switch operation by the Mustard technique (n = 115), between 1976 and 1985 (Trusler et al., 1986).

Overall Results

Among the 245 patients in the Congenital Heart Surgeons Society Transposition Study, for all of whom we have follow-up information, 42 had died by July 1, 1986. Although the usual morphological categories are represented, neither by simple anal-

Table 2

Congenital Heart Surgeons Society Transposition Study (January 1, 1985–June 1, 1986)

Age at entry (days)

≤ <	No.	% of 245	
1	111	45%	⎫ 77%
1----2	77	31%	⎭
2----3	15	6%	
3----4	6	2%	
4----5	8	3%	
5----6	4	2%	
6----7	5	2%	
7----8	6	2%	
8----9	1	0.4%	
9----10	3	1%	
10----11	4	2%	
11----12	0	0%	
12----13	2	1%	
13----14	2	1%	
14----15	1	0.4%	
Total	245	100%	

cal category any more than could be explained by chance.

One hundred and seventy-five of the patients underwent balloon atrial septostomy one or more times, 154 underwent a repair of one sort or another, 54 underwent preliminary or palliative operations, and 6 underwent no procedures during the period of observation (Table 4).

Survival at one month was 90% and at 12 months was 80%, considerably less than that of an age-, sex-, or race-matched general population (Fig. 1). If other factors are taken into account, the survival was less among patients in 2 of the 20 institutions (Table 5). Low birth weight was an incremental risk factor for death, but the survival (in percentage) has improved during the 18 months covered by the study to date.

Twelve patients died before repair was performed; 8 of these in the first two weeks of life.

ysis (Table 3) nor by multivariate analysis was the prevalence of death within this follow-up period affected by the morphologi-

The Arterial Switch Repair

The arterial switch repair was performed in 87 patients, 17 of whom died

Table 3

Congenital Heart Surgeons Society Transposition Study (January 1, 1985–June 1, 1986; $n = 245$; deaths = 42)*

Morphological category	n	All deaths		
		No.	%	CL
Simple TGA	187	29	16%	13%–19%
Essentially intact VS with important PS	2	0	0%	0%–61%
Important VSD	36	9	25%	17%–35%
VSD with important PS	15	3	20%	9%–36%
Unknown	5	1	20%	3%–53%
Total	245	42	17%	15%–20%
$p(\chi^2)$			0.65	

PS = pulmonary stenosis; TGA = complete transposition; VS = ventricular septum; VSD = ventricular septal defect.

Note: $p(\chi^2)$ for the difference between prevalence of deaths in patients with simple transposition and those with important ventricular septal defects was 0.17; in the hazard function domain, p for difference was 0.4 for both early and constant phase.

* The confidence intervals (limits) in this and all other tables are 70% confidence limits (CL).

Table 4
Procedures Performed Prior to July 1986 in Patients with Complete Transposition Entered into the Congenital Heart Surgeons Society Transposition Study
(January 1, 1985–June 1, 1986; n = 245; deaths = 42)

Procedures	n	All deaths		
		No.	%	CL
Balloon atrial septostomy	175	26	15%	12%–18%
Arterial switch (planned)	94	20	21%	17%–27%
Executed	87	17	20%	15%–25%
Aborted	7	3	43%	20%–68%
Atrial switch (planned)	60	6	10%	6%–16%
Intraventricular repair	1	1	100%	15%–100%
Rastelli operation	1	0	0%	0%–85%
Preliminary or palliative operations	54	14	26%	19%–34%
Operation of completely unknown type*	1	1	100%	15%–100%
None	6	4	67%	38%–88%

* Since completion of the analysis, this has been determined to be an atrial (Senning) switch repair, performed at age 2 days.

during the period of observation. Seven additional patients were taken to the operating room for the purpose of performing an arterial switch repair but this intention was aborted after the heart was exposed (Table 6); five were aborted to an atrial switch repair and of these three died, which suggests that aborting an arterial switch repair to an atrial switch repair has considerable hazard.

The survival at one month after the arterial switch repair was 82%, and at 12 months was 80% (Fig. 2). The hazard function for death had a single rapidly declining early phase, which nearly reached zero within six months of the operation. This hazard function for death after the arterial switch repair in North America is nearly identical to that in the much longer experience in Leiden, Holland (Quaegebeur et al., 1986).

The multivariate analysis indicated that survival was less after the arterial switch repair in institutions where that operation was used sporadically and not regularly by protocol (Table 7). It also indicated that in protocol institutions, a small number of patients or operations was not a risk factor for death. In protocol institutions, the survival has

been increasing even over the short time of this study. This is also evident in simple analysis (Table 8).

The length of the period of global cardiac ischemia (that is, the aortic cross-clamp time) is a risk factor for death after the arterial switch repair in the Congenital Heart Surgeons Society experience, but the effect is not a strong one (Fig. 3). Thus, using cold cardioplegic myocardial protection, there is not a certainly increased risk of death until the cross-clamp time is longer than about 130 minutes, the so-called point of evident difference. In the Leiden experience with the arterial switch operation, there was also an adverse effect of longer aortic cross-clamp time on survival, according to the multivariate analysis that was made (Quaegebeur et al., 1986). The strength of this effect in the updated Leiden experience is also rather weak, and the quantitative aspects of the relation of cross-clamp time to the risk of death early after repair are almost identical in these two experiences from different parts of the world (Fig. 3). This information indicates that the surgeon has the time required to perform a very precise operation.

The multivariate analysis of the Leiden

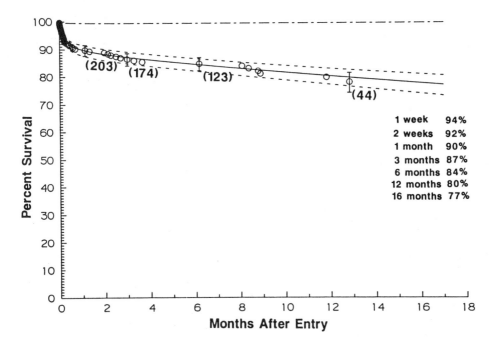

Figure 1. Percent survival among patients entered by June 1, 1986 into the Congenital Heart Surgeons Society Transposition Study (January 1, 1985–June 1, 1986, n = 245, deaths = 42). Date of follow-up was July 1, 1986. Each circle, positioned by actuarial analysis, represents a death; the vertical bars indicate the actuarially determined 70% confidence intervals. The solid line is the parametrically determined percent survival, and the dashed lines enclose the 70% confidence intervals. The numbers in parentheses are the number of patients traced at that time interval. The dash-dot-dash line is the survival of an age-sex-race–matched general population (U.S. Life Tables, 1977). The depictions are similar in the other figures in this presentation. (Equations, coefficients, and p values for this and other figures and tables are available from the authors.)

experience had indicated a steady decline across time in the early risks of the arterial switch operation (Fig. 4) (Quaegebeur et al., 1986). The multivariate analysis of the Congenital Heart Surgeons Society also indicated that the results of the arterial switch operation had already improved across the short time of the study in institutions using a standardized protocol of arterial switching (Table 7). Thus, in January 1985, at a time when the early mortality in the Leiden experience had been reduced to about 5%, that in the North American experience of the Congenital Heart Surgeons Society was 40% (Fig. 5). By about October 1985, however, in institutions in the North American experience which used a standardized protocol of arterial switching, the risk had al-

ready fallen to the Leiden level. Since that time, the risks of death early after repair in the two experiences have been the same and are predicted to approach zero by early 1987 (Fig. 5).

In summary, the arterial switch repair for patients with transposition has become very safe. The output of scientific information from the experiences of the Leiden and other centers has allowed a rapid improvement in results in institutions in the Congenital Heart Surgeons Society which use a consistent protocol of arterial switching. Furthermore, the results are similar for simple transposition and for transposition with ventricular septal defect. Survival is adversely affected by birth weight and by aortic cross-clamp time, but the latter is a weak

Table 5

Incremental Risk Factors for Death at Any Time After Entry in Patients with Complete Transposition in the Congenital Heart Surgeons Society Transposition Study (January 1, 1985–June 1, 1986; n = 245; Deaths = 42)*

Incremental risk factors for death	Early hazard phase		Constant hazard phase	
	Coefficient	p value	Coefficient	p value
(Lower) Birth Weight (kg)	−1.1 ± 0.30	0.0003	—	—
(Earlier) Date of Entry				
(months since 1/1/85)	−0.07 ± 0.042	0.095	—	—
Institution 70	1.7 ± 0.46	0.0002	—	—
Institution 81	1.3 ± 0.68	0.05	—	—

Note: Demographic and morphological variables, date of entry, the institution, and individual institutional case loads were entered into the analysis. Investigation of possible spurious correlations were negative.
* The multivariate equations incorporating these risk factors, and those for all other risk factor analyses presented, are available upon request from the authors.

effect. Importantly, the hazard function for death after the arterial switch repair has, to date, only a single rapidly declining early phase. And, to date, no constant phase of hazard has been observed extending into the late postoperative period.

The Atrial Switch Operation

Among the 245 patients in the study, 60 underwent a planned atrial switch repair. The two-week survival after that operation

Table 6

Death at Any Time After Repair, Including Hospital Deaths, in Patients in the Congenital Heart Surgeons Society Transposition Study Who Underwent an Arterial Switch Repair (January 1, 1985–June 1, 1986)

Arterial switch repair	n	All deaths		
		No.	%	CL
Executed	87[a]	17	20%	15%–25%
Aborted	7	3	43%	20%–68%
to exploration only (no CPB)	1	0	0%	0%–85%
to BH operation	1[b]	0	0%	0%–85%
to atrial switch repair	5[c]	3	60%	29%–86%
Total	94	20	21%	17%–27%

BH = Blalock-Hanlon; CPB = cardiopulmonary bypass.
[a] In 1 (who died) of the 87 patients, the arterial switch repair was completed and then taken down and an atrial switch performed at the same operation.
[b] 3 months later a planned atrial switch repair was done.
[c] None since 1/2/86 (that patient died).

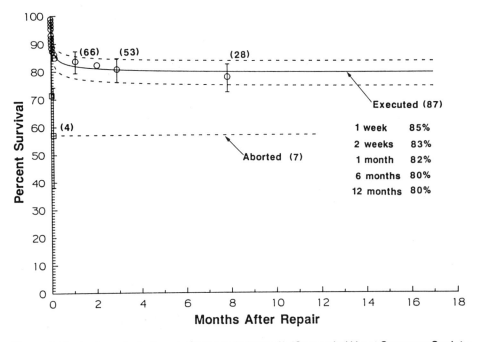

Figure 2. Percent survival after an arterial switch repair. (Congenital Heart Surgeons Society; January 1, 1985–June 1, 1986; n = 94, deaths = 20).

was 93% and the one-year survival was 89% (Fig. 6). The hazard function after the atrial switch operation had a single phase, but the follow-up is too short to be useful in framing inferences. According to analysis of the experience in Toronto (Trusler et al., 1986), the hazard function for patients followed out to 10 years after a protocol including atrial switching at 6 to 12 months of age has two phases. The constant phase continues out as long as the patients have been followed. Presumably, most of the late

Table 7

Incremental Risk Factors for Death at Any Time After an Arterial Switch Repair in Patients in the Congenital Heart Surgeons Society Transposition Study
(January 1, 1985–June 1, 1986, n = 87; deaths = 17)

	Single hazard phase	
Incremental risk factors for death	*Coefficient*	*p value*
(Earlier) date of operation (months since 1/1/85)	−0.17 ± 0.061	0.004
Nonprotocol institution	3.1 ± 0.64	<0.0001
(Longer) aortic cross-clamp time (minutes)	0.020 ± 0.0109	0.06

Note: Variables entered into the analysis were demographic and morphological, the institution of repair, individual institution number of arterial switch operations, protocol versus nonprotocol institution (institution 86 considered a protocol institution), date of operation, total circulatory arrest versus cardiopulmonary bypass, total circulatory arrest time (minutes), lowest temperature during operation, aortic cross-clamp time, ventricular septal defect, and/or patent arterial duct repair.

Table 8

Deaths at Any Time After The Arterial Switch Repair (Congenital Heart Surgeons Society Transposition Study, January 1, 1985–June 1, 1986, n = 87; deaths = 17)

Date of operation		Protocol institution							
		No				Yes			
		All deaths				All deaths			
≤	<	n	No.	%	CL	n	No.	%	CL
Jan. 1, 1985---July 1, 1985		2	2	100%	39%–100%	19	4	21%	11%–35%
July 1, 1985---Jan. 1, 1986		5	2	40%	14%–71%	27	5	19%	11%–29%
Jan. 1, 1986---June 1, 1986		6	4	67%	38%–89%	28	0	0%	0%–7%
Total		13	8	62%	43%–77%	74	9	12%	8%–17%
p (logistic)				0.4				0.004	

deaths are related to loss of sinus rhythm and a resultant tendency to die suddenly.

Only one institution in the Congenital Heart Surgeons Society study, and a low birth weight, were risk factors after the atrial switch repair (Table 9). Of course, great in-

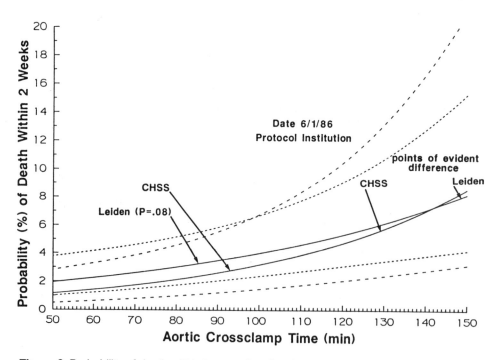

Figure 3. Probability of death within two weeks after the arterial switch repair, according to the aortic cross-clamp (global ischemic) time. These are nomograms of solutions of the multivariate equations from the Congenital Heart Surgeons Society (see Table 7; date of operation was entered as June 1, 1986 and nonprotocol institution as NO); and from the updated Leiden experience (n = 90; date of operation entered as June 1, 1986).

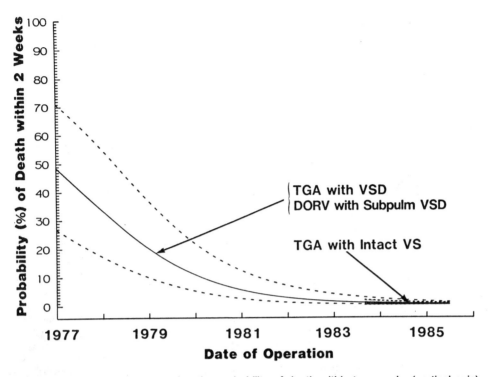

Figure 4. Nomogram representing the probability of death within two weeks (vertical axis) after an arterial switch repair, according to the date of operation (Leiden, 1977–July 1985, n = 66). DORV = double outlet right ventricle; TGA = complete transposition; VS = ventricular septum; VSD = ventricular septal defect. (Reproduced with permission from Quaegebeur et al., *J Thorac Cardiovasc Surg*, in press.)

terest attaches to the probability of survival after an atrial switch repair by the Senning technique compared with that by the Mustard technique. The simplest comparisons suggest that survival is better with the Mustard than with the Senning technique (Table 10). However, a number of detailed multivariate analyses failed to disclose an advantage of one over the other (all *p* values > 0.2).

In summary, the atrial switch operation has had an early mortality of 7%. There has been no difference to date in the results in simple transposition and transposition with ventricular septal defect. Low birth weight adversely affects survival. Although the survival after the atrial switch repair has not increased across the time of the study, the survival of all those entering a *protocol*

leading to atrial switching has improved; the improvement results largely from improvement in the prerepair management of the patient. The 12-month survival of 92%, predicted in the current era for a neonate weighing 3.4 kg at birth entering a protocol leading to atrial switching is the same as for one entering a protocol leading to arterial switching.

Simple Complete Transposition

The remainder of the discussion deals with simple complete transposition, which was the diagnosis in 189 of the 245 patients entered into the study of the Congenital

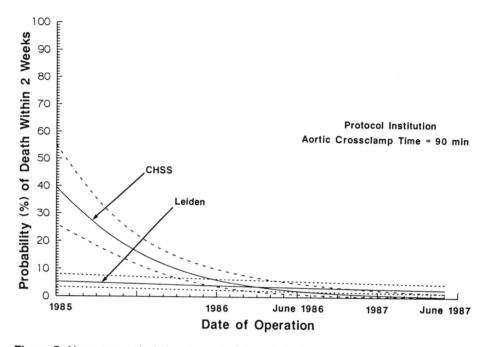

Figure 5. Nomograms depicting the probability of death within two weeks of an arterial switch repair for complete transposition with or without an important ventricular septal defect. The nomogram for the Congenital Heart Surgeons Society (CHSS) experience is a solution of the multivariate equation (see Table 7), with aortic cross-clamp time entered as 90 minutes and protocol institution as yes. The Leiden nomogram is from the multivariate equation based on their updated experience (n = 90), with the same cross-clamp time entered. Note that the nomograms present past, current, and future dates of operation, and therefore are comparing and predicting.

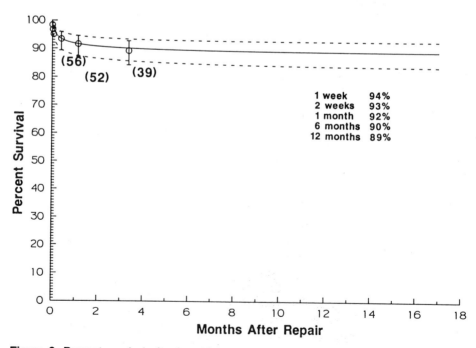

Figure 6. Percent survival after an atrial switch repair for complete transposition with or without an important ventricular septal defect (Congenital Heart Surgeons Society Transposition Study, January 1, 1985–June 1, 1986, n = 60, deaths = 6).

Table 9

Incremental Risk Factors for Death at Any Time After an Atrial Switch Repair for Complete Transposition With or Without an Important Ventricular Septal Defect (Congenital Heart Surgeons Society Transposition Study, January 1, 1985–June 1, 1986, n = 60, deaths = 6)

	Single hazard phase	
Incremental risk factors for death	Coefficient	p value
(Lower) birth weight (kg)	-1.1 ± 0.48	0.02
Institution 86	1.8 ± 0.85	0.03

Note: Variables entered into the analysis were the same as were entered into the arterial switch analysis. Senning versus Mustard type of repair could not be entered (no deaths after Mustard repair).

Heart Surgeons Society through June 1, 1986. Twenty-nine deaths have occurred among these 189 patients.

Seventy-eight patients were entered into a patient management program leading to an arterial switch repair, and 104 into one leading to an atrial switch repair (Table 11). At a glance, survival appears to be better after a program leading to atrial switching, particularly by the Mustard technique. To conclude this without a more detailed analysis would be an error, in view of the complexity of the problem. A more detailed analysis began with generation of the survivorship (Fig. 7), and the hazard function for death (not presented). Then a multivariate analysis was made. The resultant equation is the single most important part of this

Table 10

Deaths After the Atrial Switch Repair According to the Use of the Senning or Mustard Technique, and Death in Patients in a Patient Management Program (PMP) Including Either the Senning or Mustard Technique (Congenital Heart Surgeons Society Transposition Study, January 1, 1985–June 1, 1986)

		All deaths		
Category	n	No.	%	CL
Atrial switch repair	60	6	10%	6%–16%
Senning	39	6	15%	9%–24%
Mustard	21	0	0%	0%–9%
p (Fisher)			0.07	
Atrial Switch PMP in Simple TGA	104	9	9%	6%–12%
Senning	49	7	14%	9%–21%
Mustard	43	2	5%	2%–11%
Unknown	12	0	0%	0%–15%
p (Fisher)			0.11	

Table 11

Deaths in Patients with Simple Complete Transposition, According to the Repair Operation in the Patient Management Program (PMP) Into Which They Were Entered (Congenital Heart Surgeons Society Transposition Study, January 1, 1985–June 1, 1986, Simple Transposition n = 187; deaths = 29)

Repair operation	n	All deaths		
		No.	%	CL
Arterial switch	78	16	21%	16%–26%
Atrial switch	104	9	9%	6%–12%
Mustard	43	2	5%	2%–11%
Senning	49	7	14%	9%–21%
Unknown	12	0	0%	0%–15%
p (Fisher)			0.11	
Total	182	25	14%	11%–17%
$p(\chi^2)$			0.02	

Note: 5 of the 187 patients (4 of whom died) could not be assigned a PMP and are not included; 4 of the 5 are from nonprotocol hospitals.

evaluation (Table 12). It indicates that patient management programs of arterial switching, and of atrial switching by the Mustard or Senning technique in institutions following a regular protocol result in similar percentages of survival within the

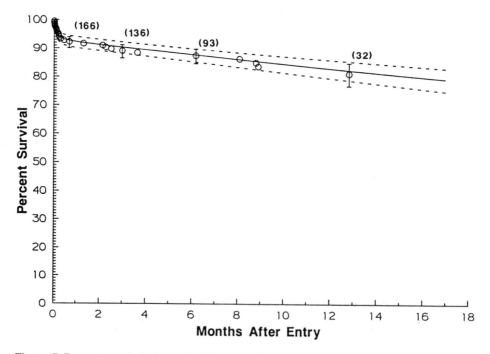

Figure 7. Percent survival after entry into the study of patients with simple complete transposition (Congenital Heart Surgeons Society Transposition Study, n = 182; deaths = 25).

Table 12

Incremental Risk Factors for Death at Any Time After Entry in Patients with Simple Complete Transposition (Congenital Heart Surgeons Society Transposition Study, January 1, 1985–June 1, 1986, n = 182, deaths = 25)

Incremental risk factors for death	Early hazard phase		Constant hazard phase	
	Coefficient	p value	Coefficient	p value
(Lower) birth weight (kg)	−1.2 ± 0.39	0.001	—	—
(Earlier) date of entry (months since 1/1/85)	−0.11 ± 0.061	0.08	—	—
Arterial switch PMP in a nonprotocol institution	3.0 ± 0.53	<0.0001	—	—

Note: Variables entered were those in Table 5, plus protocol versus nonprotocol institution for both arterial and atrial switch repair, arterial versus atrial switch protocol, arterial switch versus atrial switch patient management program (PMP), and Senning PMP versus Mustard PMP. Senning (versus Mustard) PMP as a risk factor p = 0.4 (early phase) and 0.24 (late phase).

follow-up period of this study. It also indicates that the results have improved over the relatively short time of this study. A comparison of these patient management programs with those of a program leading to an atrial switch repair at The Toronto Hospital for Sick Children, and with a program of arterial switch repair in Leiden shows the power of the effect of birth weight (Fig. 8). The 12-month predicted survival in patients weighing 3.4 kg and currently entering for treatment is 92%. This number is essentially the same in the three experiences.

Summary of Current Knowledge and Inferences Concerning Survival in Neonates Born with Transposition

There is no demonstrable difference so far in survival in patients with transposition, whether or not there is a coexisting important ventricular septal defect, in the Congenital Heart Surgeons Society transposition study. The same conclusions were reached in a study of the results of the arterial switch repair in Leiden, Holland (Quaegebeur et al., 1986). This all suggests that patients with transposition, with and without an important ventricular septal defect, should have repair very early in life, and probably (for other reasons) by an arterial switch repair.

Survival after an arterial switch repair has improved in the recent part of the Congenital Heart Surgeons Society experience. Likewise, the prevention of death before an atrial switch repair has improved. There is no evidence in this study to date of a relationship between survival and the interval between entry and repair, but this should not be considered final information in this regard.

There is as yet no demonstrable superiority of one patient management program over another (that is, no demonstrated superiority of a program of arterial switching or one of atrial switching and no evidence of superiority of the Senning or Mustard technique for atrial switching). Currently, 12-month survival in protocol institutions of patients with simple transposition and transposition and important ventricular septal defect entering at birth is predicted to be 92% in those with a birth weight of 3.4 kg. This figure is the same whether an atrial

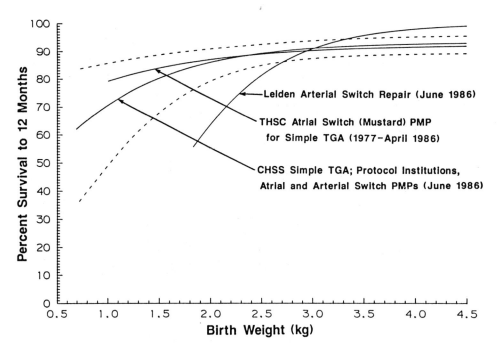

Figure 8. Nomograms of predicted percent survival to 12 months of patients with simple complete transposition entering currently into a treatment program in the first few days of life, according to birth weight. That for the patients in the Congenital Heart Surgeons Society (CHSS) study is a solution of the multivariate equation in Table 12 for protocol institutions with date of entry June 1, 1986; the nomogram is applicable to both atrial and arterial switch patient management programs. Those for Leiden and Toronto Hospital for Sick Children (THSC) are solutions of similar multivariate equations, again with date of entry entered as June 1, 1986. The 70% confidence intervals of the Leiden and THSC experience (not shown) and of those of the CHSS experience are all overlapping.

or arterial switch patient management program is used. It would be premature to suggest that the summary and inferences will be similar after the study has been in progress longer.

In all patient management programs in the studies of the Congenital Heart Surgeons Society, low birth weight was a risk factor for death before or after repair. There was no suggestion, as yet, from the study that one patient management program is superior to another in low birth weight infants. Results have, however, improved in the low birth weight group. With increased safety of the arterial switch repair, this may prove to be the most satisfactory method for low birth weight infants.

The neonatal heart may be more tolerant of global ischemia than older hearts as a group, but not more than older hearts with minimal secondary cardiomyopathy. In any event, there is little relationship between aortic cross-clamp time and survival in the experience of either the Congenital Heart Surgeons Society or the Leiden group.

Comment

By January 1988, over 500 neonates will have been entered into the study of complete transposition organized by the

Congenital Heart Surgeons Society. The plan is to follow them for 10 years. The gathering of data is a formidable task, both for the individual institutions and for the Data and Analysis Center. The analyses are time-consuming and complex, and will become more so. But, after 20 years of active treatment of patients with complete transposition, there are many unanswered questions. This study will provide some useful answers to many of these questions. Probably, it has already improved results in the participating institutions.

References

Quaegebeur JM, Rohmer J, Ottenkamp J, et al. The arterial switch operation. An eight-year experience. *J Thorac Cardiovasc Surg* 1986;92:361–384.

Trusler GA, Williams WG, Blackstone EH, Kirklin JW. Unpublished data, 1986.

V

The Left Valve in
Atrioventricular Septal Defect

5.1

Anatomical and Echocardiographic Features of the Left Valve in Atrioventricular Septal Defect

Robert H. Anderson, Tjark J. Ebels, James R. Zuberbuhler, and Norman H. Silverman

Although Peacock, as long ago as 1846, clearly described the trifoliate arrangement of the left atrioventricular valve in lesions unified by a lack of normal atrioventricular septation (atrioventricular canal malformations, endocardial cushion defects), controversies continue concerning the optimal description and surgical repair of this structure. Many of the disagreements stem from the traditional approach of classifying lesions in terms of their presumed embryogenesis. Thus, arguing from developmental premises, Di Segni et al. (1983a, 1983b) hold that "isolated" clefts of the mitral valve are a form of "endocardial cushion defect." A similar stance had been adopted by Feldt et al. (1976), who classified the isolated cleft along with "atrioventricular canal" variants of isolated ventricular septal defect, with the more classic examples of "atrioventricular canal malformations." This line of thinking leads to consideration of the left atrioventricular valve in all these lesions as being of mitral morphology, with or without a "cleft" of variable extent and structure. Such an approach, in turn, leads inexorably to the surgical concept of valve repair by means of closure of the presumed "cleft."

More recently, the trifoliate concept of the left valve in atrioventricular septal defect, described so clearly by Peacock (1846), has been revitalized by Carpentier (1978), with emphasis on its surgical significance. Stimulated by Carpentier's observations, which seem to provide a more tangible explanation of the anatomy in these lesions,

From: Anderson, RH, Neches, WH, Park, SC, Zuberbuhler, JR, eds: *Perspectives in Pediatric Cardiology*: Mount Kisco, New York, Futura Publishing Co., © 1988.

we and our colleagues have studied in depth the morphological features of hearts unified by lack of normal atrioventricular septation (Becker and Anderson, 1982; Penkoske et al. 1985; Piccoli et al., 1979; Silverman et al, 1984). Our observations show, unequivocally to our eyes, that hearts with deficient atrioventricular septation differ fundamentally in several readily recognizable ways from those other hearts that have normal atrioventricular septal structures. Furthermore, our research has shown that, in those hearts with deficient atrioventricular septal structures, the left atrioventricular valve bears scant resemblance to the bifoliate structure described appropriately as "mitral" in those hearts with normal atrioventricular septation. In this chapter, thus, we review the anatomical and echocardiographic findings that underscore our contention that this structure is best described as a three-leaflet left atrioventricular valve. Even should future research demonstrate an embryologic link between these lesions and "isolated" cleft of the mitral valve in terms of failure of fusion of endocardial cushion tissues, the lesions are as dissimilar anatomically as chalk and cheese. It is anatomy (rather than embryology) that dictates diagnosis and surgical repair. It is for this reason that we maintain our stance (Anderson et al., 1985) that understanding of the function and repair of the valve in atrioventricular septal defects is optimized by recognition of its trifoliate nature.

again irrespective of their leaflet structure. Such argumentation is specious. The aortic, pulmonary, and truncal valves are so described because they guard the entrances to aortic, pulmonary, and common trunks. The mitral valve, in contrast, although always found within the morphologically left ventricle, was not described as "mitral" for that reason. Instead, it received its mitral adjective because it resembles a bishop's hat (a "mitre"), in contrast to the valve with three leaflets (tricuspid) which guards the morphologically right atrioventricular junction. The original alternative name for the mitral valve was the bicuspid valve. It makes little sense, therefore, to describe a valve guarding the morphologically left junction as "mitral" if it has more than two leaflets and bears no resemblance to the bishop's hat. It could be confusing if it possessed three leaflets to describe it as a tricuspid valve, since no distinction would then be made from the valve guarding the morphologically right junction. If the left-sided valve found in atrioventricular septal defects does differ from a normal mitral valve, as we contend to be the case (Penkoske et al., 1985; also see below), then the valve is better not described as a mitral valve. Rather, it is both simple and accurate to describe it as a left valve. This is, of course, only justified when the valve in question is found in a left-sided location. The comparable valve in an individual with complete mirror-image arrangement ("situs inversus") would simply and accurately be described as a right-sided atrioventricular valve.

The Naming of Cardiac Valves

It is important that we state clearly our reasons for describing the left valve in atrioventricular septal defects as a trifoliate structure rather than an abnormal mitral valve. It may be argued that an aortic or pulmonary valve is thus described irrespective of the number of its leaflets. This approach, so the argument goes, is equally applicable to valves in the "mitral" position,

Morphology of the Left Atrioventricular Valve in Hearts with Normal Atrioventricular Septation

In order to describe the left atrioventricular valve in atrioventricular septal defects appropriately, we must first be fully cognizant of the morphological features of

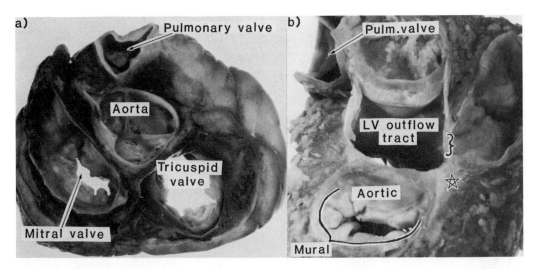

Figure 1. Illustrations of the anatomy of the aortic valve and its relationships to the atrioventricular valves. The photographs are viewed from above. *a* shows the valves after removal of the arterial trunks and atrial chambers. *b* shows the extensive "posterior" diverticulum of the subaortic outflow tract revealed by removal of the noncoronary leaflet of the aortic valve. The bracket shows the site of the membranous atrioventricular septum, while the star marks the position of the normal muscular atrioventricular septum.

the valve in hearts with normal atrioventricular septation which prompted the "mitral" (or bicuspid) appellation. It is also essential to understand the normal relationships between this valve, the aortic valve, and the subaortic outflow tract from the morphologically left ventricle. When seen from above in anatomical orientation (Fig. 1), the aortic valve is deeply wedged between the left and right atrioventricular orifices, the latter structures being guarded by the mitral and tricuspid valves, respectively. The mitral orifice has a very limited connection with the ventricular septum. The overall orientation of its orifice is oblique, most of its apparently "septal" circumference being separated from the septum by the subaortic outflow tract (Fig. 1b). This arrangement can be equally well demonstrated in short-axis echocardiographic cuts, which confirm the oblique arrangement of the fishmouth opening in the valve (Fig. 2). Such cuts taken deeper in the ventricles show the oblique orientation of the papillary muscles supporting the commissures of the valve, these being located in the anterolateral and posteromedial positions (Fig. 3). Long-axis

cuts at right angles to the inlet part of the ventricular septum (so-called four-chamber cuts) then show the influence of this normal "wedged" arrangement of the subaortic outflow tract on atrioventricular septation.

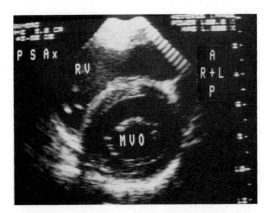

Figure 2. The anatomy of the normal mitral valve is well seen echocardiographically. This shows the bicommissural arrangement of the normal valves with the aortic leaflet oriented more or less parallel to the ventricular septal surface and separated from it by the posterior extension of the outflow tract. A = anterior; L = left; P = posterior; R = right.

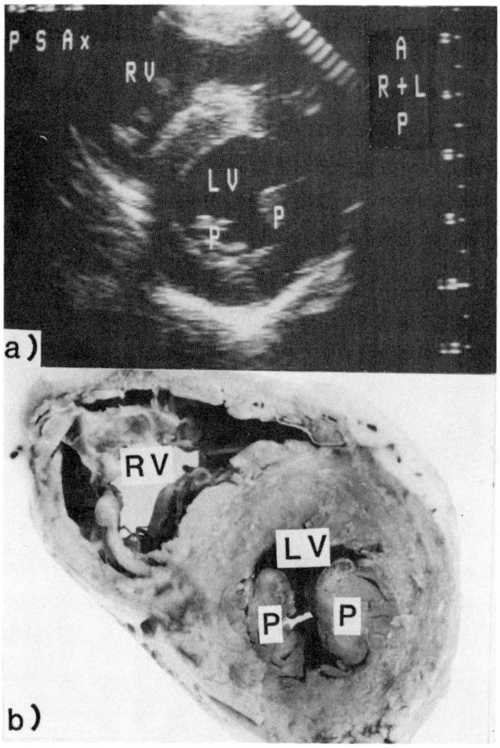

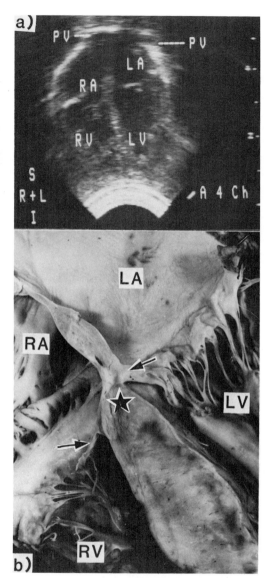

Figure 3. The arrangement of the papillary muscles of the normal mitral valve. The echocardiographic parasternal short-axis (PSAX) section is from the same patient shown in Fig. 2. Note that the papillary muscles lie directly underneath the commissures at 4 and 7 o'clock. It must be appreciated that the echocardiographic orientation may seem different from that seen anatomically because the transducer is applied to the chest in such a manner that there is some rotation of the image with respect to its true anatomical plane. The anatomical section chosen for comparison (b) has itself been rotated to match the echocardiographic section. LV = left ventricle, RV = right ventricle.

Cuts taken close to the diaphragmatic surface of the heart, through that short area in which the mitral orifice has a direct septal attachment, show that the mitral attachment is closer to the base than the more apically located orificial attachment of the septal leaflet of the tricuspid valve (Fig. 4). It is this offsetting of the orificial attachments of the mitral and tricuspid valves that produces the normal muscular atrioventricular septum. Cuts taken more anteriorly (Fig. 5)

Figure 4. This echocardiogram in four-chamber plane (a), together with a comparable anatomic section (b) demonstrates the arrangement in the normal heart which produces the atrioventricular muscular septum (star). Note the offset between the levels of the proximal septal attachment of the mitral and tricuspid valves (arrows). LA = left atrium; RA = right atrium; PV = pulmonary vein; I = inferior; L = left; R = right; S = superior.

show how the wedged subaortic outflow tract of the left ventricle "lifts" the mitral valve away from the septum. The septal surface of the outflow tract is then, rather

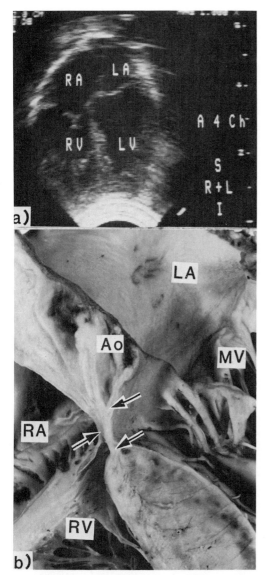

Figure 5. These echocardiographic (a) and anatomical (b) sections, from the same series shown in Fig. 4, demonstrate the atrioventricular membranous septum in the normal heart. Note how the subaortic outflow tract separates the mitral valve from the septum, and how the tricuspid valve separates the membranous septum into interventricular and atrioventricular components.

than being a muscular structure, a fibrous partition that separates the left ventricle from the right atrium. This is the membranous atrioventricular septum.

Examination of the mitral valve from above (Fig. 1) shows that the commissures between the leaflets, located anterolaterally and posteromedially, divide the valve circumference into two grossly dissimilar segments. The shorter segment, making up one-third of the overall circumference, is guarded by a deep, semicircular leaflet which is in fibrous continuity on the ventricular aspect with the leaflets of the aortic valve. If an artificial cut is made through this leaflet (a "cleft" of the mitral valve), the cut leads directly into the subaortic outflow tract (Becker and Anderson, 1982). So does an "isolated" cleft of a mitral valve in a heart with normal atrioventricular septation, as can be shown both anatomically and echocardiographically (Fig. 6). It is our preference, therefore, to describe this leaflet of the normal mitral valve as "aortic." The other leaflet occupies two-thirds of the annular circumference of the mitral orifice and is attached throughout its extent to the parietal atrioventricular junction. It is a long, narrow structure which we describe as "mural." Usually this mural leaflet is divided into a series of "scallops," most frequently three in number. Some would describe these "scallops" as individual leaflets, promoting the concept of a four-leaflet valve (Yacoub, 1975), but the arrangement is insufficiently constant to warrant such an approach.

In keeping with the arrangement of aortic and mitral valves described above, in which the ventricular inlet overlaps and is separated from the septum by the subaortic outflow tract, the inlet and outlet dimensions of the left ventricular aspect of the septum are more or less equal (Penkoske et al., 1985). From all this morphology, we can extract the fundamental features of hearts with normal atrioventricular septation. These are separate right and left atrioventricular junctions; a deeply wedged position of the subaortic outflow tract; a left atrioventricular valve in which the mural leaflet makes up two-thirds of the annular circumference; inlet-outlet ventricular dimensions of unity; and the presence of septal struc-

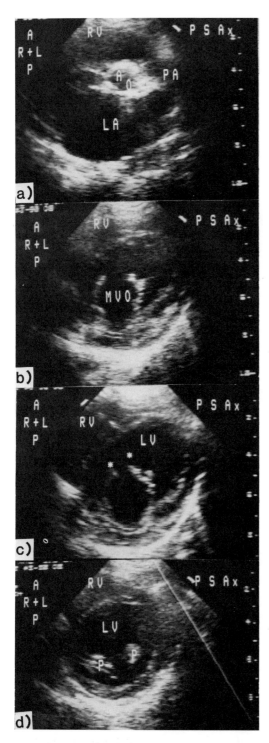

tures separating the cavity of the left ventricle from that of the right atrium.

The Morphological Stigmata of Hearts with Abnormal Atrioventricular Septation

When a heart lacks any atrioventricular septal structure, it exhibits features in addition to a simple communication between the atrial and ventricular chambers. Rather, it differs fundamentally from hearts with normal atrioventricular septation in all of the features enumerated above. First, irrespective of whether there are common or separate right and left atrioventricular orifices, there is a common atrioventricular junction (Fig. 7). Second, there is unwedging of the aortic valve, such that a "snowman" appearance is present rather than the "clover leaf" arrangement of the normal heart (Fig. 1). Third, the left atrioventricular valve has a trifoliate arrangement, to which we will return in our next section. Fourth, the inlet-outlet dimensions of the septum differ markedly from unity with the outlet measurement being significantly longer (Fig. 8). If large numbers of hearts are studied, then the inlet-outlet disproportion is comparable, irrespective of the arrangement of the valve leaflets guarding the common atrioventricular junction and their relation to the ventricular septal crest (in other words, regardless of whether there is a

Figure 6. This composite series of figures taken in the parasternal short-axis plane (PSAx) demonstrates the anatomy of "isolated" cleft of a normally structured mitral valve. Atrioventricular septation is normal in this heart. The top frame is taken at the level of the aortic root and demonstrates the normal right ventricle, pulmonary trunk (PA), and aorta (AO). The second frame is a more caudal cut showing the cleft in the aortic leaflet of the mitral valve (MVO) communicating with the normally wedged subaortic outlet. The next frame shows a slightly lower cut and again demonstrates the cleft (asterisks). The bottom frame demonstrates the papillary (P) muscle arrangement, which is that of the normal heart (compared with Fig. 3).

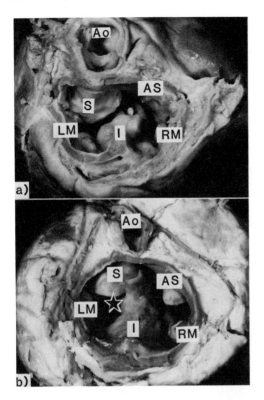

Figure 7. These dissections of the short axis of hearts with deficient atrioventricular septation are viewed from above and should be compared with Fig. 1. They show the common atrioventricular junction and "unwedged" position of the aortic valve found irrespective of whether there is a common valve orifice (upper panel, "complete defect") or separate right and left orifices (lower panel, "partial defect" or "ostium primum defect"). AO = aorta; S = superior bridging leaflet; I = inferior bridging leaflet; LM = left mural leaflet; AS = anterosuperior leaflet; RM = right mural leaflet; star = so-called "cleft" in the space between the bridging leaflets.

"complete" defect or an ostium primum defect; Penkoske et al., 1979; Piccoli et al., 1979). Using echocardiograph measurements, however, Gutgesell and Huhta (1986) have shown that the degree of "scooping" of the ventricular septum is greater in hearts with a common atrioventricular valve ("complete" defects). Further studies on the specimens in the Pittsburgh collection endorse this observation when the two groups are compared (Fig. 9), al-

though there is considerable overlap. Thus, while it remains correct to state, qualitatively, that atrioventricular septal defects are indistinguishable among themselves once the atrioventricular valve leaflets have been removed, it is also correct quantitatively to state that, as a group, those with common valve orifices have a greater deficiency of the central part of their ventricular septal structures. The fifth and final way in which atrioventricular septal defects differ from the normal is that they have no septal structures separating the cavity of the left ventricle from that of the right atrium. There is almost always a large hole present at the anticipated site of these structures (the atrioventricular septal defect). Rarely, hearts will be encountered with all the anticipated stigmata of atrioventricular septal defects but with intact septal structures (Silverman et al., 1984). Careful examination of these hearts (Fig. 10) will show that the septal structures separate atrium from atrium or ventricle from ventricle but never an atrial from a ventricular chamber.

The Left Atrioventricular Valve in Atrioventricular Septal Defects

The morphology of this valve is conditioned by the fact that it guards the left half of a common atrioventricular junction. This is so whether the left valve is a discrete and separate structure (as in so-called "ostium primum" defects; Fig. 7b) or whether it is the left half of a common orifice (as in so-called "complete" defects; Fig. 7a). The leaflet morphology is, therefore, determined by the five-leaflet arrangement of the common atrioventricular junction. Two of these leaflets are located anterosuperiorly and murally (inferiorly) entirely within the right ventricle. One further leaflet is exclusively within the left ventricle. This leaflet, as with the mural leaflet of the mitral valve, is attached to the parietal component of the left

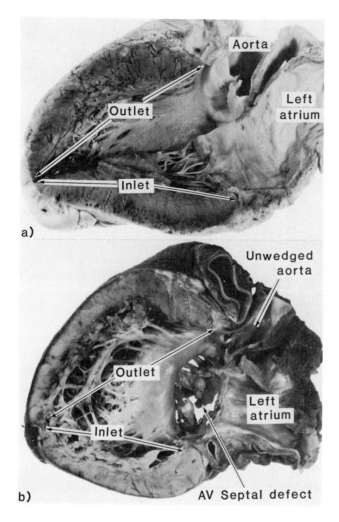

Figure 8. These two dissections of a normal heart (a) and one with deficient atrioventricular septation and common valve orifice (b) demonstrate the fundamental differences in septal morphology and dimensions found in the setting of an atrioventricular septal defect.

atrioventricular junction. Unlike the mural leaflet of the mitral valve, however (which occupies two-thirds of the overall circumference of the mitral orifice), the mural leaflet of the left valve in an atrioventricular septal defect occupies less than one-third of its orificial circumference. The precise portion depends upon the method of measurement used (Penkoske et al., 1985). Irrespective of the measurement technique, there is a statistically significant difference between the size of the mural leaflet in hearts with deficient and those with normal atrioventricular septation. Hearts with "isolated" clefts of the mitral valve, those with so-

called "atrioventricular canal type" ventricular septal defect, and those with straddling tricuspid valve all have values for the mural leaflet of their left valve which are normal and which point to the presence of normal atrioventricular septation. This inference is borne out by examination of the other features of these hearts, such as the inlet-outlet septal dimensions, these confirming the presence of normal atrioventricular septation.

In the left valve of atrioventricular septal defects, therefore, one leaflet is somewhat reminiscent of the mitral valve in that it occupies a mural position. Its dimensions,

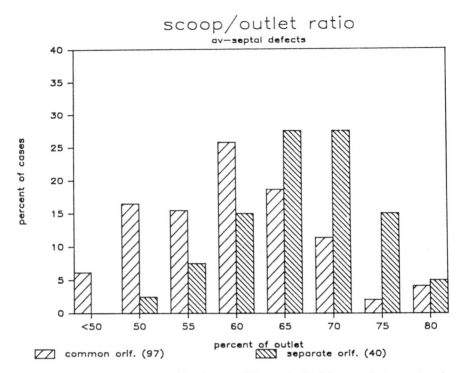

Figure 9. A bar graph showing the degree of "scooping" of the ventricular septum in hearts from the Pittsburgh collection with atrioventricular septal defect. The differences between the groups are statistically significant ($p < 0.00003$).

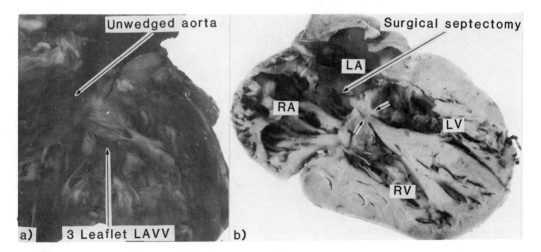

Figure 10. These sections show a heart with deficient atrioventricular septation but intact septal structures. The atrial septum had been removed at surgery. The left ventricular outflow (a) is typical of an atrioventricular septal defect while the four-chamber section (b) shows the valve leaflets attached to the septum at the same level (arrows).

however, distinguish it unequivocally from the mural leaflets of the mitral valve. The other leaflet tissue has no counterpart in the normal mitral valve, being made up of paired components of two leaflets which bridge the ventricular septum, their other parts being in the right ventricle. This arrangement is most obvious in those lesions that have a common valve orifice ("complete" defects; Fig. 7b). In this setting, it can be seen that the space between the bridging leaflets is part of the valve orifice. During ventricular systole, this space is closed by apposition of the bridging leaflets. In strictly literal terms, therefore, the space is the commissure (junction) between the leaflets, even though the space is not supported by a fan-shaped commissural cord arising from papillary muscle (the conventional criterion for a "commissure" in an atrioventricular valve; Lam et al., 1970). Indeed, the commissural cords of each of the bridging leaflets, as may be expected because of the

bridging, are positioned one in the left and one in the right ventricle (Fig. 11). The space between the facing surfaces of the bridging leaflets in the setting of a common orifice is unequivocally part of the orifice of the valve. It is just as much a part of the orifice when the common valve is divided in two by a connecting tongue of leaflet tissue. Usually in this setting, the bridging leaflets, together with the tongue, are firmly adherent to the crest of the ventricular septum. This is the arrangement seen in the so-called "ostium primum" defect. As Peacock (1846) observed, and as Carpentier (1978) emphasized, the left valve in this setting is a structure with three leaflets (Fig. 12). Conventionally it is described as a mitral valve having a cleft in its anterior (aortic) leaflet (Feldt, 1976). Controversy then surrounds the question of whether the so-called "cleft" truly represents the space between the cloven components of an anterior leaflet, or whether it is a commissure between two

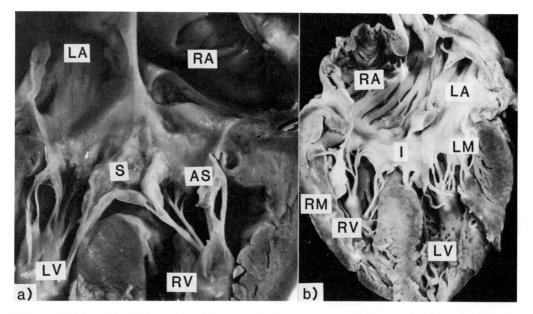

Figure 11. These illustrations show the anatomical arrangement of the superior (a) and inferior (b) bridging leaflets in two separate hearts with atrioventricular septal defect and common valve orifice. The heart shown in (a) has been sectioned in a four-chamber plane and is seen from behind. The superior bridging leaflet (s) is tethered between papillary muscle in the two ventricles. The heart shown in (b) is seen from the front and illustrates the biventricular tethering of the inferior bridging leaflet.

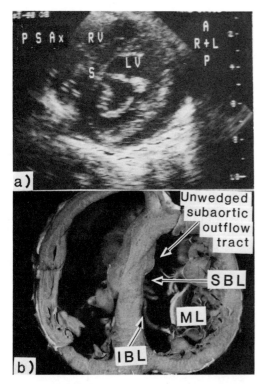

Figure 12. These echocardiographic and anatomical sections demonstrate the parasternal short-axis view (PSAX) at the level of the left atrioventricular valve in atrioventricular septal defect. They show the three-leaflet arrangement, with left ventricular components of the bridging leaflets together with the mural leaflet.

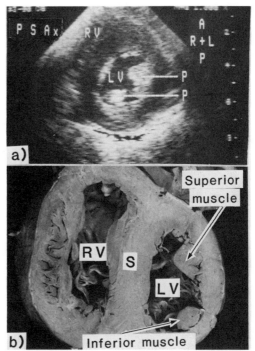

Figure 13. These echocardiographic and anatomical sections, taken in the parasternal short-axis plane, show the arrangement of the papillary muscles beneath the commissures (from the same series shown in Fig. 11) in atrioventricular septal defect. The arrangement differs from that seen in the normal heart (compared with Fig. 3).

leaflets of a three-leaflet valve. One argument advanced against the structure being a commissure is that it is *not* supported by a fan-shaped commissural cord. But, as discussed above, this criterion was designed for use in postmortem study of valves. The logic underscoring such use does not bear rigorous examination when used in the context of the functioning left atrioventricular valve. In the living heart, the space between the left ventricular components of the bridging leaflets is part of the orifice of the valve. Thus, the left valve in an atrioventricular septal defect is morphologically dissimilar from the mitral valve in a heart with normal atrioventricular septation, be that valve normally structured or cloven. Dis-

similarity is also seen in the subvalve supporting apparatus. The papillary muscles of the mitral valve in the heart with normal atrioventricular septation are located in anterolateral and posteromedial position (Fig. 3). In contrast, those in atrioventricular septal defects are found superiorly and inferiorly (Fig. 13), the distance between the inferior leaflet and the septum ranging with the extent of bridging of this leaflet into the left ventricle. Insufficiency and regurgitation through this left valve must be assessed in the light of this three-leaflet arrangement. It does not follow that such regurgitation must occur through the so-called cleft which, as we have shown, is in reality the functional commissure (using this word in the sense of the junction) between the left ventricular components of the bridging leaflets. It may well be that this junction is inadequate and that the valve leaks at this site. It is equally possible that regurgitation can occur through either of the commissures between the bridging leaflets and the mural leaflet. Indeed, there is some evidence to show that regurgitation through the inferior commissure is related to the size of the mural leaflet (Meijboom et al., 1986).

Conclusions

It can be said with confidence that the left atrioventricular valve in atrioventricular septal defects is a three-leaflet structure that bears only superficial resemblance to a mitral valve. If this is understood, then the words used for description of the valve are relatively unimportant. It does seem, nonetheless, that injudicious application and inaccurate definition of terms such as "cleft," "commissure," and "mitral" have contributed markedly to the confusion that undoubtedly exists with regard to this valve. It is our belief that, at present, use of the simple descriptive phase, "three-leaflet left atrioventricular valve," will ameliorate if not eradicate such problems.

References

Anderson RH, Zuberbuhler JR, Penkoske PA, Neches WH. Of clefts, commissures and things. *J Thorac Cardiovasc Surg* 1985;90:605–610.

Becker AE, Anderson RH. Atrioventricular septal defects. What's in a name? *J Thorac Cardiovasc Surg* 1982;83:461–469.

Carpentier A. Surgical anatomy and management of the mitral component of atrioventricular canal defects. In Anderson RH, Shinebourne EA (Eds): *Paediatric Cardiology 1977.* Edinburgh: Churchill Livingstone, 1978; pp 477–486.

Di Segni E, Bass JL, Lucas RV, Einzig S. Isolated cleft mitral valve: A variety of congenital mitral regurgitation identified by 2-Dimensional Echocardiography. *Am J Cardiol* 1983a;51:927–931.

Di Segni E, Edwards JE. Cleft anterior leaflet of the mitral valve with intact septa. A study of 20 cases. *Am J Cardiol* 1983b;51:919–926.

Feldt RH. In Feldt RH (Ed): *Atrioventricular Canal Defects.* Philadelphia: WB Saunders, 1976;

Gutgesell HP, Huhta JC. Cardiac septation in atrioventricular canal defect. *J Am Coll Cardiol* 1986;8:1421–1424.

Lam JHC, Ranganathan N, Wigle ED, Silver MD. Morphology of the human mitral valve. I. Chordae Tendineae:A new classification. *Circulation* 1970;41:449–458.

Meijboom EJ, Ebels TJ, Anderson RH, et al. Left atrioventricular valve after surgical repair in atrioventricular septal defect with separate valve orifices ("ostium primum atrial septal defect"):An echo-Doppler study. *Am J Cardiol* 1986;57:433–436.

Peacock TB. Malformation of the heart consisting in an imperfection of the auricular and ventricular septa. *Trans Pathol Soc* (London) 1946;1:61–62.

Penkoske PA, Neches WH, Anderson RH, Zuberbuhler JR. Further observations on the morphology of atrioventricular septal defects. *J Thorac Cardiovasc Surg* 1985;90:611–622.

Piccoli GP, Gerlis LM, Wilkinson JL, et al. Morphology and classification of atrioventricular defects. *Br Heart J* 1979;42:621–632.

Silverman NH, Ho SY, Anderson RH. Atrioventricular septal defect with intact atrial and ventricular septal structures. *Int J Cardiol* 1984;5:567–572.

Yacoub M. Anatomy of the mitral valve chordae and cusps. In Kalmanson D (Ed): *The Mitral Valve.* London: Edward Arnold, 1976; pp 15–20.

A Review of Those Morphological Variables Influencing Competence of the Valve and Modalities of Clinical Investigation

Robert M. Freedom and Jeffrey F. Smallhorn

The atrioventricular orifice, whether common or partitioned, in atrioventricular septal defect may be regurgitant. Such regurgitation may be clinically trivial or very severe (Brandt et al., 1972; Somerville and Jefferson, 1968; Studer et al., 1982). Furthermore, the function of the atrioventricular orifice is seemingly independent of its disposition relative to the interventricular septum. Thus, whether the form of the atrioventricular septal defect is balanced, dominant right, or dominant left (Bharati and Lev, 1973), the atrioventricular orifice may function abnormally (Jarmakani et al., 1978; Mehta et al., 1979). One might anticipate, however, that in patients with left ventricular hypoplasia complicating the atrioventricular septal defect, the left component of the common atrioventricular orifice would be more obstructive than regurgitant (Freedom et al., 1978).

In the previous chapter, the basic distortion of the atrioventricular junction in atrioventricular septal defect has been reviewed. Allwork (1982), Anderson and his colleagues, in this and in other presentations (1983), and Becker and Anderson (1982) have all presented persuasive evidence why the left atrioventricular valve in atrioventricular septal defect is unlike a mitral valve, and why they eschew its designation in the conventional way (Freedom et al., 1978).

From: Anderson, RH, Neches, WH, Park, SC, Zuberbuhler, JR, eds: *Perspectives in Pediatric Cardiology*: Mount Kisco, New York, Futura Publishing Co., © 1988.

Yet, convention has a long history, and some still vigorously adhere to "mitral" terminology (Lee et al., 1985).

Mechanisms Responsible for Regurgitation of the Left Atrioventricular Orifice

We all have evolved considerably in our understanding and appreciation of the complex morphology of the atrioventricular orifice in atrioventricular septal defect, despite a somewhat dissonant chorale in nomenclature. Irrespective of what we call it, the regurgitation does not result from a so-called "cleft in the mitral valve." Indeed, the so-called "isolated" cleft of the aortic leaflet of the mitral valve in hearts with normal atrioventricular septation does not share any of the morphological stigmata of the atrioventricular septal defect. Rather, in an atrioventricular septal defect, regurgitation occurs in the space between the superoanterior and inferoposterior bridging leaflets, whether or not a connecting tongue of tissue joins them—this resulting in partitioning of the atrioventricular orifice. Dysplasia or relative deficiency of atrioventricular valve tissue, cordal malattachments, annular dilation, and Ebstein's malformation can all contribute to the functional status of the valve (Caruso et al., 1978; Edwards, 1960). The presence of left ventricular papillary muscle abnormalities (such as parachute deformity) may also alter valve function. Similarly, the presence of associated left ventricular outflow tract obstruction may aggravate valve regurgitation. In addition, left-to-right shunting at the ventricular level with right atrioventricular valve regurgitation (such as dysplasia or Ebstein's malformation) can also mimic regurgitation through the left valve (Caruso et al., 1978, Handler et al., 1981, Roach et al., 1984).

The functional status of the atrioventricular orifice in atrioventricular septal defect is predicated on one's understanding of the morphology of these defects. While selective left ventricular angiography may illuminate some of the mechanisms responsible for regurgitation, cross-sectional echocardiography is mandatory in the evaluation of these patients. In the discussion that follows, we illustrate the important conjunction of echocardiographic and angiographic evaluation of selected structural and functional aspects of the atrioventricular junction.

Assessment of the Severity of Regurgitation Through the Left Atrioventricular Valve

Although clinical auscultation and invasive hemodynamic recordings may provide some basis for assessing the severity of left atrioventricular valve regurgitation, more precise information can be gleaned from Doppler echocardiographic and angiocardiographic investigations.

Those features of selective left ventricular angiography that provide the diagnosis of atrioventricular septal defect, whether partial or complete, are well recognized, and there is an extensive literature documenting the pertinent angiographic features (Baron et al., 1964; Brandt et al., 1976; Soto et al., 1981). Somerville and Jefferson in 1968 suggested that the direction of the jet (of the regurgitant stream) and the relative density of opacification of the right atrium and left atrium may provide some direction in the assessment of severity (Figs. 1–4). Because the so-called cleft in the left atrioventricular valve points toward the interventricular septum (Smallhorn et al., 1982), it is not surprising that relatively mild regurgitation seemingly opacifies the right before the left atrium. With more severe regurgitation, passage of contrast from the left ventricle opacifies both the left atrium as well as a portion of the right atrium. Okamura and his associates (1974) have extended these observations, providing a qualitative scoring

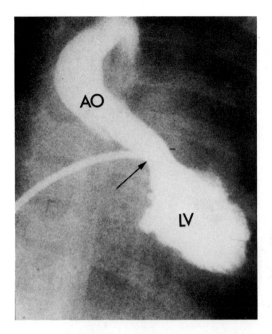

Figure 1. Left ventriculogram (LV) in ostium primum atrioventricular septal defect in diastole and systole. The elongated nature or "gooseneck" deformity of the left ventricular outflow tract (arrow) is seen. One can also recognize the disproportion between the left ventricular inlet and outlet dimensions. The left valve is not regurgitant as demonstrated by the left ventriculogram with the catheter positioned across the valve.

system to assess the severity of regurgitation based on the presence or absence of regurgitant jet; the degree of opacification of both atria and the pulmonary trunk; and comparison of the degree of opacification of both atria and the pulmonary trunk with that of the ascending aorta.

Such angiocardiographic mapping of the magnitude of regurgitation through the left valve can now be done noninvasively using a color Doppler technique. Again, whether the assessment is angiocardiographic or Doppler, the determination of the severity of regurgitation remains qualitative. The various components of an atrioventricular septal defect (including the size of the atrial and ventricular components; the attachments of the superior and inferior bridging leaflets to the ventricular septum;

whether the atrioventricular orifice is partitioned or common; the morphological mechanisms responsible for subaortic stenosis; and the displacement of the atrioventricular valve) can all be imaged by cross-sectional echocardiography (Chin et al., 1983, Silverman et al., 1984; Smallhorn et al., 1982a, 1982b). The magnitude of regurgitation can be enhanced by associated left ventricular outflow tract obstruction. The left atrium may not opacify even in the presence of severe regurgitation if the atrial septum is malaligned and malattached to the left, producing one variant of double-outlet right atrium. And the ability to deal with the regurgitation will be affected by the degree of valvular dysplasia; the presence or absence of ventricular dominance; the presence of a potentially parachute left atrioventricular valve; and the presence of a double-orifice. We will examine these factors as well.

Left Ventricular Outflow Tract Obstruction (Figs. 5–7)

Jue and Edwards (1967) pointed out the potential for subaortic stenosis in atrioventricular septal defect, but fortunately this potential is usually more apparent than real. The elongation of the left ventricular outflow tract and the characteristic unwedging of the aorta are both consequences of the basic deficiency in atrioventricular septation. Indeed, they reflect the discrepancy between the left ventricular inlet and outlet dimensions (Allwork, 1982; Becker and Anderson, 1982, Penkoske et al., 1985). Those mechanisms responsible for obstruction of this elongated outflow tract include an abnormal position of the papillary muscles; malattachment of the left-sided component of the atrioventricular valve; left ventricular hypoplasia (so-called dominant right form); fibromuscular obstruction; accessory tissue tags; and combinations of the above (Ebels et al., 1984, 1986; Lappen et al., 1983; Pic-

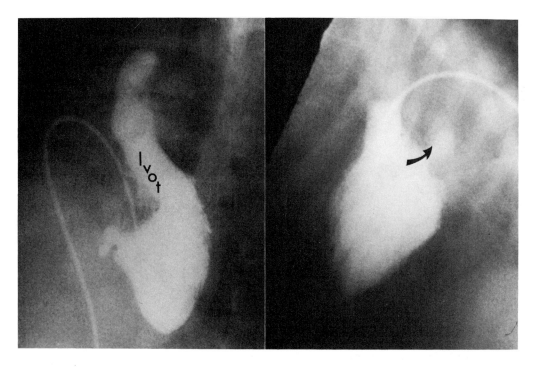

Figure 2. Mild central regurgitation through the left valve demonstrated by this hepatoclavicular four-chamber left ventriculogram. (*left*) The left ventricular outflow tract (lvot) is elongated, but is not obstructive. (*right*) In this reciprocal view, one can appreciate a central jet of regurgitation.

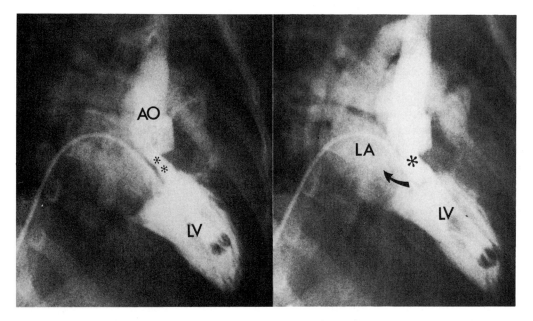

Figure 3. The left atrioventricular valve in a patient with a complete form of atrioventricular septal defect, previously banded pulmonary trunk, and subaortic stenosis. Note the severely compromised nature of the left ventricular outflow tract (asterisk) in this patient. There is moderately dense regurgitation (curved arrow) through the left valve.

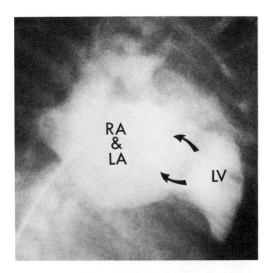

Figure 4. Severe regurgitation in a neonate with an ostium primum defect. This left ventriculogram (LV) filmed in a shallow right anterior oblique projection shows florid regurgitation (arrow) into both right and left atria (LA and RA).

coli et al., 1982). Any or all of these factors tend to potentiate the severity of regurgitation through the left valve whether the atrioventricular orifice is partitioned or not.

The So-called Parachute Deformity of the Left-Sided Atrioventricular Valve

Schiebler and his associates (1961) first designated an anomaly of the mitral valve as the "parachute deformity" when all of the tendinous cords inserted into one papillary muscle group. This concept was then extended by Shone and his colleagues (1963) to include insertion of the mitral valve and its cords onto immediately adjacent papillary muscle groups. David and his

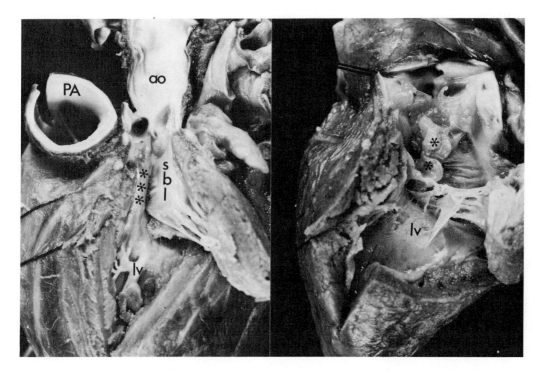

Figure 5. Pathological appearances of left ventricular outflow tract obstruction in atrioventricular septal defect. (*left*) Diffuse narrowing of the left ventricular outflow tract (asterisk) produced by anomalous insertion of the superior bridging leaflet. This baby also had a small left ventricle (lv) and aorta (ao). (*right*) Diffuse subaortic stenosis secondary to accessory tissue tags (asterisk).

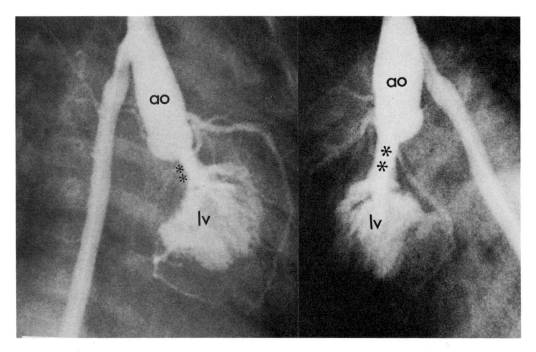

Figure 6. Dominant right ventricle, a small left ventricle, and "tunnel" form (asterisks) of subaortic stenosis. As in most patients with a dominant right ventricular form of atrioventricular septal defect, the interventricular communication is small or nonexistent.

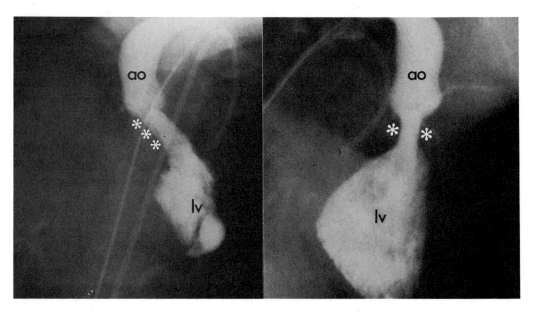

Figure 7. Diffuse left ventricular outflow tract obstruction (white asterisks) in a neonate with a partial form of atrioventricular septal defect, azygos continuation of the inferior caval vein, and left atrial isomerism.

colleagues (1982) described an essentially single focus of left ventricular cordal insertion in 23 of 164 autopsied cases of atrioventricular septal defect. They reminded us that surgical closure of the so-called cleft between the superior and inferior bridging leaflets "unmasks" the parachute potential, often with fatal surgically-produced mitral stenosis.

The disposition of the left ventricular papillary muscles in atrioventricular septal defect differs from the situation in the normal individual. The anterolateral papillary muscle is shifted posteriorly and inferiorly, whereas the posteromedial papillary muscle retains its usual location (Chin et al., 1983). This morphological obstruction is relevant

to the clinical diagnosis of parachute or parachute-like deformity in atrioventricular septal defect (Chin et al., 1983; David et al., 1982). Chin and his colleagues have recorded the role of cross-sectional echocardiography in evaluating left ventricular papillary muscle architecture and our own observations confirm their experience.

Ventricular Dominance
(Figs. 8–10)

The atrioventricular orifice can be equally disposed to the ventricular mass (so-called balanced type), or the atrioven-

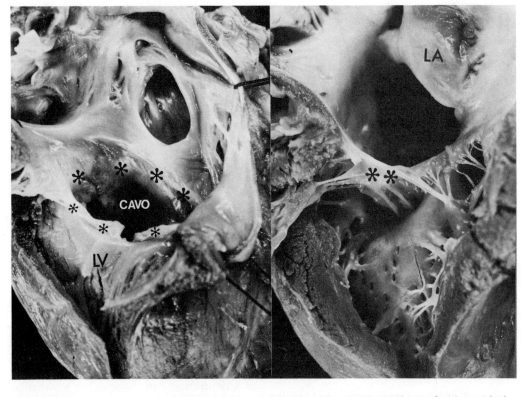

Figure 8. Two morphological expressions of the dominant right ventricular form of atrioventricular septal defect. (*left*) Internal view of left atrium and left ventricle (LV) showing the entire circumference (asterisk) of the annulus of common atrioventricular orifice (cavo). This orifice is predominately connected to the morphologically right ventricle, resulting in a very small systemic ventricle. (*right*) A similar, but less extreme, situation. LA = left atrium.

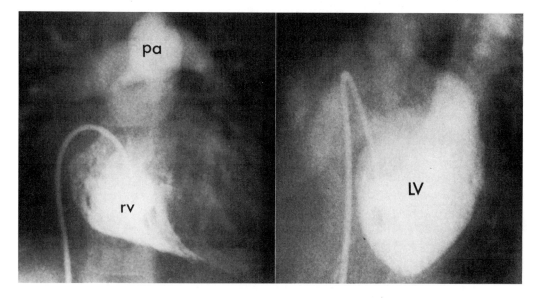

Figure 9. Dominant left ventricular form of atrioventricular septal defect in a child with associated pulmonary stenosis. Complete repair was effected with a Fontan-type approach. (*left*) Right ventriculogram (rv) demonstrates a hypoplastic right ventricle. (*right*) The four-chamber left ventriculogram (LV) shows a large systemic ventricle.

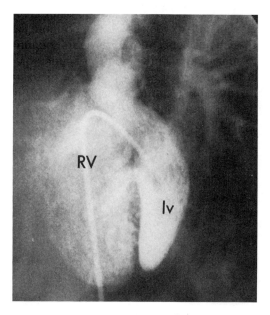

Figure 10. Dominant right ventricle in complete form of atrioventricular septal defect. This four-chamber left ventriculogram (lv) shows a slightly hypoplastic left ventricle and a much enlarged right ventricle.

tricular orifice can connect primarily with the morphologically left ventricle (dominant left form), or with the morphologically right ventricle (dominant right form) (Bharati and Lev, 1973). In patients with the dominant left form, the inlet and trabecular portions of the morphologically right ventricle exhibit varying degress of underdevelopment. When the atrioventricular orifice connects primarily with the morphologically right ventricle, then the inlet and trabecular portions of the morphologically left ventricle tend to be hypoplastic. Such patients may exhibit inlet and/or outlet obstruction of variable severity (Freedom et al., 1978).

When one ventricle is very small, and when its atrioventricular orifice connects primarily to the contralateral ventricle, there is little difficulty in recognizing ventricular dominance, or rather determining that the disposition of the atrioventricular orifice to the ventricular mass is not balanced (Freedom et al., 1978; Silverberg, 1965; Studer et al., 1982). It is when the situation is less extreme that ventricular volume determinations in concert with the echocardiographic appearance must be carefully scrutinized.

One must remember that when an atrioventricular septal defect is complicated by double outlet right ventricle, the morphologically left ventricle tends to be underdeveloped. The postmortem study by Bharati and her colleagues (1980) indicated that 41% of such patients exhibited right ventricular dominance.

Double Orifice Left Atrioventricular Valve

A double orifice valve is uncommon, and its most frequent association is with atrioventricular septal defects (Rowe et al., 1984; Wakai and Edwards, 1958; Warnes and Somerville, 1983). This anomaly is more than a pathological-morphological curiosity. Its recognition is important to surgical management. Warnes and Somerville (1983) suggest an incidence of 3% to 5% in patients with atrioventricular septal defect, with the majority occurring in patients with a partitioned atrioventricular orifice. The Mayo Clinic group recently published their experience with the double-orifice anomaly between 1961 and July 1984 (Lee et al., 1985). Twenty-five of 581 patients who underwent surgery for atrioventricular septal defects were identified as having a double orifice left atrioventricular valve (4.3%). Sixteen of these 25 patients (64%) had a partial form of the defect while in nine patients the atrioventricular septal defect was of the complete type. The Mayo Clinic group advise strongly against division or severing of the tissue bridge between the dominant and the accessory orifice. This was done in one patient, resulting in massive regurgitation. They also found that the noncleft orifice was usually competent and did not require closure.

In the setting of double orifice, complete closure of the so-called cleft can result in functional stenosis. The Mayo Clinic group advocated partial closure of the cleft to ameliorate regurgitation. Carpentier, discussing this paper and in a separate communication (1978), took a different position. He would prefer to reconstruct the regurgitant commissure rather than close it.

It is evident from the above comments that optimal surgical planning mandates preoperative recognition of the double orifice. While left ventricular angiography may provide this diagnosis, our experience would suggest that cross-sectional echocardiography is more reliable. Furthermore, one can interrogate each orifice using the Doppler technique to provide a functional correlate.

Double Outlet Atrium

Double outlet atrium embraces considerable heterogeneity in congenitally malformed hearts (Horiuchi et al., 1976, Otero Coto et al., 1981; Van Mierop, 1977). Double outlet atrium, either right or left, is when one atrium connects with both ventricles. Using this definition, a straddling atrioventricular valve can constitute one form of double outlet atrium. Another form of double outlet atrium is when there is atresia of one atrioventricular orifice, the other atrium communicating with the ventricular mass via two separate orifices without displacement of the atrial septum (Perez-Martinez et al., 1984). A very uncommon form of double outlet atrium is when one atrium opens into both ventricular cavities through two atrioventricular valves, while the other atrium has a normal connection with one ventricle. Finally, the initially described examples of double outlet atrium resulted from a malposition of the atrial septum. The cases reported by Van Mierop (1977) and Horiuchi et al. (1976) were examples of atrioventricular septal defects. Other examples of atrioventricular septal defect with a malattached atrial septum producing a double outlet atrium have subsequently been reported (Alivizatos et al., 1985; Corwin et al., 1983).

When the underlying anatomy is an atrioventricular septal defect, a leftward-deviated and malattached atrial septum results in a double outlet atrium, whether the atrioventricular orifice itself is common or partitioned. A restrictive interatrial communication may result in left atrial hypertension and may simulate the hemodynamics of mitral atresia or a divided left atrium (cor triatriatum). We can conceive of the situation when, in the setting of an atrioventricular septal defect, moderate to severe atrioventricular valve regurgitation is complicated by left atrial outlet atresia with an inadequate atrial communication.

The diagnosis of double outlet atrium has evolved from the necropsy table to recognition at surgical cardiotomy. Now the various morphological expressions of double outlet atrium can best be recognized by cross-sectional echocardiographic examination.

Echocardiographic Evaluation of the Left Atrioventricular Valve in Atrioventricular Septal Defect

In this section we will deal with the echocardiographic recognition of the left atrioventricular valve in atrioventricular septal defect and the associated abnormalities that may affect valve function. Most patients with an atrioventricular septal defect have the same basic left-sided valve morphology, namely, a short mural leaflet together with the left-sided components of the bridging leaflets (Piccoli et al., 1979a, 1979b). The existence of common or parti-

tioned valve orifices depends on the absence or presence of a connecting tongue between the bridging leaflets. The papillary muscle distribution is different in that the posteromedial muscle is situated in a more anterosuperior position. This results in a different orientation of the commisures such that the cleft in the left atrioventricular valve, which lies between the bridging leaflets, points toward the right ventricle. It does not extend toward the left ventricular outflow tract as seen in an isolated cleft associated with an otherwise normal mitral valve (Smallhorn et al., 1982). The papillary muscle distribution also has important consequences involving valve function, particularly when the mural leaflet becomes smaller owing to further anterosuperior rotation of the posteromedial group (Chin et al., 1983; Ilbawi et al., 1983; Meijboom et al., 1986).

The Echocardiographic Approach

A combined subcostal and precordial approach is necessary for complete evaluation of the left-sided atrioventricular valve. In the subcostal long-axis cut, the typical "gooseneck" deformity of the left ventricular outflow tract as described angiographically is readily appreciated (Smallhorn et al., 1982; Yoshida et al., 1980) (Fig. 11). The elongated outflow tract appears narrower during diastole owing to encroachment by the superior bridging leaflet, which is inserted into the elongated and unwedged outflow. With further clockwise rotation into a short-axis view at the left of the left atrioventricular valve, the three leaflet components are readily appreciated, as are their insertions into the papillary muscle groups. The superior bridging leaflet is seen in a more superior position, together with its insertion into the undersurface of the left ventricular outflow tract. The inferior bridging leaflet is observed with its insertions into the

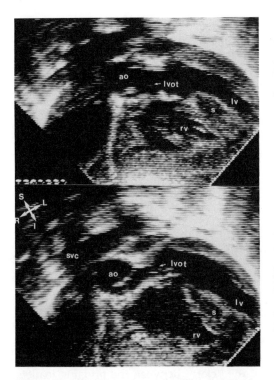

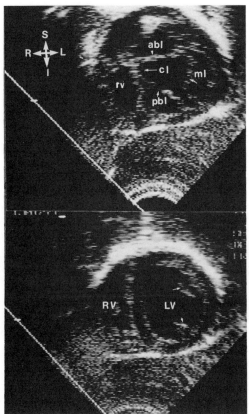

Figure 11. The upper picture is a subcostal long-axis cut in atrioventricular septal defect demonstrating the unwedged left ventricular outflow tract, along with the "gooseneck" deformity produced in part by the superior bridging leaflet during diastole (shown in the lower panel). ao = aorta; lv = left ventricle; lvot = left ventricular outflow tract; rv = right ventricle; s = septum; svc = superior caval vein.

Figure 12. The upper picture is a subcostal short-axis view at the level of the left-sided atrioventricular valve leaflets. Note the mural leaflet and the left-sided components of the bridging leaflets. The lower picture from the same patient shows the papillary muscle distrubution. Note that the posteromedial muscle is situated more laterally than in the normal heart. abl = superior bridging leaflet; cl = cleft; LV = left ventricle; ml = mural leaflet; ibl = inferior bridging leaflet; rv = right ventricle.

crest of the interventricular septum. In this position, the presence of common or partitioned orifices can be determined with the bridging leaflets appearing to fuse across the crest of the interventricular septum in the latter (Fig. 12). The relative position of the papillary muscles and size of the mural leaflet can be appreciated from this view.

If the transducer is then rotated counterclockwise into a four-chamber view, the inferior bridging leaflet can be visualized in more detail (Smallhorn et al., 1982b). In the majority of cases it is firmly adherent to the crest of the interventricular septum, unlike its superior counterpart, which frequently exhibits an interventricular communication beneath its surface.

Similar information can be gleaned from the precordium with regard to the left ventricular outflow tract, the left atrioventricular valve morphology, and the papillary muscle distribution. The advantage of this approach is related to age, the subcostal window invariably being inadequate in the older population. It also provides a more detailed assessment of the left ventricular outflow tract from another view, helping in the exclusion or diagnosis of obstruction at

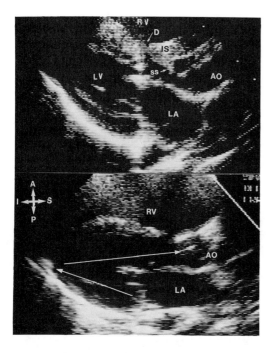

Figure 13. The upper picture is a precordial long-axis cut in atrioventricular septal defect with associated subaortic stenosis. Note that the stenosis is due to a combination of a subaortic shelf, an unwedged position of the aorta and abnormal insertion of the superior bridging leaflet. The lower picture from a different patient with an unobstructed outflow tract shows the inlet-outlet disproportion seen in atrioventricular septal defects. AO = aorta; D = ventricular septal defect; LA = left atrium; IS = infundibular septum; LV = left ventricle; RV = right ventricle.

and then move the transducer slightly posteroinferiorly to provide optimal imaging of this leaflet. If the scan starts too posteriorly, then part of the inferior leaflet may be seen, providing confusion with its superior counterpart.

Abnormalities of the Left-sided Valve in Atrioventricular Septal Defect

It is vitally important to recognize these prior to surgical intervention. Failure so to do may result in an inability to complete the repair. Echocardiography provides the optimal assessment. Probably one of the most important abnormalities to exclude is a single papillary muscle which, if present, may render the valve stenotic after partial suture of the "cleft" between the bridging leaflets (Chin et al., 1983; David et al., 1982). This, as already described, is best seen in either a subcostal or precordial short-axis cut. Care must be taken to differentiate this from a dominant papillary muscle group, where the second one is much smaller. In the former situation the single papillary muscle literally has the appearance of a solitary tooth in a mouth (Fig. 14). It is situated centrally and receives all the tension apparatus from the valve. A similar anatomical situation occurs when there are two papillary muscle groups in abnormally close proximity. More recently, Meijboom and colleagues (1986) have attempted to relate this to the presence of postoperative regurgitation, but as yet have not correlated it with severity.

As the scan continues more superiorly, a double orifice left atrioventricular valve should be seen if present. The identification of a second orifice depends in part on its size and in part on the age of the patient (Lee et al., 1985; Rowe et al., 1984; Trowitzsch et al., 1985). It is very difficult to visualize in very small infants, even in the presence of a larger second orifice. This is because the

that level (Fig. 13). Again, the inlet-outlet disproportion can be appreciated.

If the transducer is now rotated clockwise into a short-axis view, the papillary muscle distribution can be seen toward the apex of the heart, while the mural and bridging leaflets can be assessed with anterosuperior angulation. The so-called cleft, which is merely the gap between the two bridging leaflets, can be seen pointing toward the right ventricle and not the left ventricular outflow tract (Fig. 12). An apical four-chamber view probably provides the optimal image of the superior bridging leaflet. Care must be taken to start the scan at the level of the left ventricular outflow tract

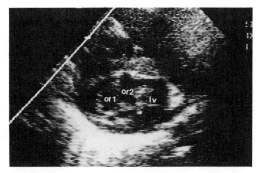

Figure 15. Precordial short-axis view in atrioventricular septal defect and a double orifice left atrioventricular valve. Note the two circles which represent the two orifices. LV = left ventricle; OR = orifice.

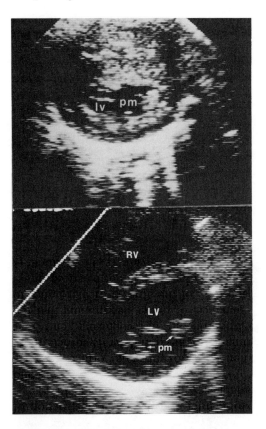

Figure 14. The upper picture is a precordial short-axis view demonstrating a solitary papillary muscle. Compare this with the lower picture from a case with atrioventricular septal defect and two papillary muscles. LV = left ventricle; PM = papillary muscle; RV = right ventricle.

echoes from the valve leaflets are often thickened and prevent an accurate assessment. When the patient is older, and the second orifice of reasonable size, the two orifices may be seen as a pair of circles (Fig. 15). Recognition is somewhat more difficult than in a double orifice mitral valve existing in a heart with normal atrioventricular septation where each orifice may be seen at different levels in the ventricle. This is the result of the orifice being divided by leaflet tissue, each orifice then being supported by its own tension apparatus. This arrangement is rarely seen in atrioventricular septal defects. Instead, the two components are usually the result of fusion of leaflet tissue

across the orifice and the subvalvular apparatus as anticipated for an atrioventricular septal defect. For this reason, the two orifices are usually only seen at one level and close to the valve's annulus. The two orifices may also be imaged from an apical four-chamber view, but again this depends on their size.

Stenosis of the left-sided atrioventricular valve may also be encountered. This may be associated with discrete annular hypoplasia in the absence of ventricular hypoplasia, but more commonly is associated with a degree of ventricular underdevelopment (Smallhorn et al., 1982b). The annular and ventricular size are best evaluated from a combination of subcostal and precordial short- and long-axis views, with the results being related to normal values for age (Fig. 16). As already mentioned, a solitary papillary muscle may result in stenosis but this is usually encountered only after surgical intervention.

What is more difficult to determine is the role of valve dysplasia in producing either stenosis or incompetence. The valve usually appears somewhat thickened, but quantifying this and relating it to the valve function is very difficult with current techniques.

The left atrioventricular valve may also play a role in the development of left ven-

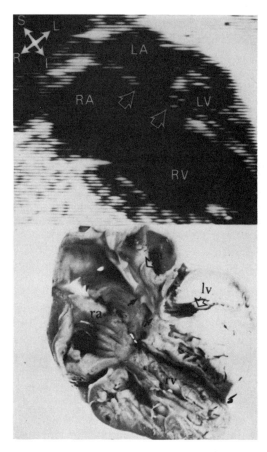

Figure 16. The upper picture is a precordial short-axis view on atrioventricular septal defect and right ventricular dominance. Note the small left ventricle. The lower picture from a different case demonstrates the anatomical features. LA = left atrium; LV = left ventricle; RA = right atrium; RV = right ventricle. (Reprinted with permission from Smallhorn et al., 1982b.)

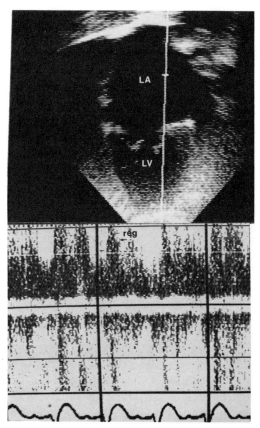

Figure 17. This montage is from a patient with atrioventricular septal defect and significant left atrioventricular valve regurgitation. Note the regurgitant jet is detected in the distal part of the left atrium. Flow mapping revealed a broad deep regurgitant jet. LA = left atrium; LV = left ventricle.

Doppler Evaluation of the Left-sided Atrioventricular Valve in Atrioventricular Septal Defect

tricular outflow tract obstruction. Although discrete fibromuscular obstruction may be encountered in this condition, more commonly it is due to a combination of the unwedging of the aorta plus encroachment by tension apparatus from the left-sided atrioventricular valve (Fig. 13). The outflow tract, as previously mentioned, is best assessed from a combined precordial and subcostal long-axis view. The obstruction has the appearance of a narrow tunnel crossed by a web of atrioventricular valve apparatus.

Doppler echocardiography has added to the preoperative evaluation of the left-sided atrioventricular valve in several ways. First, the presence of stenosis may be difficult if not impossible to assess unless the interatrial septum is intact. The Doppler velocity across the valve in this setting will be increased with evidence of turbulence distal to the orifice. A valve gradient can be calculated from the measured velocity. The same difficulty applies to the left ventricular outflow tract unless the interventricular septum is intact or the ventricular septal defect restrictive. Again, remember that the Doppler shift reflects only the relative pressure difference between the two sites.

Probably of greater significance is the evaluation of regurgitation through the left atrioventricular valve. Doppler interrogation provides only an approximation of the severity of such regurgitation related to the extent and width of the jet interrogated by flow mapping. The severity is based on the detection of a systolic jet and is not related to the volume of regurgitation (Fig. 17). Be that as it may, this feature does provide important functional information, particularly since flow mapping, unlike angiographic evaluation, can be carried out completely noninvasively. In the majority of the cases, the regurgitant jet can be traced into the right atrium across the interatrial communication. The origin of the regurgitant jet has important surgical implications. The introduction of color flow mapping will hopefully throw more light on this important topic.

References

Alivizatos P, Anderson RH, Macartney FJ, et al. Atrioventricular septal defect. Defect with balanced ventricle and malaligned atrial septum:Double-outlet right atrium:Report of two cases. *J Thorac Cardiovasc Surg* 1985;89:295–297.

Allwork SP. Anatomical embryological correlates in atrioventricular septal defect. *Br Heart J* 1982;47:419–429.

Anderson RH, Becker AE, Lucchese FA, et al. *Morphology of Congenital Heart Disease.* Baltimore: University Park Press, 1983;65–83.

Baron MG, Wolf BS, Steinfeld L, Van Mierop LHS. Endocardial cushion defects. Specific diagnosis by angiocardiography. *Am J Cardiol* 1964;13:162–175.

Becker AE, Anderson RH. Atrioventricular septal defects. What's in a name. *J Thorac Cardiovasc Surg* 1982;83:461–469.

Bharati S, Kirklin JW, McAllister HA Jr, Lev H.

The surgical anatomy of common atrioventricular orifice associated with tetralogy of Fallot, double outlet right ventricle and complete regular transposition. *Circulation* 1980;61:1142–1149.

Bharati S, Lev M. The spectrum of common atrioventricular orifice (canal). *Am Heart J* 1973;86:553–561.

Bloom KR, Freedom RM, Williams CM, et al. Echocardiographic recognition of atrioventricular valve stenosis associated with endocardial cushion defect: Pathologic and surgical correlates. *Am J Cardiol* 1979;44:1326–1331.

Brandt PWT, Clarkson PM, Neutze JM, Barratt-Boyes BG. Left ventricular cineangiocardiography in endocardial cushion defect (persistent common atrioventricular canal). *Aust Radiol* 1972;16:367–376.

Carpentier A. Surgical anatomy and management of the mitral component of atrioventricular canal defect. In Anderson RH, Shinebourne EA (Eds): *Pediatric Cardiology, 1977.* Edinburgh: Churchill Livingstone, 1978: 477–486.

Caruso G, Losekoot TG, Becker AE. Ebstein's anomaly in persistent common atrioventricular canal. *Br Heart J* 1978;40:1275–1279.

Chin AJ, Bierman FZ, Sanders SP, et al. Subxiphoid 2-dimensional echocardiographic identification of left ventricular papillary muscle anomalies in complete common atrioventricular canal. *Am J Cardiol* 1983;51:1695–1699.

Corwin RD, Singh AK, Karlson KE. Double-outlet right atrium: A rare endocardial cushion defect. *Am Heart J* 1983;106:1156–1157.

David F, Castaneda AR, Van Praagh R. Potentially parachute mitral valve in common atrioventricular canal. Pathologic anatomy and surgical importance. *J Thorac Cardiovasc Surg* 1982;84:178–186.

Ebels T, Meijboom EJ, Anderson RH, et al. Anatomic and functional "obstruction" of the outflow tract in atrioventricular septal defects with separate valve orifices ("Ostium primum atrial septal defect"):An echocardiographic study. *Am J Cardiol* 1984;54:843–847.

Ebels T, Yen Ho S, Anderson RH, et al. The surgical anatomy of the left ventricular outflow tract in atrioventricular septal defect. *Ann Thorac Surg* 1986;41:483–488.

Edwards JE. The problem of mitral insufficiency caused by accessory chordae tendineae in persistent common atrioventricular canal. *Mayo Clin Proc* 1960;35:299–306.

Freedom RM, Bini M, Rowe RD. Endocardial cushion defect and significant hypoplasia of the left ventricle:A distinct clinical and pathological entity. *Eur J Cardiol* 1978;7:263–281.

Handler JB, Berger TG, Miller RH, et al. Partial atrioventricular canal in association with Ebstein's anomaly. Echocardiographic diagnosis and surgical connection. *Chest* 1981;80:515–517.

Horiuchi T, Saji K, Osuka Y, et al. Successful correction of double outlet left atrium associated with complete atrioventricular canal and L-loop double outlet right ventricle with stenosis of the pulmonary artery. *J Cardiovasc Surg* 1976;17:157–161.

Ilbawi MN, Idriss FS, Deleon SY, et al. Unusual mitral valve abnormalities complicating surgical repair of endocardial cushion defects. *J Thorac Cardiovasc Surg* 1983;85:697–704.

Jarmakani JM, George B, Wheller J. Ventricular volume characteristics in infants and children with endocardial cushion defects. *Circulation* 1978;58:153–157.

Jue KL, Edwards JE. Anomalous attachment of mitral valve causing subaortic atresia. *Circulation* 1967;35:928–932.

Lappen RS, Muster AJ, Idriss FS, et al. Masked subaortic stenosis in ostium primum atrial septal defect:Recognition and treatment. *Am J Cardiol* 1983;52:336–340.

Lee C-N, Danielson GK, Schaff HV, et al. Surgical treatment of double-orifice mitral valve in atrioventricular canal defects. Experience in 25 patients. *J Thorac Cardiovasc Surg* 1985;90:700–705.

Mehta S, Hirschfeld S, Riggs T, Liebman J. Echocardiographic estimation of ventricular hypoplasia in complete atrioventricular canal. *Circulation* 1979;59:888–893.

Meijboom E, Ebels T, Anderson R, et al. Left atrioventricular valve after surgical repair in atrioventricular septal defect with separate valve orifices. Ostium primum atrial septal defect. *Am J Cardiol* 1986;57:433–436.

Nunez L, Gil Aquado M, Sanz E, Perez-Martinez VM. Surgical repair of double-outlet right atrium. *Ann Thorac Surg* 1984;37:164–166.

Okamura K, Kudo T, Koyanagi H, et al. Evaluation of mitral regurgitation in endocardial cushion defect with reference to surgical intervention on mitral valvular cleft. *Am Heart J* 1974;88:579–587.

Otero Coto E, Calabro R, Marsico F, Lopez Arranz JS. Right atrial outlet atresia with straddling left atrioventricular valve. A form of double outlet atrium. *Br Heart J* 1981;45:317–324.

Penkoske PA, Neches WH, Anderson RH, Zuberbuhler JR. Further observations on the morphology of atrioventricular septal defects. *J Thorac Cardiovasc Surg* 1985;90:611–622.

Perez-Martinez VM, Garcia-Fernandez F, Oliver-Ruiz J, Nunez-Gonzalez L. Double-outlet right atrium with two atrioventricular valves and left atrial outlet atresia. *J Am Coll Cardiol* 1984;3:375–380.

Piccoli GP, Gerlis LM, Wilkinson JL, et al. Morphology and classification of atrioventricular defects. *Br Heart J* 1979a;42:621–632.

Piccoli GP, Wilkinson JL, Macartney FJ, et al. Morphology and classification of complete atrioventricular defects. *Br Heart J* 1979b;42:633–639.

Piccoli GP, Yen Ho S, Wilkinson JL, et al. Left-sided obstructive lesions in atrioventricular septal defects. *J Thorac Cardiovasc Surg* 1982;83:453–460.

Roach RM, Tandon R, Moller JH, Edwards JE. Ebstein's anomaly of the tricuspid valve in persistent common atrioventricular canal. *Am J Cardiol* 1984;53:640–642.

Rowe DW, Desai B, Bezmalinovic Z, et al. Two dimensional echocardiography in double orifice mitral valve. *J Am Coll Cardiol* 1984;4:429–433.

Schiebler GL, Edwards JE, Burchell HB et al. Congenital corrected transposition of the great vessels. A study of 33 cases. *Pediatrics* 1961;27(Suppl):850–888.

Shone JD, Sellers RD, Anderson RC, et al. The developmental complex of parachute mitral valve, supravalvular ring of left atrium, subaortic stenosis and coarctation of aorta. *Am J Cardiol* 1963;11:714–725.

Silberberg B. Coexistent aortic and mitral atresia associated with persistent common atrioventricular canal. *Am J Cardiol* 1965;16:754–757.

Silverman NH, Yen Ho S, Anderson RH, et al. Atrioventricular septal defect with intact atrial and ventricular septal structures. *Int J Cardiol* 1984;5:561–572.

Smallhorn JF, de Leval M, Stark J, et al. Isolated anterior mitral cleft. Two dimensional echocardiographic assessment and differentiation from "Clefts" associated with atrioventricular septal defect. *Br Heart J* 1982a;48:109–116.

Smallhorn JF, Tommasini G, Anderson RH, Macartney FJ. Assessment of atrioventricular septal defects by two dimensional echocardiography. *Br Heart J* 1982b;47:105–121.

Somerville J, Jefferson K. Left ventricular angiocardiography in atrioventricular defects. *Br Heart J* 1968;30:446–457.

Soto B, Bargeron LM Jr, Pacifico AD, et al. Angiography of atrioventricular canal defects. *Am J Cardiol* 1981;48:492–499.

Studer M, Blackstone EH, Kirklin JW. Determinants of early and late results of repair of atrioventricular septal (canal) defects. *J Thorac Cardiovasc Surg* 1982;84:523–542.

Trowitzsch E, Bano-Rodrigo A, et al. Two dimensional echocardiographic findings in double orifice mitral valve. *J Am Coll Cardiol* 1985;6:383–387.

Van Mierop LHS. Pathology and pathogenesis of endocardial cushion defects. Surgical implications. In Davila JC (Ed): *Second Henry Ford Hospital International Symposium on Cardiac Surgery.*

New York: Appleton-Century-Crofts, 1977;201–207.

Wakai GS, Edwards JE. Pathologic study of persistent common atrioventricular canal. *Am Heart J* 1958;56:779–794.

Warnes C, Somerville J. Double mitral valve orifice in atrioventricular defects. *Br Heart J* 1983;49:59–64.

Yoshida H, Funabashi T, Nakaya S, et al. Subxiphoid cross-sectional echocardiographic imaging of the "goose-neck" deformity in endocardial cushion defect. *Circulation* 1980;62:1319–1323.

5.3

The Management of the Valve in the Repair of Atrioventricular Septal Defects

John W. Kirklin, Albert D. Pacifico,
James K. Kirklin, Eugene H. Blackstone,
and Lionel M. Bargeron, Jr.

The closure of the interventricular and interatrial communications in patients with atrioventricular septal defects places the atrioventricular node and the atrioventricular conduction axis at risk, and in the early years of cardiac surgery heart block was occasionally present after the repair. Rather quickly, however, the location of the structures important to the maintenance of sinus rhythm was determined (Lev, 1958). More recently, additional studies have confirmed and amplified the earlier observations (Thiene et al., 1981). As a result, heart block has disappeared as a complication of the repair of atrioventricular septal defects (Kirklin et al., in press; Studer et al., 1982).

The importance during the postrepair period of residual, recurrent, and/or iatrogenic left atrioventricular valve incompetence and/or stenosis has long been debated. Thoughtful and objective evaluation of results, however, such as was done at the University of Alabama in Birmingham between 1969 and 1980, gives convincing evidence that all of these have occurred in the past and are important (Table 1, Fig. 1). The recognition of this, and the studies that have been performed to generate knowledge that minimizes the risk (Barratt-Boyes, 1973; Carpentier, 1978; Dubost et al., 1959; Katz et al., 1981; Kirklin and Barratt-Boyes, 1986; Piccoli et al., 1979; Studer et al., 1982), have had excellent although not perfect early and intermediate-term results of the repair in the current era of atrioventricular septal defects (Kirklin et al., 1986). Those previous studies which focused on the morphology of the atrioventricular valve are particularly rele-

From: Anderson, RH, Neches, WH, Park, SC, Zuberbuhler, JR, eds: *Perspectives in Pediatric Cardiology*: Mount Kisco, New York, Futura Publishing Co., © 1988.

Table 1
Incremental Risk Factors (Hazard Function Domain) for Death in the Early and in the Constant Phases after Repair of AV Septal Defects (UAB, 1967–1982, $n = 310$, Deaths $= 70$)

	Time of influence (hazard phase)	
Incremental risk factors for death	Early and decreasing	Throughout and constant
Demographic variables		
Younger age (months)	•	
Clinical variables		
NYHA Class (I–V)	•	•
Severity of preoperative AV valve incompetence (Grade 0–5)		•
Morphological variables		
Interventricular communication	•	
Accessory valve orifice		•
Major associated cardiac anomalies	•	
Surgical Variables		
Earlier date of operation (months since 1/1/67)	•	
Interaction with age	•	

Modified from Kirklin et al. 1986.
Note: Risk factors with units in parentheses are variable ones, with the coefficient being multiplied by the appropriate unit in solving the equation.

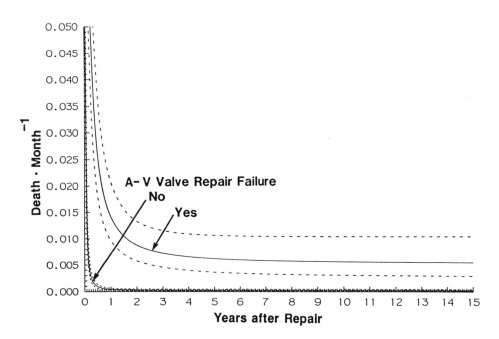

Figure 1. Hazard functions for death after the repair of atrioventricular septal defects in patients known to have had failure of the atrioventricular valve repair ($n = 32$; deaths $= 19$) and in those without valve repair failure ($n = 278$; deaths $= 51$). (Reproduced with permission from Kirklin et al., 1986.)

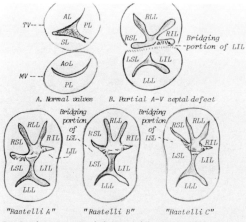

Figure 2. Schematic representation of the normal atrioventricular valve(s) and those present in atrioventricular septal defects. AL = anterior leaflet; LIL = left inferior leaflet; LLL = left lateral leaflet; LSL = left superior leaflet; PL = posterior leaflet; RIL = right inferior leaflet; RLL = right lateral leaflet; RSL = right superior leaflet; SL = septal leaflet. (Reproduced with permission from Kirklin JW, Pacifico AD, Kirklin JK: The surgical treatment of atrioventricular canal defects. In Arciniegas E (ed): *Pediatric Cardiac Surgery*. Chicago: Year Book Medical Publishers, Inc., 1985.)

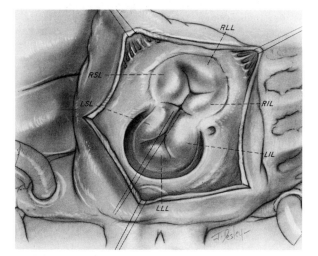

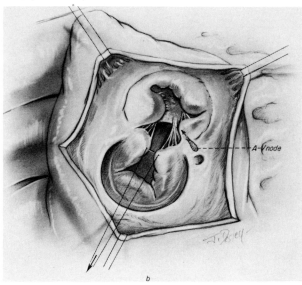

Figure 3. (*Top*) The atrioventricular valve leaflets are first viewed in the closed position as in systole, which may require injecting a bolus of saline through the valves into the ventricles. A 7-0 Prolene stitch is then placed at the most anterior (or annular) aspect of the coapting surfaces of the left superior and inferior leaflets. This guides the trimming of the Dacron and pericardial patches so that the newly created portion of the left atrioventricular valve orifice (the "annulus") will be of correct length. It helps also in the proper placement of the patch suture lines along the anterior aspect of the leaflets. (*Bottom*) Appearance of the leaflets in an open position, as in diastole. (Reproduced with permission from Kirklin and Barratt-Boyes, 1986.)

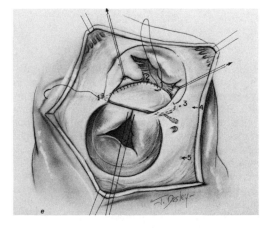

Figure 4. The Dacron patch, which closes the interventricular communication, is being sutured to the right side of the ventricular septum. It lies in a harmonious relation to the anterior surfaces of the left superior and left inferior leaflets along the line of the to-be-created portion of the orifices (the "annulus") of the newly partitioned right and left atrioventricular valves. (Reproduced with permission from Kirklin and Barratt-Boyes, 1986.)

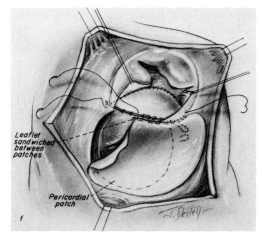

Figure 5. The creation of the new part of the "annulus" is nearly complete. Currently, this is done with interrupted mattress sutures only, positioned as shown in the drawing and using the "sandwich technique." After the annulus has been made, the posterior portion of the pericardial patch is elevated and the left atrioventricular valve is again studied. If further annuloplasty is needed, a suture is placed at the commissure between left lateral and left superior leaflets; and if necessary (uncommon) between the left lateral and the left inferior leaflets. (Reproduced with permission from Kirklin and Barratt-Boyes, 1986.)

Table 2

First-Time Repair of Atrioventricular Septal Defects (UAB, 1984–September 1, 1985)

Category	n	Hospital deaths			
		No.	%	CL	
Isolated	58	1	2%	0.2%–6%	
Complete	41	1	2%	0.3%–8%	
Partial	17	0	0%	0%–11%	
Complete AV septal defect with TF					
Complete AV septal defect with DORV	6	0	0%	0%–27%	⎫ 1/14 hosp. deaths,
	3	1	33%	4%–76%	⎬ 7% (CL
Complete AV septal defect with atrial isomerism	3	0	0%	0%–47%	⎬ 0.9%–22%)
Partial AV septal defect with major associated cardiac anomaly	2	0	0%	0%–61%	⎭
Total	72	2	3%	1%–6%	
$p(\chi^2)$			.03		

AV = atrioventricular; CL = 70% confidence limits; DORV = double outlet right ventricle; TF = tetralogy of Fallot.

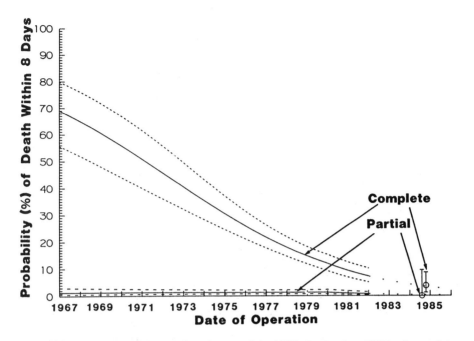

Figure 6. Actual hospital mortality after repair in 1984–September 1985, of complete and partial atrioventricular septal defects with or without major associated cardiac anomalies. The mortality is shown as circles and the vertical bars represent the 70% confidence limits. Note that the actual mortalities lie on the nomogram lines representing a solution of the multivariate equation based on the 1967–1982 experience. The solid line represents the eight-day mortality and the dashed lines enclose the 70% confidence limits. The widely dotted depiction extends the solid line of probability estimate into a time period (1982–1986) not included in the experience used for derivation of the equations and coefficients. (Reproduced with permission from Kirklin et al., 1986.)

vant to the concepts discussed in this chapter (Rastelli et al., 1966; Piccoli et al., 1979; Studer et al., 1982; Kirklin and Barratt-Boyes, 1986) (Fig. 2).

Technique

The repair of most atrioventricular septal defects is performed in infancy. Repair during cardiopulmonary bypass rather than during total circulatory arrest is preferable. This provides the time needed for thoughtful evaluation of the morphology of the defect (particularly of the leaflets) and for a precise repair. The technique of cold asan-

Table 3

Repair of Isolated Atrioventricular Septal Defects (UAB, 1984–*September* 1985)

Age (months)		n	Hospital deaths		
≤	<		No.	%	CL
	1	1	0	0%	0%–85%
1----	3	—	—	—	—
3----	6	13	1	8%	1%–24%
6----	12	16	0	0%	0%–11%
12----	24	4	0	0%	0%–38%
24		24	0	0%	0%–8%
Total		58	1	2%	0.2%–6%
$(P\chi^2)$				.5	

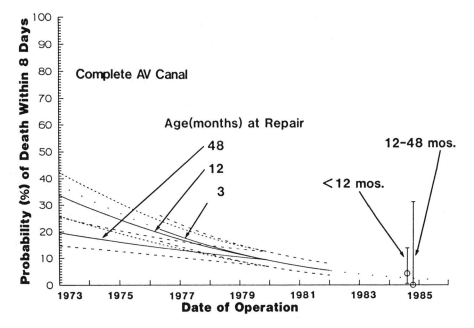

Figure 7. Depiction as in Fig. 6 of actual hospital mortality after repair in 1984–September 1985 of isolated complete atrioventricular septal defects in patients less than 12 months of age (n = 23, deaths = 1) and in those 12 to 48 months of age (n = 5, deaths = 0). Note that both actual mortalities lie within the 70% confidence limits of the mortality predicted for the repair of complete atrioventricular septal defects by the multivariate equation derived from the 1967–1982 experience. (Reproduced with permission from Kirklin et al., 1986.)

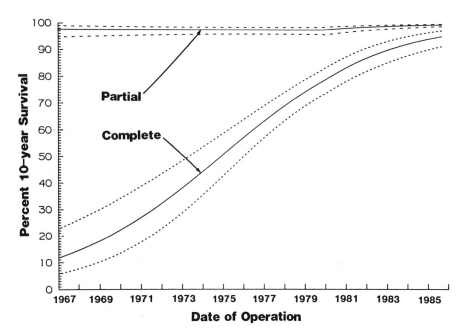

Figure 8. Nomogram representing the predicted 10-year survival (including hospital deaths) after the repair of partial and complete atrioventricular septal defects with or without major associated cardiac anomalies, according to the year in which the operation was performed. (Reproduced with permission from Kirklin et al., 1986.)

guinous cardioplegia (Conti et al., 1978) and controlled reperfusion into the isolated aortic root (Kirklin JK, personal communication, 1986) are strongly recommended for myocardial protection, although others might recommend another technique.

After arrest of the heart, and suitable exposure of the septal defect, all details of the morphology are examined. As regards the valve, this is studied with the leaflets closed, as in systole, and then open as in diastole (Fig. 3). When there is a typical so-called "complete atrioventricular septal defect," in other words, presence of the potential for both interatrial and interventricular shunting, the interventricular communication is closed with a Dacron patch (Fig. 4). The patch should be trimmed to a size that will result in a correct length of the surgically created portion of the left atrioventricular valve orifice, using the previously placed marking suture (see Fig. 3) as a guide. The new portion of the orifice is then created by enclosing the anterior (or peripheral or annular) portions of the left superior and left inferior bridging leaflets between the Dacron and pericardial patches ("sandwich technique") (Fig. 5). Interrupted mattress sutures of 6-0 Dacron are used for this.

The pericardial patch used to close the interatrial communication is elevated without tension before the repair is completed so that a final evaluation can be made of the left atrioventricular valve. If an accessory orifice is present (which surgically can be considered as an incomplete commissure), it is left undisturbed. Such dual orifices are not a source of incompetence. Attempts to "do something" with the accessory orifice nearly always result in stenosis or incompetence of the left atrioventricular valve. Should the coaptation of the left superior and left inferior bridging leaflets be imperfect (which is unusual at this stage), a few additional interrupted sutures are placed between the coapting surfaces of the two leaflets near the newly created annulus in order to correct this. Should there appear to be residual central incompetence, annuloplasty sutures are placed (see the legend for Fig. 5) unless the measured diameter of the valve orifice is smaller than normal for size.

The remainder of the operation is completed in the usual manner.

Results

Currently, the hospital (or eight-day) mortality following the repair of so-called partial atrioventricular septal defects (that is, those defects with the potential only for interatrial shunting) approaches zero and that after the repair of complete defects about 2% (Table 2; Figure 6). These low

Table 4
Summary of the Important Features in the Management of the Atrioventricular Valve(s) in the Repair of Atrioventricular Septal Defects

- When the common atrioventricular valve, or the divided left atrioventricular valve, with or without an accessory orifice, is competent, *avoid* distorting or narrowing it in the repair.
- Create a new part of the left atrioventricular valve orifice of precisely the correct length by measuring the length of the peripheral portions of the left superior and left inferior leaflets.
- Create this new part of the annulus with the "sandwich technique."
- When the valve is incompetent, study the morphology and select
- Realignment by sutures of the coapting surfaces of the left superior leaflet and left inferior leaflet, without producing stenosis.
- When incompetence remains, measure the orifice and when large, narrow it by annuloplasty at the commissure between the left lateral and the left superior leaflet and, when necessary, between the left lateral and the left inferior leaflet.
- Be alert postoperatively to possible residual incompetence.

mortalities pertain to infants as well as to older patients (Table 3). The currently good results represent the final phases of a steady improvement in the results of the repair of these lesions (see Figs. 6 and 7). These improvements have resulted from the gradual accumulation of the new knowledge referred to previously together with the training of young surgeons.

Currently, the 10-year survival, including hospital deaths, of patients undergoing repair of partial atrioventricular septal defects is predicted to be about 99.5%, and after repair of the complete form about 95%. This again represents a steady improvement across time (Fig. 8).

Summary

The technical aspects of the management of atrioventricular valve leaflets in surgery for atrioventricular septal defect are summarized in Table 4. With these facts, and with proper application of current knowledge concerning the location of the conduction tissue, proper management of cardiopulmonary bypass, and proper myocardial protection, the early and intermediate-term results of atrioventricular septal defects of all kinds are excellent, although still not perfect.

References

Barratt-Boyes BG. Correction of atrioventricular canal defects in infancy using profound hypothermia. In Barratt-Boyes BG, Neutze JM, Harris EA (Eds): *Heart Disease in Infancy: Diagnosis and Surgical Treatment*. Edinburgh: Churchill Livingstone, 1973:110.

Carpentier A. Surgical anatomy and management of the mitral component of atrioventricular canal defects. In Anderson RH, Shinebourne EA (Eds): *Pediatric Cardiology*. London: Churchill Livingstone, 1978:477–490.

Conti VR, Bertranou E, Blackstone EH, et al. Cold cardioplegia vs. hypothermia as myocardial protection: Randomized clinical study. *J Thorac Cardiovasc Surg* 1978;76:577–589.

Dubost C, Blondeau P. Canal atrio-ventriculaire et ostium primum. *J Chir* 1959;78:241.

Katz NM, Blackstone EH, Kirklin JW, et al. Suture techniques for atrioventricular valves: An experimental study. *J Thorac Cardiovasc Surg* 1981;81:528–536.

Kirklin JW, Blackstone EH, Bargeron LM Jr, et al. The repair of atrioventricular septal defects in infants. *Int J Cardiol* 1986;13:333–351.

Kirklin JW, Barratt-Boyes BG. *Cardiac Surgery*. New York: John Wiley and Sons, 1986: Chap. 19.

Lev M. The architecture of the conduction system in congenital heart disease. I. Common atrioventricular orifice. *AMA Arch Pathol* 1958;65:174–191.

Piccoli GP, Gerlis LM, Wilkinson JL, et al. Morphology and classification of atrioventricular defects. *Br Heart J* 1979;42:621–632.

Rastelli GC, Kirklin JW, Titus JL. Anatomic observations on complete form of persistent common atrioventricular canal with special reference to atrioventricular valves. *Mayo Clin Proc* 1966;41:296–308.

Studer M, Blackstone EH, Kirklin JW, et al. Determinants of early and late results of repair of atrioventricular septal (canal) defects. *J Thorac Cardiovasc Surg* 1982;84:523–542.

Thiene G, Wenink ACG, Frescura C, et al. Surgical anatomy and pathology of the conduction tissues in atrioventricular defects. *J Thorac Cardiovasc Surg* 1981;82:928–937.

VI

Aortic Coarctation: Morphology and Investigation

6.1

Aortic Coarctation: Anatomy of the Obstructive and Associated Lesions

Robert H. Anderson and Siew Yen Ho

Morphology of the Obstructive Lesions

Coarctation translated literally means a "drawing together." This is an apt description of the type of lesion found in the aortic arch harboring this anomaly. When the coarctation is an isolated finding, the walls of the aorta are pinched in waist-like fashion, the ascending and descending portions of the arch expanding above and below the site of coarctation. This pattern is seen most frequently in children and adults rather than infants. The arterial duct is almost always closed in this former setting and is converted into a ligament. The waist lesion is then usually found extending from the site of insertion of the arterial ligament. Almost always, however, there is an additional obstructive lesion within the waist-like aortic segment. The added lesion is a diaphragmatic shelf of fibrous tissue, often with a pinhole meatus representing the only communication between ascending and descending aortic segments (Fig. 1). This type of coarctation, often described in the past as the "adult" form, is usually found as an isolated lesion apart from the well-recognized association with a bifoliate aortic valve. Histology in these cases shows the obstructive shelf to be composed of fibrous tissue. Collateral circulation tends to be well-developed, the intercostal arteries feeding a well-formed anastomotic network formed particularly around the scapula. It is the enlarged intercostal arteries that produce the rib-notching seen in chest radiographs of older children with this lesion.

A markedly different arrangement is usually found when coarctation is found in infancy. Most frequently the arterial duct is open. The obstructive lesion then tends to be found at the junction of the aortic

From: Anderson, RH, Neches, WH, Park, SC, Zuberbuhler, JR, eds: *Perspectives in Pediatric Cardiology*: Mount Kisco, New York, Futura Publishing Co., © 1988.

During the course of this investigation, RHA was supported by the Patrick Dick Memorial Fund.

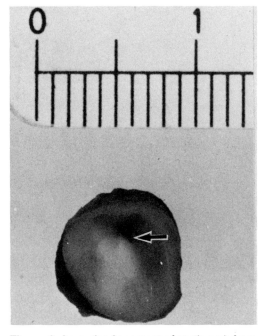

Figure 1. An excised segment of aortic arch from a patient with coarctation in the setting of a closed arterial duct. It shows the pinhole connection across the fibrous obstructing lesion (arrow).

isthmus with the duct and the descending aorta. The obstruction itself can, in some circumstances, simply be a waist lesion. It is then formed from the infolded aortic wall at the junction point (Fig. 2a). More usually there is an additional shelf-like lesion within the junctional lumen (Fig. 2b). The tissue making up the shelf is directly continuous with the wall of the duct, and encircles the junction of the isthmus with the descending aorta (Fig. 3). There is no agreement about the best description of the position of this lesion. It has become fashionable to account for its "juxtaductal" location (Rudolph et al., 1972). This is less than precise. What is needed is a description of its site relative to the flow pathway from the duct to the aorta. There are three possibilities, which can be considered pre-, para-, and postductal (Fig. 4). When studied at autopsy, almost all lesions are then seen to be in preductal position (Fig. 2) with only rare examples of para- and postductal obstructions (Becker et al., 1970).

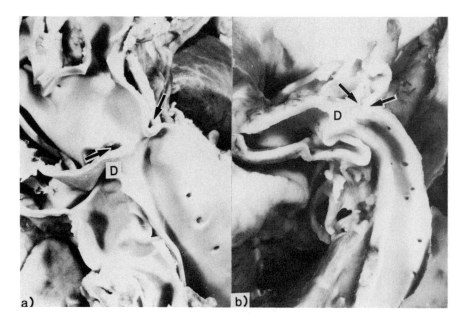

a)   b)

Figure 2. Dissections showing the difference between (a) a waist lesion and (b) a shelf lesion superimposed on isthmus hypoplasia (both between arrows) in the setting of a patent arterial duct (D).

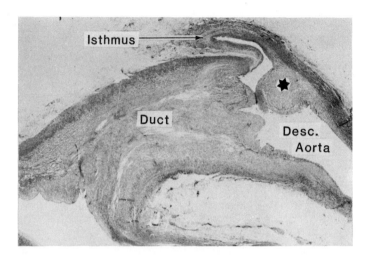

Figure 3. A histologic section through the junction of duct, isthmus, and descending aorta in a case of aortic coarctation with a shelf lesion (asterisk). The shelf is composed of ductal tissue.

In cases observed in infancy, there is the likelihood of finding a third obstructive lesion superimposed on the waist and shelf anomalies (if both these are present). This is hypoplasia of the terminal segment of the aortic arch. Such hypoplasia is most usually a gradual narrowing down, or extended waisting, from the take-off of the left sub-clavian artery to the site of discrete coarcta-

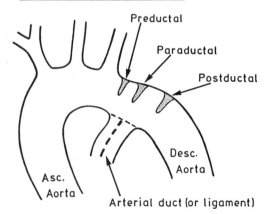

Figure 4. Diagram showing the potential sites for the coarctation lesion when the arterial duct is patent.

tion. This type of narrowing is usually termed isthmal hypoplasia. Sometimes the narrowing is more uniform, and the entire segment of the arch from the subclavian ar-tery to the duct is equally narrowed. This arrangement is described as tubular hypo-plasia. Tubular hypoplasia can also affect the segment of arch between the left com-mon carotid and left subclavian arteries (Fig. 5a). More rarely, it can involve the segment between the brachiocephalic and left com-mon carotid arteries. It is the arrangement of tubular hypoplasia which forms the start-point for the spectrum of anatomical mal-formations leading to interruption of the aortic arch. It is an easy matter to appreciate how a segment of arch narrowed by tubular hypoplasia can become increasingly nar-rowed until the lumen is occluded. The arch is then represented by a fibrous strand (Fig. 5b). It is then equally easy to appreciate how the strand can disappear resulting in the complete interruption of the aortic arch. This spectrum of hypoplasia, atresia and interruption can be observed both at the isthmus and in the arch segment be-tween the left common carotid and subcla-vian arteries.

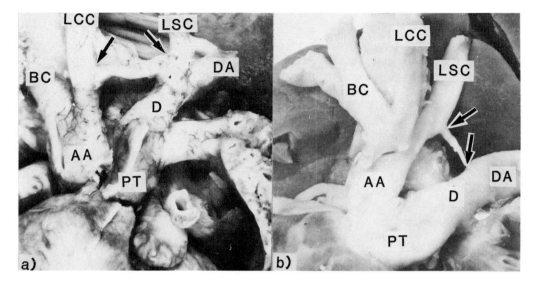

Figure 5. These specimens show the spectrum between tubular hypoplasia (*a*) and atresia (*b*) of segments of the aortic arch (between arrows). The hypoplastic segment is between the left common carotid (LCC) and subclavian (LSC) arteries while the atretic segment is the isthmus. AAO = ascending aorta; PT = pulmonary trunk; BC = brachiocephalic artery; D = arterial duct; DA = descending aorta.

The Associated Lesions

The most common anomalies associated with aortic coarctation are an arterial duct or a bifoliate aortic valve. Anomalies of the subclavian arteries are also highly significant. The aortic isthmus itself is intimately related to the origin of the left subclavian artery. Indeed, the isthmus is defined as the segment of aortic arch between the left subclavian artery and the duct. Examination of large numbers of hearts shows marked variability in the length of this segment. Usually the isthmus has considerable length and then is often hypoplastic, either as a tapering (Fig. 6a) or as a tubular lesion as discussed above. Sometimes the isthmus is very short (Fig. 6b) and then the orifice of the left subclavian artery is itself associated with and sometimes surrounded by duct tissue. Alternatively, the subclavian artery can arise at the junction of the arterial duct with the descending aorta and the isthmus can then be said to be absent.

Another significant malformation of the subclavian arteries is retroesophageal origin. The right artery is anomalously attached when the aortic arch itself is left-sided while the left artery will be involved when retroesophageal origin is found in the setting of a right arch. Retroesophageal origin places the artery beyond the site of obstruction with obvious clinical implications concerning blood pressure measurements and palpation of the radial pulses. Coarctation, irrespective of its site, has a fundamental effect on the left ventricle, involving the production of subendocardial fibrosis. This is less marked than occurs with aortic stenosis but remains highly significant (Cheitlin et al., 1980). The degree of fibrosis increases with age.

The other malformations that are of such importance in the setting of coarctation, and perhaps more so with interruption, are those occurring within the heart over and above a bifoliate aortic valve. Shone and his colleagues (1963) pointed to the significance of lesions of the mitral valve. This feature was endorsed by Rosenquist (1974).

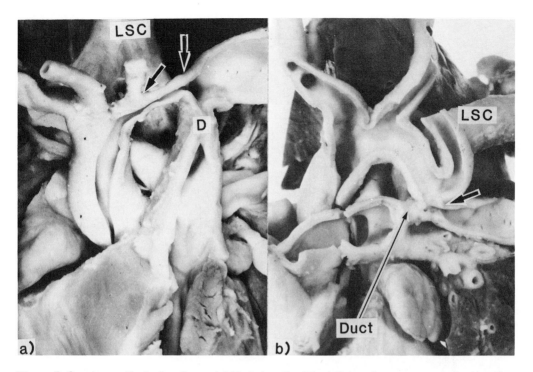

Figure 6. Specimens illustrating the variability in length of the isthmus (between arrows) according to the site of origin of the left subclavian artery (LSC). In specimen b, the isthmus is virtually nonexistent.

There is usually stenosis of the valve, either because of fusion and hypoplasia of the papillary muscles or because one papillary muscle is absent and the corresponding commissure is narrowed. Both of these anomalies have been described as "parachute" lesions by different investigators (Rosenquist 1974; Ruckman and Van Pragh, 1978). Shone and his colleagues (1963) also pointed to the association with a supravalvular stenotic ring within the left atrium. The other frequent associated defect is a ventricular septal defect (Anderson et al., 1983). In some cases with coarctation, but in many more with aortic interruption, this defect is itself associated with deviation of the outlet septum into the subaortic outflow tract and overriding of the pulmonary trunk (Fig. 7). In the majority of hearts with coarctation, however, the defect is perimembranous and associated with overriding of the aortic valve. The right ventricular margin is often closed or narrowed by tricuspid tissue tags (Anderson et al., 1984; Smallhorn et al., 1983). In many hearts, nonetheless, central muscular defects are found that do not interfere with aortic flow. All of these lesions affect the heart with coarctation in the setting of normal chamber connections. There are often anomalies of connections found in the hearts which are the harbingers of coarctation. Most, but by no means all, have an arrangement that potentiates reduced flow through the ascending part of the aorta. The typical lesion is univentricular connection to a dominant left ventricle (whether double inlet, absent right, or absent left connection), together with a discordant ventriculoarterial connection and a restrictive ventricular septal defect (Fig. 8). Alternatively, there may be double outlet right ventricle or complete transposition with the pulmonary trunk overriding an outlet ventricular septal defect

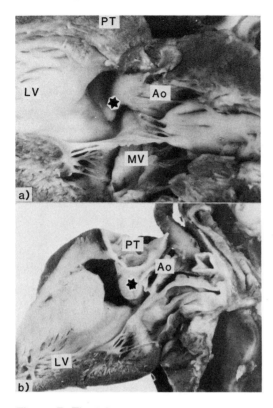

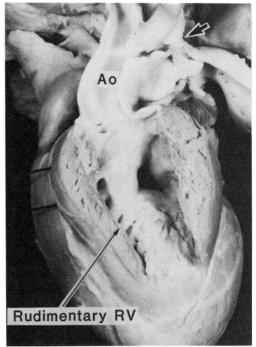

Figure 7. The left ventricular aspect (*a*) and a long-axis section (*b*) of a heart with gross obstruction of the subaortic (AO) outflow tract due to posterior deviation of the outlet septum (asterisk). PT = pulmonary trunk; LV = left ventricle; MV = mitral valve.

Figure 8. The typical pattern of aortic coarctation (arrowed) in a heart with univentricular atrioventricular connection to a dominant left ventricle (double inlet in this case) with rudimentary right ventricle (RV) and discordant ventriculoarterial connection. AO = aorta.

in the setting of a restrictive subaortic infundibulum (the Taussig-Bing malformation; Fig. 9). Other associated lesions can be found, but it is extremely rare to observe any that reduce flow through the pulmonary trunk. This is not an absolute rule since coarctation has been observed rarely in the setting of tetralogy of Fallot (Bullaboy et al., 1984).

Flow Theory versus the Skodaic Hypothesis

It would be inappropriate to close this discussion of the anatomy of aortic coarctation without devoting some words to the presumed etiology of the obstructive lesions. Many years ago, Bonnet (1903) suggested that ductal tissue was involved in the production of the coarctation lesion. This concept of the aortic wall being "lassoed" by a ductal circle as the arterial duct closed came subsequently to be known as the "Skodaic hypothesis." The concept seemed to fall from grace when Edwards et al. (1948) studied coarctation from "adult" cases using histologic techniques and showed the obstructive shelves to be formed of fibrous rather than ductal tissue. Persuaded by these studies and their endorsement by Hutchins et al. (1971), Rudolph and his colleagues (1972) discarded the Skodaic theory as being without foundation. Instead, they promoted the concept based on inequality of flow through the aortic and pulmonary pathways during fetal

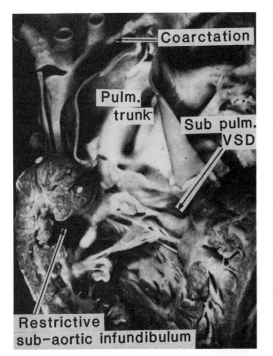

Figure 9. The restrictive subaortic infundibulum in a heart with double outlet right ventricle and subpulmonary ventricular septal defect (Taussig-Bing heart) which promotes aortic coarctation. Pulm. = pulmonary; VSD = ventricular septal defect.

life. They argued that diameters of vessels were proportional to flow through them. They showed that the isthmus was significantly narrower than either the adjacent transverse or descending segments of the aorta. They then hypothesized that any lesion that further reduced aortic flow during fetal life would potentiate to the development of significant isthmal hypoplasia. As discussed, the anatomical findings strongly support the notion that lesions potentiating to reduced aortic flow are important in the development of coarctation. But, in promoting the importance of flow, the role of the ductal tissue should not be dismissed. This is the more so when it is remembered that many patients with isolated coarctation do not have anatomical evidence of lesions which have obviously reduced aortic flow during development. Furthermore, atten-

tion should be directed to an important study performed by Wielenga and Dankmeier (1968). These workers from Leiden had compared, using serial reconstructions, aortic arches studied microscopically from normal patients and from those with coarctation. The majority of the latter group had died during infancy. They showed conclusively that in the normal arches, the ductal wall had a very discrete junction with the aorta and did not extend around the isthmal-aortic junction. In contrast, in the arches with coarctation, the isthmus inserted into a luminal sling composed of ductal tissue. These findings were subsequently confirmed by Rosenberg (1973), by Ho and Anderson (1979), and by Elzenga and Gittenberger-de-Groot (1983). The latter workers further showed that while the coarctation lesions in young specimens were composed unequivocally of ductal tissue, in older hearts they were made up of fibrous tissue. The implication of this observation is that the shelf lesion becomes converted into fibrous tissue with age. If correct, this then reconciles the apparently conflicting observations of, on the one hand, Edwards et al. (1948) and the "fibrous tissue" school and, on the other hand, Wielenga and Dankmeier (1968) and the "Skodaic" school. Taken together, the various findings show that the patterns of fetal flow are important in the setting of coarctation. They do not, however, explain all examples of coarctation, nor do they rule out the additional factor of retraction of a sling of ductal tissue during closure of the arterial duct.

References

Anderson RH, Lenox CC, Zuberbuhler JR. Morphology of ventricular septal defect associated with coarctation of the aorta. *Br Heart J* 1983;50:176–181.

Anderson RH, Lenox CC, Zuberbuhler JR. The morphology of ventricular septal defects. *Perspect Pediatr Pathol* 1984;8:235–268.

Becker AE, Becker MJ, Edwards JE. Anomalies associated with coarctation of the aorta. Particular reference to infancy. *Circulation* 1970; 41:1067–1075.

Bonnet LM. Sur la lesion dite stenose congenitale de l'aorte dans la region de l'isthme. *Rev Med (Paris)* 1903;23:108.

Bullaboy ChA, Derkac WN, Johnson DH, Jennings RB. Tetralogy of Fallot and coarctation of the aorta: Successful repair in an infant. *Ann Thorac Surg* 1984;38:400–401.

Cheitlin MD, Robinowitz M, McAllister H, et al. The distribution of fibrosis in the left ventricle in congenital aortic stenosis and coarctation of the aorta. *Circulation* 1980;62:823–830.

Edwards JE, Christensen NA, Clagett OT, McDonald JR. Pathologic considerations in coarctation of the aorta. *Proc Staff Meet Mayo Clin* 1948;23:324–332.

Elzenga NJ, Gittenberger-de-Groot AC. Localized coarction of the aorta. An age dependent spectrum. *Br Heart J* 1983;317–323.

Ho SY, Anderson RH. Anatomical closure of the ductus arteriosus. *J Anat* 1979;128:829–836.

Hutchins GM. Coarctation of the aorta as a branch-point of the ductus arteriosus. *Am J Pathol* 1971;63:203–209.

Rosenberg HS. Coarctation of the aorta: Morphology and pathogenic considerations. *Perspect Pediatr Pathol* 1973;1:339–368.

Rosenquist GC. Congenital mitral valve disease associated with coarctation of the aorta. A spectrum that includes parachute deformity of the mitral valve. *Circulation* 1974;49:985–993.

Ruckman RN, Van Praagh R. Anatomic types of congenital mitral stenosis: Report of 49 cases with consideration of diagnosis and surgical implications. *Am J Cardiol* 1978;42:592–601.

Rudolph AM, Heymann MA, Spiznas V. Haemodynamic considerations in the development of narrowing of the aorta. *Am J Cardiol* 1972; 30:514–525.

Shone JD, Sellers RD, Anderson RC, et al. The developmental complex of "Parachute Mitral Valve", supravalvular ring of left atrium, subaortic stenosis, and coarctation of the aorta. *Am J Cardiol* 1963;11:714–725.

Smallhorn JF, Huhta JC, Adams PA, et al. Cross-sectional echocardiographic assessment of coarctation in the sick neonate and infant. *Br Heart J* 1983;50:349–361.

Wielenga G, Dankmeijer J. Coarctation of the aorta. *J Path Bact* 1968;95:265–274.

6.2

Coarctation of the Aorta: Significance of Aortic Flow

Julien I. E. Hoffman, Michael A. Heymann, and Abraham M. Rudolph

Two obstructive aortic lesions should be distinguished (Sinha et al., 1969). One is a long tubular hypoplasia of the aortic isthmus or the transverse arch between the brachiocephalic (innominate) and right carotid arteries or between the right and left carotid arteries. The other is a localized shelf that has been described as "an obstructive curtain suspended from the anterior, superior and posterior aspects of the aortic wall with its apex directed towards the insertion of the ductus" (Ho and Anderson, 1979a). The two lesions may be combined.

Tubular hypoplasia of the aortic arch or isthmus is almost never an isolated lesion. It is usually part of a complex of lesions that are likely in fetal life to decrease left ventricular output. Examples are the Taussig-Bing anomaly, ventricular septal defect and subaortic stenosis, and some forms of atrioventricular septal defects (Ho and Anderson,

1979b; Moulaert et al., 1976; Rudolph et al., 1972; Sinha et al., 1969; Smallhorn et al., 1983). The reason for the lack of adequate development of the arch or isthmus is likely to be a reduction in flow across it during fetal life. About 12% of the combined ventricular output in the fetal lamb passes from the ascending to the descending aorta across the isthmus (Heymann et al., 1973; Rudolph, 1974). This explains why the isthmus is normally the narrowest part of the aorta. The ascending aorta receives about 35% and the descending aorta beyond the arterial duct (ductus arteriosus) receives about 75% of the combined ventricular output in the lamb fetus near term. In lesions like pulmonary atresia, the total combined ventricular output is ejected into the aorta so that flow across the aortic arch and isthmus is the total output less the amount that goes to the head and upper limbs. In children with

From: Anderson, RH, Neches, WH, Park, SC, Zuberbuhler, JR, eds: *Perspectives in Pediatric Cardiology*: Mount Kisco, New York, Futura Publishing Co., © 1988.

Supported in part by Program Project Grants HL 24056 and 25847 from the United States Public Health Service and by BRSG Grant SO7 RR05355 awarded by the Biomedical Research Support Program, Division of Research Resources, National Institutes of Health.

such lesions, the isthmus is always wide in response to the increased flow (Bruins, 1978; Moulaert et al., 1976; Rudolph et al., 1972; Shinebourne and Elseed, 1974). Conversely, it is likely that hypoplasia of the transverse arch or isthmus reflects a reduced flow across it in fetal life, the reduction being due to diversion of flow away from the ascending aorta. In extreme situations, development of the isthmus is so affected that complete interruption of the aortic arch occurs.

Ho and Anderson (1979a, 1979b) have shown that the hypoplastic isthmus may insert into the arterial duct so that ductal tissue surrounds the distal orifice of the tubular segment. It is possible that the reduced flow causes both the tubular hypoplasia and the displacement of the junction between the isthmus and the descending aorta. As Ho and Anderson have suggested, if the ductal tissue constricts, it will add to the increased resistance to flow offered by the narrow segment. The mechanism of formation of the coarctation shelf is still disputed. As summarized by Ho and Anderson (1979a), three main theories have been proposed: First, ductal tissue extends around the aorta, and when it contracts postnatally the aortic wall is infolded. Second, the narrowing in some way is related to the migration of the seventh intersegmental artery from its postductal position to a more proximal preductal position where it becomes the left subclavian artery. Third, there is an altered balance of flows from the aorta and pulmonary trunk in fetal life.

The first theory, proposed originally by Craigie (1841) and Skoda (1855), is supported by histologic studies of the region of the arterial duct and the coarctation. The coarctation shows an infolding of the aortic wall and, in most instances, there is an extension of pale ductal tissue forming a sling around the infolded wall (Elzenga and Gittenberger-de Groot, 1983; Ho and Anderson, 1979a, 1979b; Wielenga and Dankmeijer, 1968). With this anatomy, it is easy to understand how contraction of ductal muscle can cause a constriction at this site in the aorta. In fact, there may not need to be an abnormality of extension of ductal tissue, because Gillman and Burton (1966) observed that oxygen would regularly cause constriction of the preductal aorta in normal newborn guinea pigs.

In its simplest form, this theory implies that the coarctation should not be present in the fetus when the duct is relaxed. Allan et al. (1984), however, detected a coarctation and right ventricular hypertrophy in a 21-week-old fetus. By birth, severe tubular hypoplasia of the aortic isthmus had also developed, and there was a small ventricular septal defect. This report shows that a coarctation can develop when the duct is, presumably, relaxed and that other abnormalities are present when the coarctation is first seen.

The theory about cranial migration of the seventh intersegmental artery has some support because the migration of the left subclavian artery is abnormal in about two out of three patients with coarctations or tubular hypoplasia (Bruins, 1978). Furthermore, during embryogenesis, this region undergoes extensive remodeling as the branchial arch system begins to assume its final form (Netter and van Mierop, 1969). Beyond knowing that this migration must be complex and related to intrinsic control mechanisms as well as to external forces, there is little that can be done to prove or disprove this theory.

The theory about abnormalities of flow has much recent support. Hutchins (1971) regarded the coarctation as being the branch point of the arterial duct much like the ridge that divides the two iliac arteries where they branch from the aorta. He argued that if there was relatively greater pulmonic than aortic flow, there would be a predisposition to coarctation when the ductal flow divided into proximal and distal streams. There is no evidence for such proximal retrograde flow in normal fetuses, but retrograde flow might occur with abnormal flow patterns. No experiments of this type have been done. Rudolph et al. (1972) pointed out that the junction between the ascending aorta and the arterial duct normally formed an acute angle. They believed that when aortic isthmic flow decreased, the angle between the arterial duct and the descending aorta would alter. This, plus the resulting turbulence, might cause formation of the posterior shelf of the coarctation. They also pointed out that it was not necessary to have a sling of ductal muscle around the aorta to produce a symptomatic coarctation. If there already were a posterior shelf, then constriction of the normal ductal ampulla would suffice to produce severe aortic obstruction. In experiments on fetal lambs with surgically created posterior aortic indentations, Rudolph et al. (1972) showed that postnatal closure of the duct produced a pressure gradient between the ascending and descending aorta. The pressure gradient went away as the arterial duct relaxed. Similar observations have been made in neonates with coarctations in whom the obstruction can be abolished or minimized by infusing prostaglandin E_1 (Freed et al., 1981; Heymann et al., 1979; Talner and Berman, 1975). These findings in humans, however, are equally supportive of the Skodaic theory of a ring of contractile ductal muscle and the theory that the obstruction is due only to shrinking of the region of the ductal ampulla. The animal experiments (Rudolph et al., 1972) merely show that rings of ductal muscle are not essential for obstruction to occur. In no way do they exclude such rings in the pathological coarctations that occur in children.

The possibility that altered flow patterns cause the coarctation is supported by the association of coarctations with other lesions that might divert blood flow from the ascending aorta during fetal life. Coarctation of the aorta, although often an isolated lesion, frequently is associated with obstruction to left ventricular inflow or outflow or with ventricular septal defects (Becker et al., 1970; Bruins, 1978; Moulaert et al., 1976; Smallhorn et al., 1983). It is found with a bifoliate aortic valve in about 50% of patients (Becker et al., 1970; Tawes et al., 1969). The coarctation described in a 21-week-old fetus by Allan et al. (1984) was associated with a ventricular septal defect and right ventricular hypertrophy, thereby suggesting that excessive right ventricular flow was occurring early in fetal life. Possibly even a bifoliate valve or delayed closure of the fetal interventricular communication may have enough influence on fetal flow patterns to decrease flow in the ascending aorta and increase it through the arterial duct thereby leading to the formation of a coarctation.

Studies of the anatomy of the coarctation at various ages after birth show that usually the apex of the infolding of the coarctation points toward the duct or the arterial ligament (Hutchins, 1971). With increasing age, the edge of the coarctation moves relative to the walls of the duct (Elzenga and Gittenberger-de Groot, 1983). In neonates the edge of the shelf is opposite the proximal wall of the duct (which they call the preductal position). Then, with age, it moves distally to be opposite the middle of the duct or ligament (paraductal position) or opposite the distal edge of the duct or distal to the ligament (postductal position). The preductal position, which presumably also occurs in utero, might indicate reduced isthmic flow or an altered angle between the duct and the descending aorta. All of these findings argue strongly for a major role of flow patterns in the genesis of coarctations. Nevertheless, the occurrence of ductal tissue in the infolded wall indicates that either the coarctation is a primary lesion with secondary effects from or on fetal flows or else altered fetal flow patterns are responsible for the extension of ductal tissue around the coarctation. It has become clear in recent years that growth depends greatly on the production of growth factors from many cells, including endothelial cells and platelets (Antoniades and Owen, 1982; D'Ercole and Underwood, 1985). Furthermore, endothelial cell activity can be altered by mechanical and chemical stimuli (Ross and Glomsett, 1976; Ryan, 1986; Ryan and Ryan, 1984). It would not be surprising to find that altered flow patterns at the point where the arterial duct joins the aorta can induce structural changes in the adjacent vessels in fetal life. These changes may even include extension of specialized ductal tissue around the aorta. Perhaps the Skodaic and the altered flow pattern theories are, in reality, part of the same mechanism of formation of coarctations. If so, the distinction between physiological and anatomical causes of coarctations will be abolished.

References

Allan LD, Crawford DC, Tynan M. Evolution of coarctation of the aorta in intrauterine life. *Br Heart J* 1984;52:471–473.

Antoniades HN, Owen AJ. Growth factors and regulation of cell growth. *Ann Rev Med* 1982;33:445–463.

Becker AE, Becker MJ, Edwards JE. Anomalies associated with coarctation of the aorta. Particular reference to infancy. *Circulation* 1920; 41:1067–1075.

Bruins C. Competition between aortic isthmus and ductus arteriosus; Reciprocal influence of structure and flow. *Eur J Cardiol* 1978;8:87–97.

Craigie D. Instance of obliteration of the aorta beyond the arch, illustrated by similar cases and observation. *Edin Med J* 1841;56:427–462.

D'Ercole AJ, Underwood LE. Regulation of fetal growth by hormones and growth factors. In Falkner F, Tanner JM (Eds): *Human Growth*. New York: Plenum Publishing, 1985;327–338.

Elzenga NJ, Gittenberger-de Groot AC. Localised coarctation of the aorta. An age dependent spectrum. *Br Heart J* 1983;49:317–323.

Freed MD, Heymann MA, Lewis AB, et al. Prostaglandin E₁ in infants with ductus arteriosus-dependent congenital heart disease. *Circulation* 1981;64:899–905.

Gillman RG, Burton AC. Constriction of the neo-

natal aorta by raised oxygen tension. *Circ Res* 1966;19:755–765.

Heymann MA, Berman W Jr, Rudolph AM, Whitman V. Dilatation of the ductus arteriosus by prostaglandin E₁ in aortic arch abnormalities. *Circulation* 1979;59:169–171.

Heymann MA, Creasy RK, Rudolph AM. Quantitation of blood flow patterns in the foetal lamb in utero. In Comline KS, Cross KW, Dawes GS, Nathanielsz PW (Eds): *Foetal and Neonatal Physiology: Proceedings of the Sir Joseph Barcroft Centenary Symposium*. Cambridge: Cambridge University Press, 1973:129–135.

Ho SY, Anderson RH. Coarctation of the aorta. In Godman MJ, Marquis RM (Eds): *Paediatric Cardiology, Volume 2, Heart Disease in the Newborn*. Edinburgh: Churchill Livingstone, 1979a:173–186.

Ho SY, Anderson RH. Coarctation, tubular hypoplasia, and the ductus arteriosus. Histological study of 35 specimens. *Br Heart J* 1979b;41:268–274.

Hutchins GM. Coarctation of the aorta explained as a branch-point of the ductus arteriosus. *Am J Pathol* 1971;63:203–209.

Moulaert AJ, Bruins CC, Oppenheimer-Dekker A. Anomalies of the aortic arch and ventricular septal defects. *Circulation*, 1976;53:1011–1015.

Netter FH, van Mierop LHS. Embryology. In Yonkman FF (Ed): *The Ciba Collection of Medical Illustrations, The Heart*. New Jersey: Ciba Pharmaceutical Company, 1969;5:112–130.

Ross R, Glomsett JA. The pathogenesis of atherosclerosis. *New Engl J Med* 1976;295:369–377, 420–425.

Rudolph AM. *Congenital Diseases of the Heart*. Chicago: Year Book Medical Publishers, 1974.

Rudolph AM, Heymann MA, Spitznas U. Hemodynamic considerations in the development of narrowing of the aorta. *Am J Card* 1977;30:514–525.

Ryan US, and Ryan JW. (1984) Cell biology of pulmonary endothelium. *Circulation* 1984; 70(Suppl III):46–62.

Ryan US. The endothelial surface and responses to injury. *Fed Proc* 1986;45:101–108.

Shinebourne EA, Elseed AM. Relation between fetal flow patterns, coarctation of the aorta and pulmonary blood flow. *Br Heart J* 1974;36:492–498.

Sinha SN, Kardatzke ML, Cole RB, et al. Coarctation of the aorta in infancy: Pathologic and angiographic measurements. *Circulation* 1969; 40:385–398.

Skoda J. Protokoll der Sections—Sitzung fur Physiologie und Pathologie. *Wochenblatt der Zeitschrift der kaiserlichkoniglichen Gesellschaft der Aerzte zu Wien* 1855;1:710–722.

Smallhorn JF, Anderson RH, Macartney FJ. Morphological characterisation of ventricular septal defects associated with coarctation of aorta by cross-sectional echocardiography. *Br Heart J* 1983;49:485–494.

Talner NS, Berman MA. Postnatal development of obstruction in coarctation of the aorta: Role of the ductus arteriosus. *Pediatrics* 1975;56:562–569.

Tawes RL Jr, Berry CL, Aberdeen E. Congenital bicuspid aortic valves associated with coarctation of the aorta. *Br Heart J* 1969;31:127–128.

Wielenga G, Dankmeijer J. Coarctation of the aorta. *J Pathol Bacteriol* 1968;95:265–274.

Coarctation of the Aorta: Investigative Techniques and Unusual Variants

Lee B. Beerman and Sang C. Park

The classic clinical approach including history, physical examination, chest x-ray, and electrocardiogram allows the certain diagnosis of coarctation of the aorta in almost all patients with this abnormality. The diagnosis alone, however, is not sufficient information for referring an individual for surgical correction if optimal long-term results are desired. Without a precise anatomical definition of the type and severity of the aortic obstruction as well as its location, the operative approach may be compromised. The purpose of this chapter is to describe the investigative techniques currently used for preoperative evaluation of coarctation of the aorta and to discuss common and unusual variants that could affect the operative management. The laboratory techniques helpful in the management of this abnormality are shown in Table 1. The electrocardiogram and chest x-ray will not be discussed further since the use of these

tests has been standard for many years. The application of echocardiography, Doppler studies, and angiography to coarctation of the aorta will be emphasized. The new modalities of digital subtraction angiography and magnetic resonance imaging may prove

Table 1

Coarctation of the Aorta:
Investigative Techniques

ECG: RVH in infancy, LV predominance
  emerges >1 year
CXR: "3" or "E" sign, rib notching >5 years
Echocardiography
Doppler
Angiography
Digital subtraction angiography
Magnetic resonance imaging

ECG = electrocardiogram; CXR = chest radiograph; RVH = right ventricular hypertrophy; LV = left ventricle.

From: Anderson, RH, Neches, WH, Park, SC, Zuberbuhler, JR, eds: *Perspectives in Pediatric Cardiology*: Mount Kisco, New York, Futura Publishing Co., © 1988.

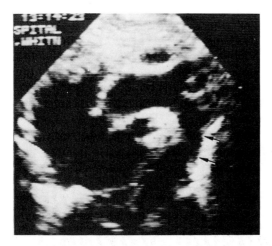

Figure 1. Normal aortic arch as demonstrated from a suprasternal echocardiogram. Note the widely patent region of the isthmus (arrows).

to be beneficial in future years, but currently these techniques are still in the process of evaluation.

Diagnostic Tools

Echocardiography

Cross-sectional echocardiography has proven to be extremely valuable in evaluating coarctation of the aorta (Huhta et al., 1984; Smallhorn et al., 1983). This procedure allows visualization of the critical area of the aorta at the junction of the isthmus, arterial duct, and descending aorta. The echocardiographic planes that are most helpful include those obtained from high left parasternal and suprasternal approaches. Figure 1 demonstrates a normal aortic arch as visualized from a suprasternal view. The entire arch is well visualized and no narrowing of the isthmus or descending aorta is apparent. Excellent visualization of a coarctation is demonstrated in Figure 2A. The left subclavian artery has a low take-off and there is a waisting of the aorta as well as

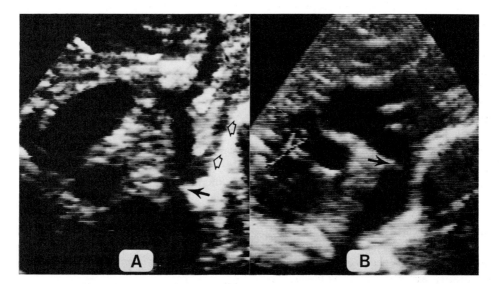

Figure 2. Echocardiograms from suprasternal view. (*A*) Coarctation of the aorta (large arrow) is seen with a low take-off of the left subclavian artery (open arrows) and a discrete *posterior* obstructing ridge and waisting of the aorta. (*B*) False-positive demonstration of aortic obstruction. The anterior ridge of echos (arrow) is caused by overlap of the ductal diverticulum and the aorta.

a discrete posterior ridge at the junction of the isthmus and descending aorta. A false-positive echocardiographic demonstration of a coarctation may occur (Fig. 2B). The apparent narrowing of the aorta is caused by an anterior ridge of dense echos. This finding may be caused by overlapping of the ductal diverticulum and the aortic isthmus. The patient illustrated had a patent arterial duct but no coarctation. These two figures show the importance of defining a true coarctation by the presence of a *posterior* ridge of obstructing tissue with or without associated waisting of the aorta.

In addition to visualization of the coarctation, echocardiography provides invaluable information for assessment of left ventricular function and associated cardiac malformations. This is particularly important when an infant presents with congestive heart failure and clinical signs of aortic obstruction. These patients almost invariably have intracardiac shunts, a patent arterial duct, left ventricular dysfunction, or more complex anomalies associated with the coarctation.

Doppler Evaluation

Doppler techniques are useful in evaluation of the coarctation. The actual peak systolic gradient across the coarcted segment can be accurately assessed using the continuous-wave Doppler technique. The suprasternal approach is most useful in demonstrating the different flow velocities in the pre- and post-coarctation segments of aorta (Fig. 3). Marx and Allen (1986) have shown an excellent correlation between the Doppler-estimated coarctation gradient and the gradient measured during catheterization. This correlation was even closer when the velocity in the aorta proximal to the coarctation was included with the distal velocity in the modified Bernoulli equation. There are potential pitfalls in using non-

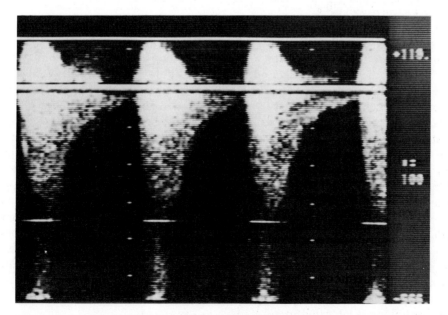

Figure 3. Continuous-wave Doppler velocities obtained from suprasternal view. Note that a lower-velocity envelope produced by flow proximal to the coarctation is contained within the high-velocity signals obtained from flow distal to the coarctation.

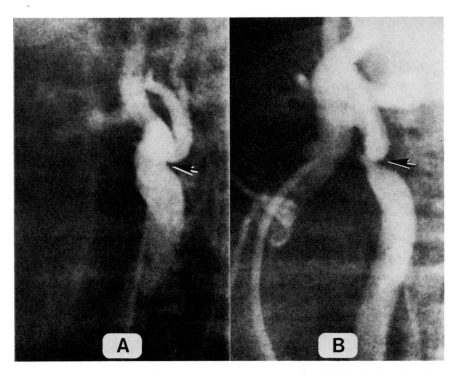

Figure 4. Aortograms in lateral view. (A) Angiogram obtained within the first few days of life demonstrates a posterior indentation (arrow) without aortic obstruction. (B) Repeat angiogram one week later in the same infant shows severe aortic narrowing (arrow) has developed.

imaging continuous-wave Doppler techniques. Lesions other than coarctation may produce high-velocity jet streams in the left posterior chest, including pulmonary valve stenosis, peripheral pulmonary arterial stenosis, stenosis of the origin of the left subclavian artery and a patent arterial duct. Pulsed Doppler echocardiography can avoid the problem of sampling a jet velocity unrelated to a coarctation by localizing the sample volume with simultaneous imaging. A gradient cannot be quantitated by these techniques, however, as the distal velocity usually exceeds the resolution capabilities of this modality. This results in aliasing. Despite these quantitative limitations, pulsed Doppler technique is of value in substantiating qualitatively the diagnosis of aortic coarctation. The presence of a high-velocity turbulent jet stream with aliasing can be detected by placing the sample volume in the descending aorta just distal to the suspected coarctation. Shaddy et al. (1986) recently demonstrated that additional valuable information about the qualitative disturbance of blood flow in the descending aorta of patients with coarctation can be obtained by using pulsed Doppler echocardiography. Antegrade flow time and acceleration time are both increased in the descending aorta of affected patients compared to normal control subjects. Thus, it is apparent that carefully performed echocardiographic and Doppler studies help in confirmation of the diagnosis of coarctation and definition of the anatomic abnormality.

Angiography

The coarctation syndrome is associated with a wide spectrum of morphological variations, some of which are common and

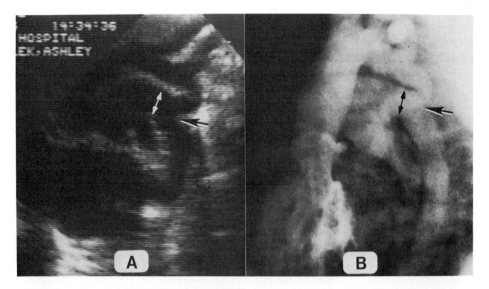

Figure 5. Coarctation of the aorta with a patent arterial duct (double-headed arrow) is shown by echocardiography (A) from the suprasternal approach and angiography (B) in the left anterior oblique view. The patent arterial end of the duct allows partial bypass of the narrowing caused by the coarctation lesion (arrow).

others that are unusual. Angiography remains the definitive technique for defining precisely the location and nature of the aortic obstruction. Several features that must be carefully assessed include the relationship of the coarctation to the arterial duct in infants, abnormalities and variants of the isthmus, anomalies of the arch and great vessels, and unusual sites of obstructive lesions.

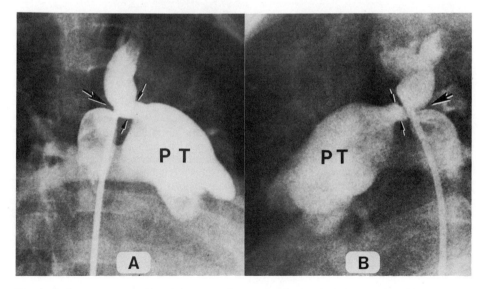

Figure 6. Severe coarctation of the aorta (large arrow) seen in right anterior oblique (A) and left anterior oblique (B) aortograms. Antegrade flow across the obstruction is virtually dependent on patency of the arterial duct (small arrow). PT = pulmonary trunk.

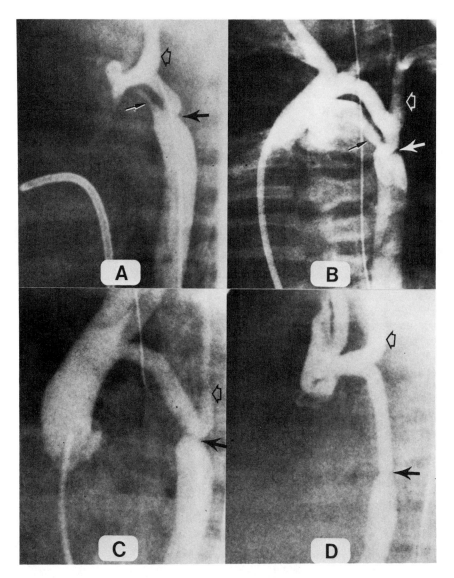

Figure 7. Marked variations of the aortic isthmus and take-off of the left subclavian artery (open arrows) in infants with coarctation of the aorta (large solid arrows) as demonstrated by angiography. (*A*) Lateral view of a normal origin of the left subclavian artery resulting in a narrow isthmus of normal length. (*B*) Anteroposterior view of a typical distal take-off of the left subclavian artery with short isthmus. (*C*) Lateral view of marked distal origin of the left subclavian artery resulting in "absence" of the isthmus. (*D*) Lateral view showing an unusually long and narrow isthmus. A patent arterial duct (small arrows) is present in (*A*) and (*B*).

Anatomical Variations and Hemodynamic Considerations

Relationship of Arterial Duct

The approach to the diagnosis and management of coarctation of the aorta requires an understanding of the intimate anatomical and physiological relationship of the arterial duct to the coarctation itself. As has been discussed in the preceding chapter, the aortic obstruction may occur in a preductal, postductal, or paraductal position. Despite these categories, in the vast majority of cases the coarctation site is within a few millimeters of the ductal insertion to the junction of the isthmus and descending aorta. The arterial duct also has a very significant physiological effect on the hemodynamic derangement that occurs when important aortic obstruction is present. This physiological effect may occur in at least two ways. First, right-to-left shunting across

the duct may provide a significant proportion of the flow in the descending aorta when the coarctation occurs in a preductal position. Second, the aortic diverticulum of the duct may allow a pathway for flow from the aortic isthmus to the descending aorta around the posterior shelf of coarctation tissue, thus permitting amelioration of the degree of actual aortic luminal narrowing. The normal process of physiological and anatomical ductal closure which occurs in the first one to two weeks of life will have a profound effect on the hemodynamic burden caused by the coarctation.

The important anatomical role that ductal constriction plays in the development of a coarctation during infancy is illustrated in Figure 4. Angiography during the first several days of life may demonstrate only a posterior notch in the descending aorta without evidence of aortic narrowing if the aortic end of the arterial duct is widely patent. Hemodynamic studies usually show no significant gradient across the eventual

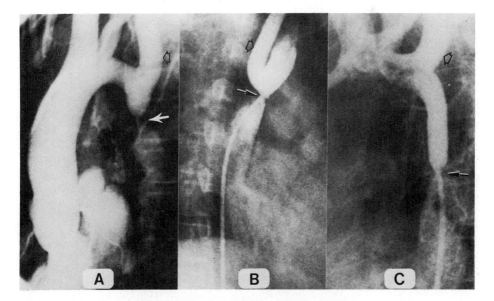

Figure 8. Aortograms demonstrating variations of the isthmus and site of origin of the left subclavian artery (open arrows) in patients with coarctation (solid arrows) presenting in later childhood or adulthood. Severe coarctation with mildly distal origin of the left subclavian artery and a typical isthmus is shown (A). Unusually short (B) and long (C) isthmic segments are also illustrated. (A) and (C) are left anterior oblique views; (B) is a right anterior oblique projection.

coarctation site. A repeat angiogram within days to weeks may reveal severe aortic obstruction associated with progressive constriction and closure of the arterial duct. The relationship of the duct to the obstructing lesion in the aorta as well as the close correlation between echocardiography and angiography is shown in Figure 5. The widely patent aortic end of the duct allows a partial bypass of flow around the posterior ridge of coarctation tissue. In the patient represented in Figure 6, the patent duct allows virtually the only communication between the isthmus and descending aorta. If this duct had closed spontaneously, complete aortic interruption almost certainly would have occurred.

Variations of the Aortic Isthmus

It is widely appreciated that considerable variations in the length and size of the isthmus are seen in infants presenting with

coarctation of the aorta. Furthermore, hypoplasia of the transverse aorta is often present in this group of patients (Morrow et al., 1986). The length of the isthmus is determined by the variable site of origin of the left subclavian artery. A relatively long isthmus associated with a severe preductal coarctation results when the left subclavian artery has a normal take-off from the aorta (Fig. 7A). In contrast to this, it is more common to have a short isthmus due to a distal origin of the left subclavian artery (Fig. 7B). Hypoplasia of part of the transverse aorta was mild in this case. In extreme cases, the isthmus can be lacking when there is marked distal displacement of the origin of the left subclavian artery (Fig. 7C). Conversely, in other cases the isthmus may be unusually long and narrow (Fig. 7D).

Although there is more uniformity of the isthmus in patients who present with coarctation in later childhood or as adults, important variations still may occur. A typical severe coarctation with a mildly distal origin of the left subclavian artery is shown

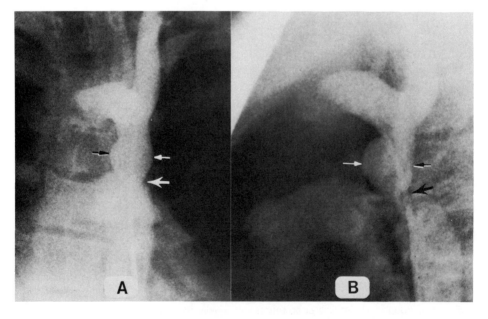

Figure 9. A congenital aneurysm of the isthmus (opposing arrows) with coarctation of the aorta (large arrows) is shown in the anteroposterior (A) and lateral (B) views. A patent arterial duct is present.

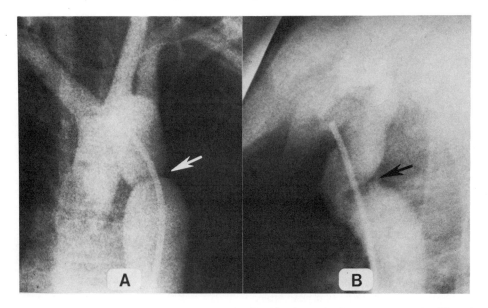

Figure 10. Pseudo-coarctation of the aorta (arrows) is shown in the anteroposterior (*A*) and lateral (*B*) views.

in Figure 8A. The variants illustrated in Figures 8B and 8C show unusually short and long isthmic segments, respectively. Other abnormalities of the isthmus are very uncommon but include a congenital aneurysm of the isthmus (Fig. 9) and pseudo-coarcta-

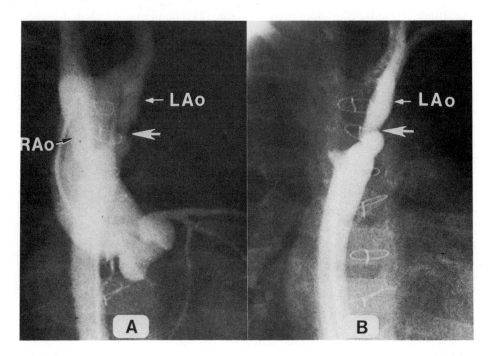

Figure 11. A double aortic arch is associated with coarctation (large arrow) in the smaller left arch as illustrated in the anteroposterior view (*A*). A selective injection in the left arch is shown in the same view (*B*). RAo = right aortic arch; LAo = left aortic arch.

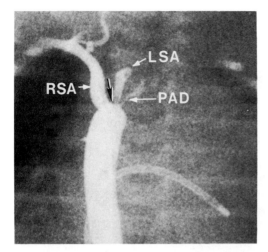

Figure 12. A right aortic arch with coarctation of the aorta (arrow) is shown in the anteroposterior view. An anomalous distal left subclavian artery (LSA), right subclavian artery (RSA), and a patent arterial duct (PAD) are visualized, but there is no reflux of contrast media into the aorta proximal to the severe coarctation from the injection into the descending aorta.

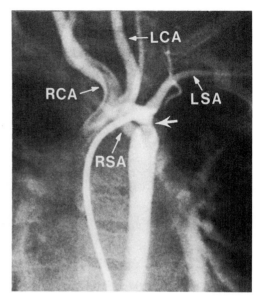

Figure 13. An anomalous right subclavian artery (RSA) arising distal to the coarctation (arrow) is shown in anteroposterior view. RCA = right carotid artery; LCA = left carotid artery; LSA = left subclavian artery.

tion (Fig. 10). In the latter condition, there is tortuosity of the isthmus which gives the appearance of a coarctation in the anteroposterior view. The lack of any discrete narrowing, however, is shown in the lateral view. Although there may be as much as a 10 to 15 torr gradient across this segment, long-term adverse effects are not expected and surgical intervention is generally not indicated.

Abnormalities of Aortic Arch

Abnormalities of the aortic arch and great vessels may be associated with coarctation of the aorta. Although rare, aortic constriction may occur in the presence of a double aortic arch. An example of this is shown in Figure 11, where a discrete narrowing is present within the smaller left arch. The association of a right aortic arch and coarctation is extremely uncommon

(Fig. 12). The patient illustrated also had an anomalous distal origin of the left subclavian artery, patency of the arterial duct and a large ventricular septal defect. The right subclavian artery may arise distal to the coarctation in the setting of a left arch (Fig. 13). This anomaly may be physiologically significant if the left subclavian artery must be occluded during the repair. This could result in compromise of the perfusion of the posterior cerebral circulation because of lack of effective antegrade flow in either vertebral artery subsequent to interruption of both subclavian arteries. A coarctation may also occur in the presence of a left arch which has a retroesophageal component of the aorta crossing to descend on the right side of the vertebral column (Fig. 14).

Unusual Sites of Obstruction

The vast majority of coarctations occur within millimeters of the ductal insertion

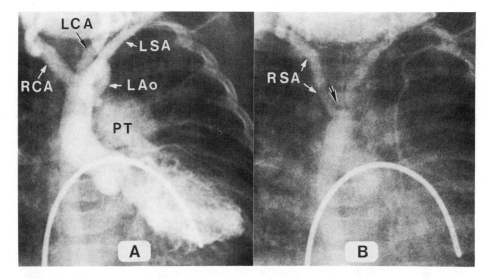

Figure 14. A left aortic arch (LAo) with a retroesophageal component and right descending aorta is shown in the anteroposterior left ventriculogram (*A*). A delayed phase demonstrates a coarctation (arrow) and the distal origin of the right subclavian artery (RSA). The pulmonary trunk (PT) is opacified because of an associated ventricular septal defect. RCA = right carotid artery; LCA = left carotid artery; LSA = left subclavian artery.

into the descending aorta. They are then found in either an immediate pre-, post-, or paraductal (or ligamentous) position. Although very uncommon, coarctation may occur in a site remote from the ductal or ligamentous insertion to the descending aorta. Uncommonly high (Fig. 15A) and low (Fig. 15B) sites of narrowing may be found. Obstruction may also occur proximal to the left subclavian artery (Fig. 15C). A coarctation of the mid- to low thoracic aorta is illustrated in Figure 16. Abdominal coarcta-

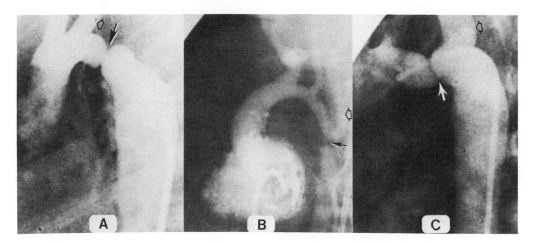

Figure 15. Lateral aortograms demonstrating unusually high (*A*) and low (*B*) sites of coarctation (solid arrows). (*C*) shows obstruction proximal to the left subclavian artery (white arrow).

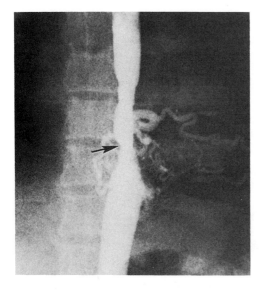

Figure 16. An anteroposterior view of a mid thoracic coarctation (arrow).

tions have been recognized for years and are known to be associated with severe hypertension. The etiology of this abnormality, which has been reported to occur in 0.5 to 2.0% of all coarctations, is different from the usual coarctation. It can have both congenital and acquired causes. Some of these are fibromuscular hypoplasia, congenital hypercalcemia, congenital rubella syndrome, neurofibromatosis, syphilis, tuberculosis, giant cell arteritis, and radiation aortitis (Calhoun et al., 1983). Abdominal coarctation may be associated with multiple peripheral pulmonary arterial stenoses (Fig. 17). This combination of abnormalities strongly suggests the diagnosis of congenital rubella syndrome.

Associated Intracardiac Malformations

Intracardiac malformations are frequently associated with a coarctation, particularly when patients present in infancy. Some of the more commonly associated lesions are shown in Table 2. A bicuspid aortic

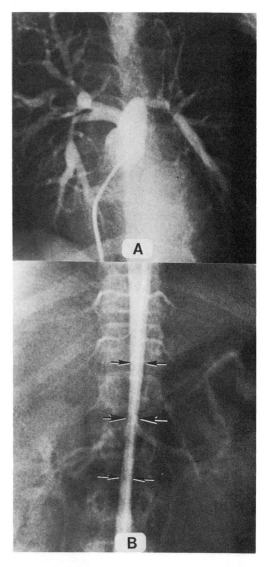

Figure 17. Multiple peripheral pulmonary arterial stenoses are shown in a pulmonary arteriogram in the anteroposterior view with cranial caudal angulation (A) in a patient with an abdominal coarctation (arrows) of the diffuse type, illustrated by an anteroposterior aortogram (B).

valve with or without associated stenosis or regurgitation probably occurs in half of the patients with aortic coarctation. This is the most common abnormality in those individuals presenting after the period of infancy. The other abnormalities tabulated fre-

Table 2
Coarctation of the Aorta: Associated Lesions

Patency of the arterial duct
Ventricular septal defect
Atrial septal defect
Mitral valve abnormality
Dysfunctional left ventricle
Complex lesions with reduced aortic outflow:
  Taussig-Bing, left heart hypoplasia,
  rudimentary subaortic ventricular
  chamber
Bicuspid aortic valve
  Aortic stenosis
  Aortic regurgitation

quently complicate the management of infants presenting with severe congestive heart failure and decreased femoral pulses.

An example of a complex lesion resulting in restricted aortic blood flow is shown in Figure 18. This patient had double inlet left ventricle with restriction of the ventricular septal defect leading to the rudimentary and hypoplastic right ventricle with resultant severe subaortic stenosis. The lateral view demonstrates hypoplasia of the isthmus, a preductal coarctation and a large arterial duct.

Conclusion

The preoperative evaluation of patients with aortic coarctation requires more than an accurate diagnosis. It is imperative that associated malformations and the precise anatomical nature of the aortic obstruction be completely defined. Only in this way can the chances for an excellent surgical repair be optimized. If this cannot be accomplished using clinical evaluation, echocardiography, and Doppler techniques, then further studies are necessary. In the future, magnetic resonance imaging and digital subtraction angiography may provide sufficient information. At the present, angiography remains the gold standard against which other investigative techniques must be measured.

Acknowledgment: We thank Susan Gainor for her help in the preparation of this manuscript.

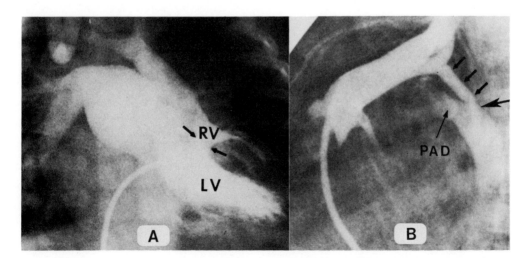

Figure 18. Double inlet left ventricle (LV) with a restrictive ventricular septal defect (opposing arrows) and hypoplastic rudimentary right ventricle (RV) is shown in the anteroposterior view of a left ventriculogram (*A*). A preductal coarctation (large arrow) associated with marked hypoplasia of the isthmus (small arrows) and a patent arterial duct (PAD) is demonstrated in the lateral view (*B*).

References

Calhoun TR, Thumwood RG, Tennyson KB, et al. Coarctation of the abdominal aorta. *Texas Heart Inst J* 1983;10:269–273.

Huhta JC, Gutgesell HP, Latson LA, Huffiness FD. Two dimensional echocardiographic assessment of the aorta in infants and children with congenital heart disease. *Circulation* 1984; 70:417–424.

Marx GR, Allen HD. Accuracy and pitfalls of Doppler evaluation of the pressure gradient in aortic coarctation. *J Am Coll Cardiol* 1986; 7:1379–1385.

Morrow WR, Huhta JC, Murphy DJ, McNamara DG. Quantitative morphology of the aortic arch in neonatal coarctation. *J Am Coll Cardiol* 1986;8:616–620.

Shaddy RE, Snider AR, Silverman NH, Lutin W. Pulsed Doppler findings in patients with coarctation of the aorta. *Circulation* 1986;73:82–88.

Smallhorn JF, Huhta JC, Adams PA, et al. Cross-sectional echocardiographic assessment of coarctation in the sick neonate and infant. *Br Heart J* 1983;50:349–361.

VII

Diseases of the Coronary Arteries

7.1

Congenital Malformations of the Coronary Arteries

Anton E. Becker

Congenital cardiac malformations may all become further complicated by abnormalities in origin and course of the coronary arteries (Parenzan et al., 1981). Basically, these abnormalities can be anticipated in all heart malformations associated with an abnormal position of the aorta relative to that of the pulmonary trunk, such as tetralogy of Fallot, double outlet ventricles, and complete transposition. From a practical stance, these abnormalities are significant since they may interfere with surgical procedures to repair the major cardiac defect. In this respect, the anomalous course of the anterior interventricular coronary artery in Fallot's tetralogy, crossing the right ventricular outflow tract, is well known. More recently, the variability in disposition of the coronary arteries in complete transposition and double outlet right ventricle with subpulmonary defect has been extensively restudied because of the growing tendency to perform an arterial switch procedure. A wide range of variations has been documented (Gittenberger-de-Groot et al., 1983; Smith et al.,

1986). As a general rule, the coronary arteries originate from the so-called facing sinuses of the aortic valve, irrespective of its position relative to the pulmonary trunk (Anderson and Becker, 1981). Moreover, the more anterior the aorta is located, the higher the chance that all or part of the left coronary arterial system originates from the proximal right coronary artery and will course either anterior or posterior to the arterial pedicle before taking up its usual epicardial course. The differences in origin and course of coronary arteries in complete transposition, nonetheless, do not hamper the surgeon in performing an adequate arterial switch procedure, except perhaps for cases in which there is a partial intramural course (Gittenberger-de-Groot et al., 1986).

Isolated congenital anomalies of coronary arteries, on the other hand, are rare. The overall reported incidence varies between 0.23% in a general autopsy series (Alexander and Griffith, 1956) and 1.2% based on a study on angiographic observations in a large number of patients without

From: Anderson, RH, Neches, WH, Park, SC, Zuberbuhler, JR, eds: *Perspectives in Pediatric Cardiology*: Mount Kisco, New York, Futura Publishing Co., © 1988.

associated congenital heart disease (Engel et al., 1975). The clinical importance of such anomalies is further limited by the fact that they form a heterogeneous group, with a large number of individual malformations that bear little or no clinical relevance. High take-off of a coronary artery may serve as one example. This condition may cause problems for the cardiologist at the time of coronary angiography, but usually has no clinical implications. Nevertheless, over the past years, experiences have taught that some innocent variations are "less innocent than others."

Classification

Isolated congenital anomalies of coronary arteries have long been divided into major and minor abnormalities, a classification proposed by Ogden (1970) (Table 1). The distinction was based on the assumption that minor abnormalities had no clinical relevance, whereas major anomalies did. It is now evident that important exceptions to this "rule" do exist. It is on these grounds that the classification of Ogden has been challenged (Becker, 1983; Vlodaver et al., 1976). An alternative descriptive approach has been advocated that takes into account the morphology of the coronary ostia within the aorta, relative to each other and the anticipated sinuses, and the presence or absence of abnormal communications.

Abnormal Morphology at Aortic Origin

The site of origin of the coronary ostia may be translocated within the aortic root to almost any site. A high take-off is defined as the situation in which the ostium arises more than 1 cm above the line of junction (the so-called aortic bar) between the aortic

Table 1
Isolated Congenital Variations of Coronary Arteries (Primary Anomalies According to Ogden 1970)

Minor forms
 High take-off
 Multiple ostia
 Anomalous origin of the circumflex artery
 Anomalous origin of the anterior
  interventricular artery
 Absent proximal ostium/single ostium in
  other aortic sinus
 Absent proximal ostium/multiple ostia in
  other aortic sinus
 Hypoplastic proximal coronary artery
 Congenital proximal stenosis
 Congenital distal stenosis
 Coronary artery from the posterior aortic
  sinus
 Ventricular origin of an accessory coronary
  artery

Major forms
 Coronary "arteriovenous" fistula
 Anomalous origin from the pulmonary trunk
  Left coronary artery
  Right coronary artery
  Both coronary arteries

sinuses and the tubular part of the aorta (Fig. 1). High take-off is considered to have no clinical significance. Nevertheless, on a theoretical basis, one may argue that the oblique take-off may cause narrowing of the lumen during aortic dilation and, hence, may lead to diminished myocardial perfusion.

On the other hand, it is now well established that translocation of coronary ostia from one sinus of Valsalva to the other is clinically important. In such instances, the left coronary artery takes origin from the right coronary sinus, together with the right coronary artery, or the right coronary artery originates from the left coronary sinus. Initially, this type of anomalous origin of coronary arteries had been classified as a "minor" congenital variation (Ogden, 1970). Experiences have taught that this is a

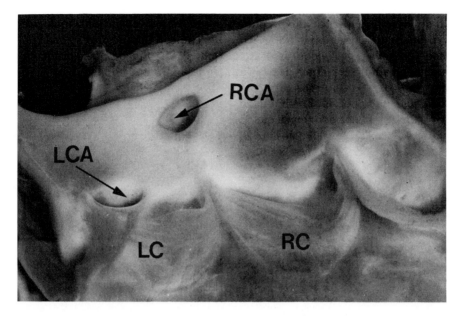

Figure 1. High take-off of the right coronary artery (RCA). The ostium is positioned above the commissure between the left (LC) and right (RC) coronary leaflets. The left coronary artery (LCA) is in its usual position.

mistake. Several authors have indicated that the condition in which the main stem of the left coronary artery passes between the aorta and the pulmonary trunk may jeopardize myocardial perfusion and should be considered as a potential cause for sudden death (Becker, 1981; Cheitlin et al., 1974; Kimbiris et al., 1978; Liberthson, 1974; McManus et al., 1981). Usually the two ostia are close together and often intimately related to a commissural site. Zijlstra et al. (1979) unequivocally demonstrated the clinical significance of this particular abnormality. They described a boy, 12 years of age, complaining of chest pain following exercise. Electrocardiographic tracings in this boy after exercise showed marked ST-segment depressions in the precordial leads. Selective left heart angiography showed an abnormal origin and course of the main left coronary artery, which was interpreted as arising from the right aortic sinus and coursing between the aorta and pulmonary trunk. The boy underwent surgery and the

diagnosis was confirmed. The main stem of the left coronary artery was reimplanted into its appropriate site. The postoperative course was uneventful and the boy recovered completely.

The reverse condition, in which the right coronary artery arises from the left sinus of Valsalva, also carries a risk of sudden death (Roberts et al., 1982).

The mechanisms that may underscore the disturbances of myocardial perfusion in these conditions have been a matter of speculation. It has been claimed that the abnormal course of the artery, sandwiched between the aorta and pulmonary trunk, could lead to compression. The affected artery, however, is deeply wedged in the groove between the aortic valve and the right ventricular outflow tract, because of the differences in height between the aortic and the pulmonary valves. Hence, although the proposed mechanism cannot be completely ruled out, it seems less likely. A more likely explanation could relate to the intrinsic

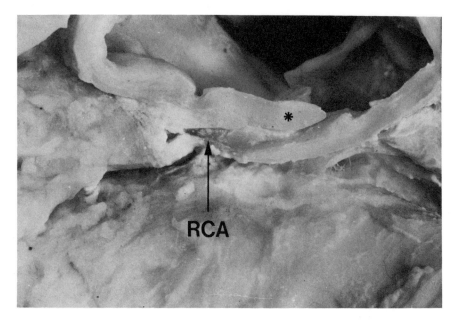

Figure 2. Detailed view of the most proximal segment of the right coronary artery (RCA). The ostium is located close to a commissure and the artery has an oblique take-off. The most proximal part is in the intramural position and the inner wall may serve as a flap (asterisk), narrowing or closing the ostium during dilation of the aortic root.

anatomy at the site of origin. The artery usually has an oblique take-off from the aortic root and its most proximal segment runs in an intramural position within the aortic wall itself (Fig. 2). This architecture, almost by necessity, dictates that dilation of the aortic root, during diastole, will cause some degree of compression of the most proximal sites of the coronary arteries and, hence, may cause myocardial ischemia. In instances, moreover, in which both ostia are closely related, an intramural course of both coronary arteries is common (Fig. 3).

The significance for sudden death in competitive athletes of these isolated congenital anomalies of the coronary arteries has recently been emphasized (Maron et al., 1986). The pathologist, confronted with the enigmatic case of sudden and unexpected death in a young individual, should be aware of this particular anatomy as a potential cause of myocardial ischemia.

Abnormal Communications

Anomalous Origin of Coronary Arteries from the Pulmonary Trunk

The pathology of this particular condition is well established. The most important situation is that in which the left coronary artery arises from the pulmonary trunk, an arrangement known as the Bland-White-Garland syndrome.

Patients with this anomaly are at jeopardy because of two pathophysiological mechanisms. First, following birth, a drop in perfusion pressure of the aberrant coronary artery occurs, accompanied by a drop in oxygen saturation. This will compromise the myocardium at a stage of postnatal growth adaptation where the left ventricular myocardial mass outgrows that of the right. Hence, myocardial ischemia develops and,

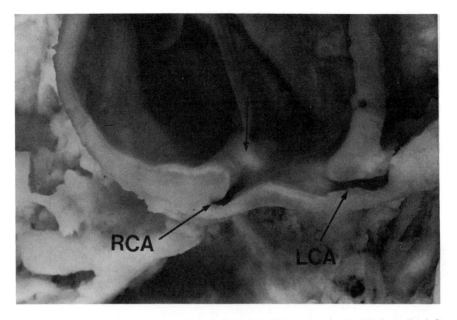

Figure 3. Origin of both the right (RCA) and left (LCA) coronary arteries from the left coronary sinus, close to the commissure and almost forming a single ostium. The most proximal parts of both arteries have an oblique intramural course.

eventually, classic infarction may occur. At that stage, the baby may present signs of left heart failure and mitral regurgitation, while the underlying anomaly may initially pass unrecognized. Indeed, it is well known to the pediatric cardiologist that any neonate who presents with left heart failure or mitral valve regurgitation should be carefully investigated for the presence of this particular coronary arterial anomaly.

Survival during the initial period of life largely depends on the development of collaterals from the right coronary artery to the jeopardized myocardium. The early critical period may pass unnoticed and the neonate may grow into infancy without signs or symptoms of the underlying anomaly. With the development of such an extensive collateral system, a second pathophysiological mechanism is introduced. Because of the connections between the right and left coronary arterial systems, a steal phenomenon can occur. Blood may then be shunted through the aberrant left coronary artery

into the pulmonary trunk. Thus, myocardial ischemia becomes increasingly important. Sudden and unexpected death is not an unusual phenomenon under these circumstances.

The pathology of the heart is dominated by extensive myocardial necrosis, with dilation of the left ventricular cavity (Fig. 4).

The pathophysiology of this condition was already clarified beautifully by Edwards in 1964. It should be pointed out, however, that there is a continuum between the two main pathophysiological mechanisms alluded to above. Terms such as infant and adult forms of the Bland-White-Garland syndrome, therefore, may be misleading.

Aberrant origin of the right coronary artery from the pulmonary trunk is extremely rare. Nevertheless, cases have been reported in which an aberrant right coronary artery was considered the cause of sudden and unexpected death in otherwise

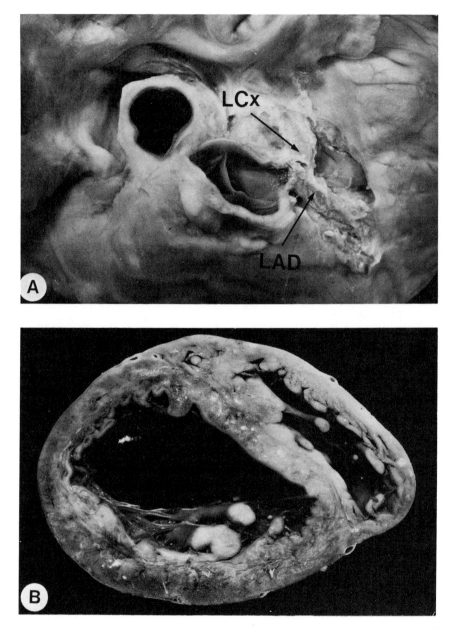

Figure 4. Anomalous origin of the left coronary artery from the pulmonary trunk. (A) Origin of the left circumflex (LCx) and anterior descending (LAD) coronary arteries, via a short main stem, from the left posterior facing valve cusp of the pulmonary trunk. (B) Cross-section of the heart showing marked dilation of the left ventricular cavity and extensive necrosis and scarring of the left ventricular myocardium. The pathology portrays the substrate for left heart failure and mitral regurgitation.

healthy individuals (Wald et al., 1971). Personal experience is limited to one instance. The patient was a 38-year-old woman with

Turner's syndrome, who died of infectious endocarditis of a two-leaflet aortic valve. The patient, however, had had a history of

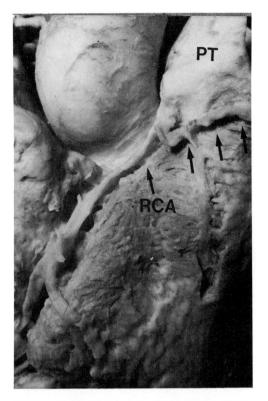

Figure 5. Aberrant origin of the right coronary artery (RCA) from the pulmonary trunk (PT). There is a large infundibular (conal) branch (arrows) connecting the left with the right coronary system.

angina pectoris for years. The reason for these complaints was never established. Autopsy revealed anomalous origin of the right coronary artery from the pulmonary trunk (Fig. 5). There was no atherosclerotic narrowing of coronary arteries. It is tempting to consider a steal phenomenon as the underlying mechanism for the anginal complaints. Indeed, Bortolotti and coworkers (1978) demonstrated an extensive collateral network between the normally arising left coronary artery and the anomalous right coronary artery with a fistulous connection into the pulmonary trunk. Hence, similar mechanisms are operative as discussed for patients with an aberrant origin of the left coronary artery.

Isolated Coronary Arterial Fistulas

Coronary arterial fistulas in the absence of additional cardiac malformations, such as pulmonary atresia with intact ventricular septum, are extremely rare. The abnormal connections can exist to any of the cardiac chambers or to other arteries and veins. Such malformations may occasionally have clinical relevance, most likely because of a "steal phenomenon" as previously described for anomalous origin of the coronary arteries from the pulmonary trunk. This may be illustrated by a patient, 61 years of age, who died accidentally. Autopsy revealed a fistulous connection between the coronary system and the pulmonary trunk, caused by a large and tortuous infundibular branch (Fig. 6). The artery connected the most proximal segment of the right coronary artery with the anterior interventricular coronary artery, but connected also with the pulmonary trunk at the site of the anteriorly positioned facing pulmonary sinus. The caliber of the anomalous branch and the size of the orifice within the pulmonary trunk suggest a functionally important connection. This impression was strengthened by the presence of myocardial scars in the absence of obstructive coronary arterial disease.

Conclusions

Isolated congenital anomalies of the coronary arteries are rare and constitute a vast and heterogeneous group. The clinical significance of anomalies such as aberrant origin of the left coronary artery from the pulmonary trunk has never been questioned. A large number of anomalies also occur, however, which have been considered of no clinical relevance and, hence, have been designated as "minor" anomalies. Past experiences have revealed that this may well be an improper qualification.

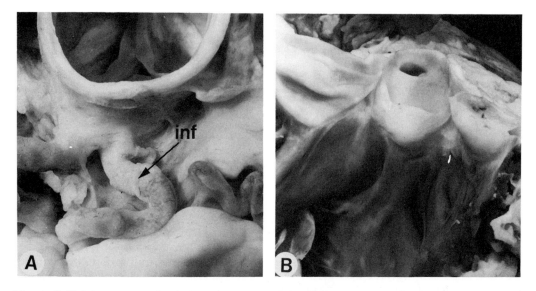

Figure 6. Fistulous connection between a tortuous infundibular artery and the pulmonary trunk. (*A*) Course of the anomalous branch (inf) originating almost from the same orifice as the main right coronary artery. The branch connects to the pulmonary trunk anteriorly (arrow) and continues to connect also with the anterior descending coronary artery. (*B*) Interior aspect of the pulmonary trunk revealing the wide orifice of the fistulous connection, suggesting its functional importance.

Translocation of coronary ostia within the aortic root itself may create a particular morphology that may cause myocardial ischemia. Anomalous origin of the left coronary artery from the right sinus of Valsalva may serve as the best example in this respect. The mechanism underlying impaired perfusion of myocardium probably does not relate to the position of the artery, sandwiched between the aorta and right pulmonary outflow tract, but rather to the oblique intramural course of the most proximal segment. The peculiar relationship may enhance a flaplike mechanism, narrowing, or closing the ostium during dilation of the aortic root. Sudden and unexpected death has been associated with this particular anatomy.

Similarly, abnormal connections between the coronary arterial systems and other vascular compartments may cause serious damage to myocardium because of a steal phenomenon. This applies not only to the classic example of the Bland-White-Garland syndrome, but also to less striking abnormalities, such as fistulous connections in the presence of coronary arteries with otherwise normal origins.

It is on this basis that a classification of minor and major anomalies seems less appropriate. The approach presently advocated takes the basic morphology as point of departure, dividing isolated congenital anomalies of coronary arteries into two main categories. These are those with abnormalities in origin within the aortic root and those with abnormal communications. This descriptive classification serves a better purpose when it comes to considering the pathophysiological implications of such isolated coronary arterial anomalies of congenital nature.

References

Alexander RW, Griffith GC. Anomalies of the coronary arteries and their clinical significance. *Circulation* 1956;14:800–805.

Anderson RH, Becker AE. Coronary arterial patterns: A guide to identification of congenital heart disease. In Becker AE, Losekoot G, Marcelletti C, Anderson RH (eds): *Paediatric Cardiology*, vol 3. Edinburgh: Churchill Livingstone, 1981:251–263.

Becker AE. Variations of the main coronary arteries. In Becker AE, Losekoot G, Marcelletti C, Anderson RH (eds): *Paediatric Cardiology*, vol 3. Edinburgh, Churchill Livingstone, 1983:263–277.

Bortolotti D, Casarotto D, Betti D, et al. Anomalous origin of the right coronary artery from the main pulmonary artery. *Eur J Cardiol* 1978; 7:451–455.

Cheitlin MD, DeCastro CM, McAllister HA. Sudden death as a complication of anomalous left coronary artery origin from the anterior sinus of Valsalva. A not-so-minor congenital anomaly. *Circulation* 1974;50:780–787.

Edwards JE. Editorial. The direction of bloodflow in coronary arteries arising from the pulmonary trunk. *Circulation* 1964;29:163–166.

Engel HJ, Torres C, Page HL Jr. Major variations in anatomical origin of the coronary arteries: Angiographic observations in 4250 patients without associated congenital heart disease. *Catheter Cardiovasc Diagn* 1975;1:157–169.

Gittenberger-de Groot AC, Sauer U, Oppenheimer-Dekker A, Quaegebeur J. Coronary arterial anatomy in transposition of the great arteries. A morphological study. *Pediatr Cardiol* 1983; 4(suppl 1):15–24.

Gittenberger-de Groot AC, Sauer U, Quaegebeur JM. Aortic intramural coronary artery in three hearts with transposition of the great arteries. *J Thorac Cardiovasc Surg* 1986;91:566–571.

Kimbiris D, Iskandrian AS, Segal BL, Bemis CE. Anomalous aortic origin of coronary arteries. *Circulation* 1978;58:606–615.

Liberthson RR, Dinsmore RE, Bharati S, et al. Aberrant coronary artery origin from the aorta. Diagnosis and clinical significance. *Circulation* 1974;50:774–779.

Maron BJ, Epstein SE, Roberts WC. Causes of sudden death in competitive athletes. *J Am Coll Cardiol* 1986;7:204–214.

McManus BM, Waller BE, Graboys TB, et al. Exercise and sudden death, part I. *Curr Prob Cardiol* 1981;6:1–89.

Ogden JA. Congenital anomalies of the coronary arteries. *Am J Cardiol* 1970;25:474–479.

Parenzan L, Baldrighi V, Baldrighi G, et al. Selective coronary angiograms in congenital heart disease. In Becker AE, Losekoot G, Marcelletti C, Anderson RH (eds): *Paediatric Cardiology*, vol. 3. Edinburgh, Churchill Livingstone, 1981:278–289.

Roberts WC, Siegel RJ, Zipes BP. Origin of the right coronary artery from the left sinus of Valsalva and its functional consequences: Analysis of ten necropsy patients. *Am J Cardiol* 1982;49:863–868.

Smith A, Arnold R, Wilkinson JL, et al. An anatomical study of the patterns of the coronary arteries and sinus nodal artery in complete transposition. *Int J Cardiol* 1986;12:295–304.

Vlodaver Z, Amplatz K, Burchell HB, Edwards JE. *Coronary Heart Disease. Clinical, Angiographic and Pathologic Profiles*. New York, Springer Verlag, 1976.

Wald S, Stonecipher K, Baldwin BJ, Nutter DO. Anomalous origin of the right coronary artery from the pulmonary artery. *Am J Cardiol* 1971;27:677–681.

Zijlstra JP, Düren DR, Tan SL, et al. Operatieve behandeling van de aberrante oorsprong van de A. coronaria sinistra bij een 12-jarige jongen. *Nederlands Tijdschrift voor Geneeskunde* 1979; 123:1681–1685.

Echocardiographic Demonstration of the Coronary Arteries in Children

Norman H. Silverman and Klaus G. Schmidt

Until recently, the display of coronary arterial anatomy had not developed as extensively as other areas of echocardiography. Continuing improvement in the resolution of ultrasound equipment and image processing as well as developments in imaging diseased coronary arteries, particularly in Kawasaki disease, has now made it possible to provide more accurate definition (Capannari et al., 1986; Satomi et al., 1984; Yoshida et al., 1982).

Methods

Because the image plane does not move concomitant with the heart during the cardiac cycle, there are only isolated moments when the coronary arteries can be seen. In order to recognize these arteries, it is necessary to use a technique that augments the time during which these arteries can be observed. This can be achieved using newer videotape recorders which allow forward and reverse playback similar to that found in cineangiographic review systems. This permits careful study of the few frames in which the artery lies in the scan plane. Augmented imaging of the coronary arteries can also be achieved directly from state-of-the-art echocardiographic equipment by means of a technique called the "cineloop." The cineloop provides the ability to reexamine short periods of imaging repeatedly through a microprocessor. Successive frames of video information are acquired in digital format and occupy a series of memory slots. The frames of this information can be recalled and replayed at the same rate as they were acquired. Alternatively, they may be reviewed at a faster or slower rate in order to appreciate the images as clearly as possible. Certain frames where no coronary artery is visible may be removed from the cycle or the frame sequence altered. The re-

From: Anderson, RH, Neches, WH, Park, SC, Zuberbuhler, JR, eds: *Perspectives in Pediatric Cardiology*: Mount Kisco, New York, Futura Publishing Co., © 1988.

Table 1
Cases of Suspected Coronary Artery Abnormalities (n = 62)

Kawasaki's Disease	52
with diffuse dilation of the coronary arteries	6
of these, additional pericardial effusion	1
with coronary arterial aneurysms	7
of these, additional pericardial effusion	1
with normal coronary arterial anatomy (echo)	39
Coronary artery fistula	2
Anomalous origin of the left coronary artery	6
Right coronary artery crossing the right ventricular outflow tract in tetralogy of Fallot	2

The coronary arteries are also difficult to image because of their curvilinear course. Several planes of echocardiographic imaging are therefore necessary for complete delineation. These include parasternal long- and short-axis views at the level of the aortic root and apical and subcostal images taken in a variety of planes. Knowledge of the direction and position of the coronary arteries is essential for precise orientation of the transducer. Using these techniques, we examined 23 patients with abnormalities of the coronary arteries. These came from a group of 62 patients who were specifically examined because of suspicion of coronary arterial malformations (Table 1).

Imaging the Normal Coronary Arteries

sulting cineloop contains the image sequence of the coronary arteries and can be examined as a cycle or as individual frames. Since the information is in digital format, it may also be manipulated to highlight the artery in a manner similar to digital techniques used in subtraction radiography. It is now possible to examine the images of the coronary arteries immediately after they have been acquired in real time with the aid of a "frame grabber" incorporated into current ultrasound machines (Ultramark 8, Advanced Technology Laboratories, Seattle, WA). A more usual and practical means of analyzing the data is when the images are captured from the videotape sometime after recording by use of a frame grabber incorporated into a video analysis review system (Microsonics, Indianapolis, IN). It is important to remember that although these techniques provide the examiner with improved opportunity to view the coronary arteries, they do not produce artificial information. Precise echocardiographic technique and imaging in multiple planes are the essential prerequisites for optimal imaging of the coronary arteries.

The coronary arteries are imaged in the parasternal short axis by scanning cranially in the sinuses of Valsalva (Feigenbaum, 1986; Silverman and Snider, 1982; Weyman et al., 1976). Although most echocardiographic images published to show coronary arterial anatomy demonstrate the main arteries together in the parasternal short-axis plane (Fig. 1), they are more frequently imaged separately. This is because they run in slightly different planes. Whereas the right coronary artery tends to run in a fairly vertical direction, the left artery runs a more horizontal course. When imaging the aortic root, therefore, slight counterclockwise (vertical) rotation of the transducer is necessary to image the right (Fig. 2), and slight clockwise (horizontal) rotation to image the left coronary artery (Fig. 3). The left coronary artery lies in the echocardiographic plane intermediate between those used for imaging the left atrial appendage and the pulmonary trunk. Cranial and caudal scanning between the above-mentioned structures is necessary to define the area within which the artery lies. The left coronary arterial length is variable and can be traced to

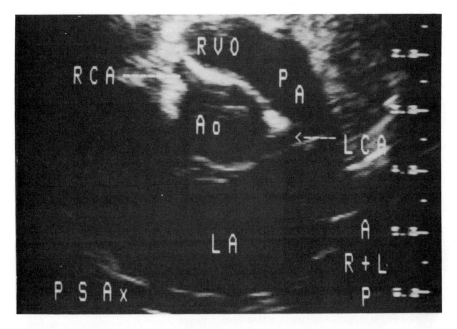

Figure 1. Parasternal short axis (P S Ax), showing the origin of both coronary arteries in a case of severe aortic stenosis. The coronary arteries are mildly enlarged and visible in one plane. RCA = right coronary artery; RVO = right ventricular outflow tract; Ao = aorta; PA = pulmonary artery; LCA = left coronary artery; LA = left atrium; A = anterior; R = right; L = left; P = posterior.

the point where it gives rise to the left circumflex artery. The left anterior descending artery can be seen for some distance, and occasionally even the first diagonal (lateral) branch (Fig. 4). With caudal angulation from the area of the aortic root, the anterior descending artery can be seen on the anterior cardiac surface at the point of junction between the right and left ventricular free walls and the septum (Fig. 5). It is most frequently seen when it is enlarged, such as where there is left ventricular hypertrophy.

The parasternal long axis has been used to image the left main stem and the anterior descending branch of the left coronary artery. The transducer is rotated into a parasternal plane parallel to the vertebrae (parasagittal plane). Here the pulmonary trunk is imaged anterior to the coronary artery. This view is of value for defining the anomalous origin of left coronary artery (see below). From this plane, the transducer is swept toward the left surface of the heart. Then, as

the area between the aortic and pulmonary roots is imaged, the left main and left anterior descending coronary arteries come successively into view (Fig. 6). With extreme leftward shift, the descending artery can sometimes be seen on the border of the heart (Fig. 7). The right coronary artery can also be seen in the high parasternal long-axis view. When the ascending aorta is imaged with the scan plane oriented in a vertical direction, the right atrioventricular groove with the coronary artery lying within it is readily demonstrated (Fig. 8). The origin and a good part of the right coronary artery can be seen. The normal coronary arteries can usually be seen over the first 2 to 5 cm from their origin. Many of these high parasternal views can be obtained with greater facility in the smaller child where the sternum is unossified and the lungs are not hyperinflated.

Several other views have been used to image the normal coronary arteries. These

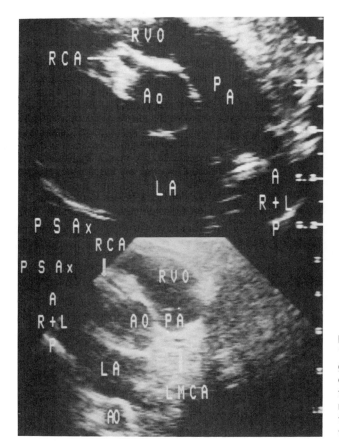

Figure 2. Parasternal short axis. *Top:* Right coronary artery at its origin from aorta. *Bottom:* Slight further counterclockwise rotation of the transducer allows visualization of its more distal course on the surface of the right ventricle. Left coronary artery not visible in this plane.

include the apical and the subcostal planes. Any coronal plane from an apical or subcostal position will show the origin of the left coronary and anterior descending arteries as they travel laterally and then descend on the anterior ventricular surface (Fig. 9). The proximal right coronary artery has also been imaged quite regularly in children from the subcostal coronal plane and can be traced for a few centimeters in the right atrioventricular groove. Occasionally, it is possible to identify the normal right coronary artery from the four-chamber plane as it lies in the posterior atrioventricular groove. The posterior four-chamber plane is identified showing the coronary sinus entering the right atrium. The transducer is then rotated slightly counterclockwise and moved slightly medially to image the artery (Fig. 10).

Mucocutaneous Lymph Node Syndrome (Kawasaki Disease)

Several studies have shown that aneurysms of the coronary arteries can be demonstrated well by echocardiography (Chung et al., 1982; Hiraishi et al., 1979; Meyer, 1984; Yoshikawa et al., 1979). We have used an eclectic multiple-plane approach to image such aneurysms. Out of 52 patients evaluated with this syndrome, we found 13 with dilation of the coronary arteries and/or aneurysms (Table 1). Most were central in position and were discovered in the right, left main stem, anterior and posterior descending coronary arteries. The coronary arterial aneurysms are easy to identify because the coronary artery is dilated and because the surrounding perivascular tissue

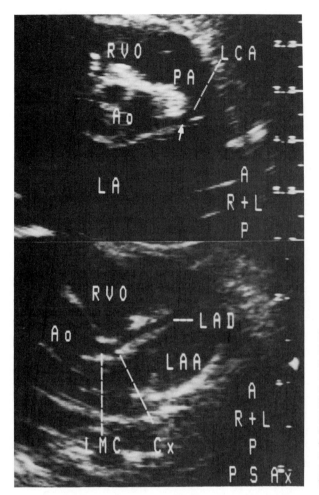

Figure 3. Parasternal short axis. *Top:* Left coronary artery arises from the aorta. Arrow indicates the site of its branching into left anterior descending and circumflex artery. *Bottom:* More horizontal imaging shows the proximal portion of the left anterior descending artery to the left of the right ventricular outflow tract. LAD = left anterior descending artery; LAA = left atrial appendage; LMC = left main coronary artery; Cx = left circumflex artery.

is echo-reflective. This echocardiographic sign of "haloing" may relate to acute and chronic inflammatory changes around the vessel. As with the echocardiographic technique in the normal patient, multiple plane imaging is required in order to image the coronary arteries.

Capannari et al. (1986) found echocardiography was a very sensitive and specific technique for defining proximal coronary arterial aneurysms when using coronary angiography as the "gold standard." Indeed, there were no patients in their series who had isolated peripheral aneurysms, suggesting that isolated peripheral aneurysms are a rare presentation. Therefore, echocardiogra-

phy may be as sensitive and specific for recognizing patients with coronary artery involvement in Kawasaki disease as coronary angiography, except for the rare patient in whom there are isolated peripheral aneurysms. It might be argued that in the setting of isolated peripheral aneurysms, the disease might be more benign and no surgical intervention need be planned. It is our conviction that unless surgical intervention is planned, echocardiography is sufficient to follow most of these patients. Coronary arteriography is indicated only when bypass surgery is contemplated. We also believe that coronary angiography should be performed by special designated centers that

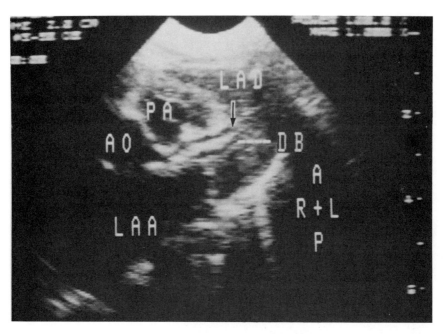

Figure 4. Similar view to that in Fig. 3, bottom; a more distal part of the left anterior descending artery and its first diagonal branch (DB) can be seen.

are actively concerned with research into the fate of the coronary arteries, but we do not subscribe to the premise that "routine angiography" is necessary in the clinical management of this disease. In a recent report on the value of prophylactic use of gamma globulin in the prevention of coronary aneurysms (Newburger et al., 1986), echocardiography, not angiography, was selected as the preferred screening test.*

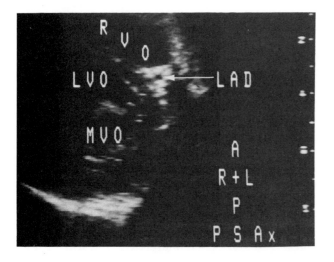

Figure 5. Parasternal short axis at the level of the mitral valve. The left anterior descending artery can be seen at the junction between the ventricular free walls and the ventricular septum. LVO = left ventricular outflow tract; MVO = mitral valve orifice; other abbreviations as above.

---

* Editor's note: It may also be argued that the study was less than optimal for this precise reason. See Chapter 7.4

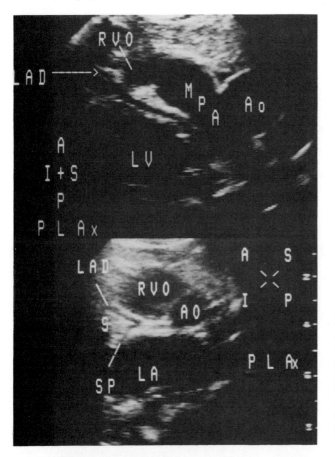

Figure 6. Parasternal long axis (P L Ax) in a more parasagittal orientation. *Top:* Left anterior descending artery between right and left ventricular outflow tracts. *Bottom:* More distal part of left anterior descending artery. A septal perforator (SP) is also demonstrated. MPA = main pulmonary artery; S = ventricular septum; I = inferior; S = superior.

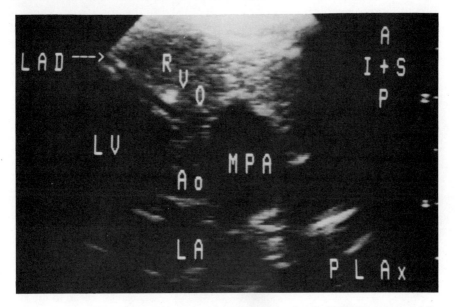

Figure 7. Parasternal long-axis view with more leftward shift. Note the course of the left anterior descending artery (arrow).

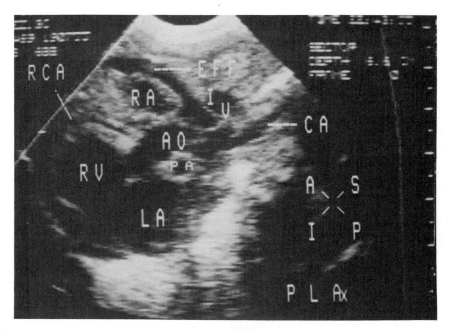

Figure 8. Parasternal long axis with some clockwise rotation of the transducer. The right coronary artery is demonstrated within the atrioventricular groove. RA = right atrium; EFF = pericardial effusion; IV = innominate vein; CA = carotid artery.

Planes of Imaging

The parasternal short-axis plane at the level of the aortic root readily shows aneurysms in the right and left proximal coronary arteries (Fig. 11). When both the coronary arteries are large, they are more easily recognized in the same short-axis view than the normal coronary arterial pattern. It is important to note that the aneurysms are seen distal to the aortic root. The orifices of the coronary arteries are most usually not involved and are, therefore, of normal size.

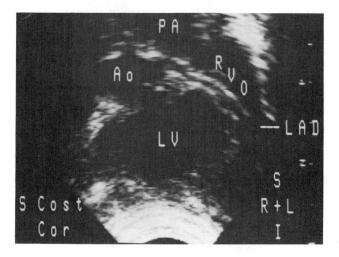

Figure 9. Subcostal coronal view (S Cost Cor). The left main coronary artery is seen at its origin from aorta and the left anterior descending artery can be traced to the left margin of the heart.

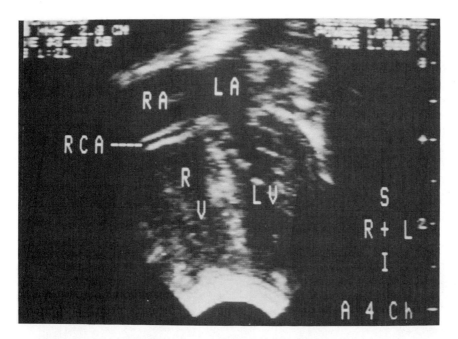

Figure 10. Apical four-chamber view (A 4 Ch). The right coronary artery travels in the posterior atrioventricular groove to the right border of the heart.

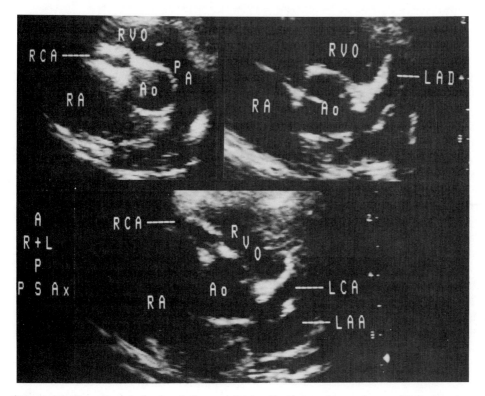

Figure 11. Parasternal short axis in a patient with Kawasaki syndrome. Note the very proximal aneurysm of the right (*top left*) and left (*top right*) coronary arteries as well as dense echoreflective tissue around them. *Bottom:* Both dilated vessels can be recognized in the same plane with repositioning of the transducer.

387

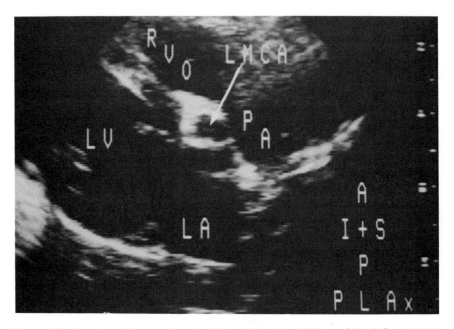

Figure 12. Parasternal long-axis orientation. Note the dilation of the left coronary artery just posterior to the pulmonary trunk. LMCA = left main coronary artery.

The "ductal cut," a high parasternal parasagittal view, is extremely valuable for imaging aneurysms of the main stem of the left and the anterior descending coronary arteries as they course behind the pulmonary trunk (Satomi et al., 1984) (Fig. 12).

Aneurysms of the proximal segment of the right coronary artery can be imaged from the parasternal long-axis view with rightward tilt of the transducer (Fig. 13, top). Aneurysms in the distal right coronary artery may also be identified posteriorly in this plane near the crux of the heart (Fig. 13, bottom).

At the level of the ventricles, the parasternal short-axis view provides the plane for imaging aneurysms of the coronary arterial branches as they pass down and across the ventricle (Fig. 14). Aneurysms or dilation of the anterior and posterior descending coronary arteries, marked by the junction of the septa with the free walls of the ventricular chambers, can be displayed (Fig. 14, top). In addition, dilation of the obtuse

marginal branch can be seen as it courses over the surface of the left ventricle (Fig. 14, bottom). It is notable that, when scanning downward from their origin, the dilated arteries may be seen to appear and then disappear. This is probably indicative of the presence of peripheral aneurysms.

The apical four-chamber view has been used to define aneurysms of the left main stem and anterior descending coronary arteries. The posterior angulated view is of value for defining aneurysms of the portion of the right coronary as it travels in the posterior atrioventricular groove toward the crux of the heart (Fig. 15). Aneurysms of the circumflex coronary artery may also be seen next to the coronary sinus. When dilated, the artery can be seen in the tissue of the left atrioventricular junction.

Following the suggestions of Yoshida et al. (1982), we have also examined all of our patients using subcostal coronal and sagittal plane imaging. We scanned the surface of the heart from the posterior to the anterior

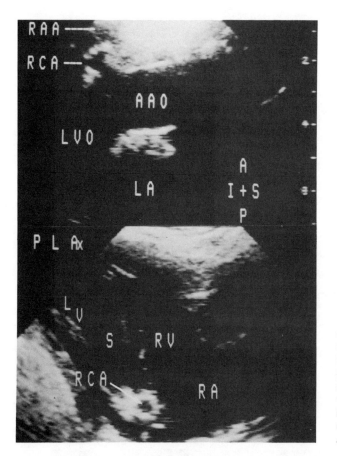

Figure 13. Parasternal long axis. *Top:* In a more parasagittal plane, the dilated right coronary artery can be recognized at its origin from ascending aorta (AAO). *Bottom:* The dilated peripheral right coronary is demonstrated in a parasternal long-axis view with rightward shift where it runs in the posterior atrioventricular groove. RAA = right atrial appendage.

and from left to right. Aneurysms, when present, can be seen in both the right and left main stems as they extend from their origin at the aortic root (Fig. 16). As the scan moves slightly anteriorly, aneurysms of the right coronary can be traced in the ventriculoinfundibular fold (Fig. 17, top) between the anterior surface of the right ventricle and the right atrial appendage. With some right posterior angulation, aneurysms of the left anterior descending artery can also be seen as traced across the obtuse margin of the heart (Fig. 17, bottom). Aneurysms of the distal portion of the right coronary artery can be seen in the subcostal coronal plane as the artery winds its way across the acute margin of the heart to its diaphragmatic surface (Fig. 17, bottom). The subcostal parasagittal views are valuable for defin-

ing the posterior descending coronary artery as it runs along the diaphragmatic surface of the heart (Fig. 18). Aneurysms of the posterior descending coronary artery are generally not easily seen with other echocardiographic projections.

It is important to consider that echocardiography is a technique that best defines dilated coronary arteries. The arterial strictures, which may be the greatest problem in Kawasaki disease, are not easily seen. The types of proximal aneurysms, however, are readily distinguished, be they saccular, fusiform, or diffusely ectatic.

There are other features of importance in Kawasaki disease which are definable by echocardiography. The first is the presence of pericardial effusions. These are frequent in the early convalescent phase of the illness

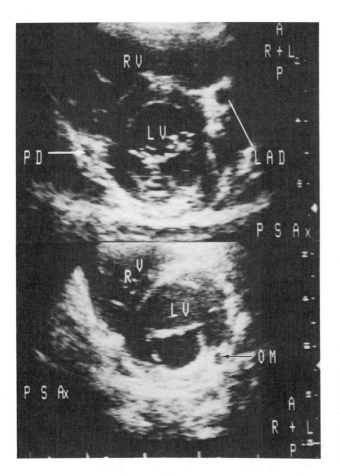

Figure 14. Parasternal short axis. *Top:* Note both dilated anterior descending (LAD) and posterior descending artery (PD) at the points of junction of ventricular septum with the free ventricular walls. *Bottom:* In a similar view the obtuse marginal branch (OM) of the circumflex artery is visualized.

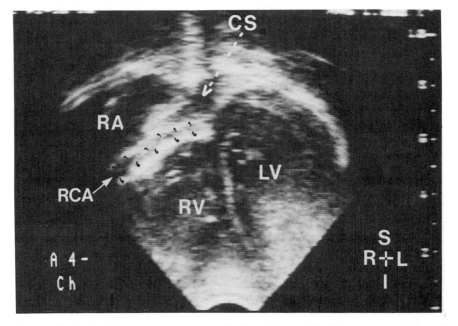

Figure 15. Apical four-chamber view with the plane shifted to a more right and posterior position. Note the echo-density around the right coronary artery (RCA) as it travels in the posterior atrioventricular groove (black commas). CS = coronary sinus.

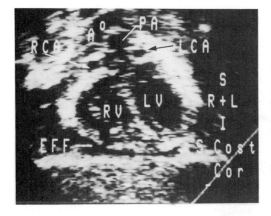

Figure 16. Subcostal coronal view. Aneurysmal dilation of the proximal right (RCA) and left (LCA) coronary arteries is seen, as well as additional pericardial effusion (EFF).

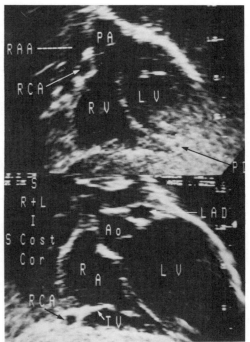

Figure 17. Subcostal coronal view. *Top:* The dilated right coronary lies between the right atrial appendage (RAA) and the infundibulum of the right ventricle. Note the posterior descending branch (PD, black arrow) at the diaphragmatic surface of the heart. *Bottom:* The dilated left anterior descending artery (LAD) is seen left to the aortic root as well as the dilated peripheral RCA in the right atrioventricular groove (black arrow). TV = tricuspid valve.

(Fig. 19). Second, ventricular function and segmental wall motion abnormalities as a reflection of impaired coronary arterial perfusion have been documented with both M-mode and cross-sectional imaging techniques (Chung et al., 1982). Finally, aortic and mitral insufficiency have also been defined by use of pulsed Doppler ultrasound (Gidding et al., 1986; Nakano et al., 1985).

Anomalous Origin of the Left Coronary Artery from the Pulmonary Trunk

This condition is uncommon and may be either quite obvious or quite subtle. We have encountered six cases, four within the last year. The echocardiographic appearance of poor left ventricular function mimics that of a cardiomyopathy. The echocardiographic definition of the anomalous origin was spearheaded by a report from Fisher et al. (1981), who described detection of the anomalous origin from the pulmonary trunk in three patients in whom the diagnosis had been established previously by angiography. These patients were all over one year

of age at the time that the anomaly was recognized by echocardiography. We had the opportunity to evaluate the coronary arteries carefully in four cases. Spurred by developments of contrast echocardiography in the cardiac catheterization laboratory, we were able to define a plane for examining the anomalous origin, which is different from those previously reported (Martin et al., 1986) (Fig. 20). The anomalous artery arises most frequently out of the posterior portion of the pulmonary trunk but may arise from the base of the right pulmonary artery. Its position in this site is not much different from the one it normally occupies

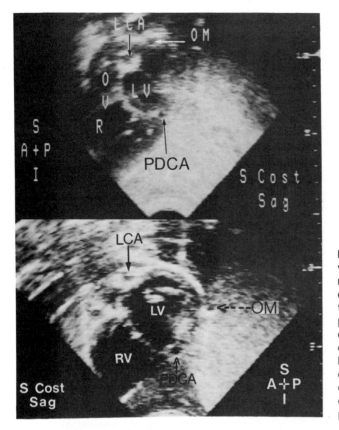

Figure 18. Subcostal parasagittal view (S Cost Sag). *Top:* Dense echo reflections around the dilated left coronary artery (LCA) and the obtuse marginal branch (OM). Note the peripheral dilation of the posterior descending coronary artery (PDCA) on the diaphragmatic surface of the heart. *Bottom:* The plane is shifted obliquely and to the right; it shows dilation of the PDCA. An enlarged obtuse marginal (OM) can be seen posteriorly.

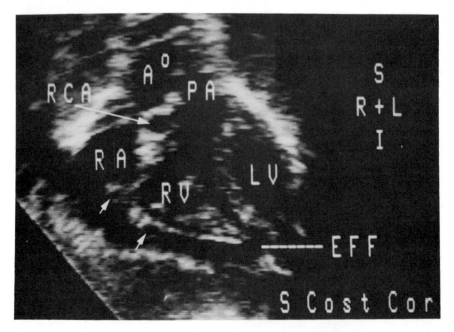

Figure 19. Subcostal coronal view. Dilated right coronary artery (RCA) is obvious; note peripheral small aneurysms of RCA (small arrows). There is substantial pericardial effusion (EFF).

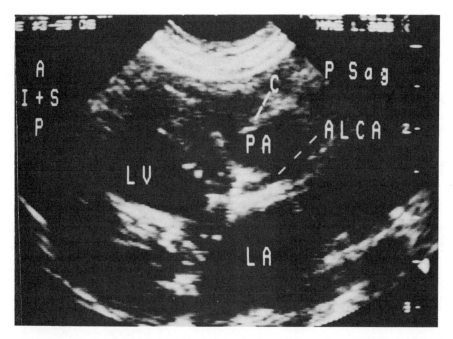

Figure 20. Parasternal long-axis view in a sagittal orientation. The anomalous origin of the left coronary artery (ALCA) is identified at the back of the pulmonary trunk. C = catheter in the PA.

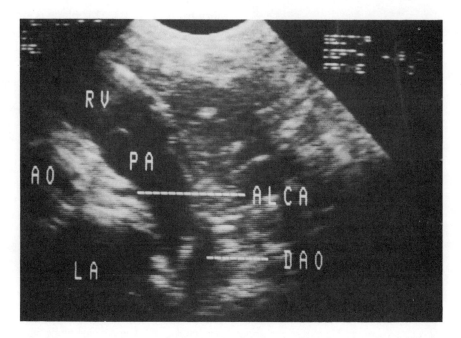

Figure 21. High parasternal parasagittal cut. At the posterior aspect of the pulmonary trunk, the abnormal origin of the left coronary can be seen. DAO = descending aorta.

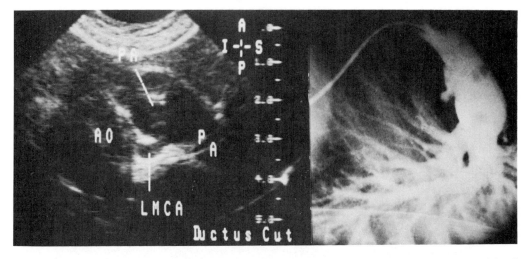

Figure 22. *Left:* High parasternal parasagittal cut (Ductal cut), demonstrating the anomalous origin of the left main coronary artery (LMCA). Note the catheter tip in the pulmonary trunk (PA). *Right:* Lateral PA-angiogram, turned into a comparable view. The aspect of the origin of LMCA from the posterior part of the pulmonary trunk resembles very much that of the echo-view.

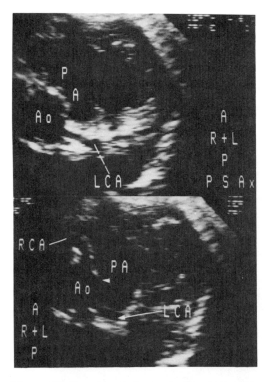

when arising from the aorta. The appropriate plane for imaging the anomalous origin, therefore, is an anterior-posterior one passing through the long axis of the pulmonary trunk (Fig. 21). This plane is similar to the one we use for defining patency of the arterial duct. It is a high parasternal plane

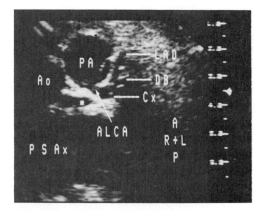

Figure 23. Parasternal short axis. *Top:* Left coronary artery (LCA) seems to arise from the aorta (Ao). *Bottom:* Similar view of the aortic root, showing dilated right coronary artery (RCA). Note dropout in the lateral wall of the aorta at 2 o'clock (arrowhead).

Figure 24. Parasternal short-axis view of the aortic root. Abnormal origin of the left coronary artery (ALCA) and its branching to left anterior descending (LAD) and circumflex (Cx) arteries is demonstrated. To the left of the aortic root (AO), the transverse sinus of the pericardium (asterisk) can be seen, and it seems to be connected to the aorta.

parallel to the vertebral bodies and running through the long axis of the right ventricular outflow tract. We prefer to call this a parasagittal cut rather than to define it as either a long- or short-axis plane. The anomalous artery can be seen arising from the posterior portion of the trunk and bears a close resemblance to the lateral cineangiogram (Fig. 22).

In contrast, the parasternal short-axis view may be quite inappropriate for detecting anomalous origin of the left coronary artery. As highlighted by Robinson et al. (1984) this view can create the erroneous impression that the left coronary artery is connected to the left aortic sinus of Valsalva (Fig. 23, top). This discrepancy may well be related to imaging of the transverse pericardial sinus in this area (Fig. 24), but there are other factors to consider that may give rise to this artifact. First, the aortic root is imaged in lateral resolution at the site of the left

sinus of Valsalva. If one observes the published images of the aortic root, it is possible to notice areas of dropout of the wall in this region (Fig. 23, bottom; Fig. 25). The second factor is the imaging of the transverse pericardial sinus while a third factor is lateral imaging of the coronary artery itself. If these three factors are aligned, then artificial dropout of the aortic root continues with the transverse pericardial sinus, which is continuous with the peripheral coronary artery. The major concern, therefore, is not about the artery or the transverse pericardial sinus itself, but about its connection to the aortic root. It is the dropout in this crucial area which is mainly responsible for that artifact. We also believe the description of Caldwell et al. (1983) to be incorrect. They suggested that three sequential frames which show a lack of continuity of the left coronary with the aorta are enough to prove the diagnosis. With more cranial angulation, it is some-

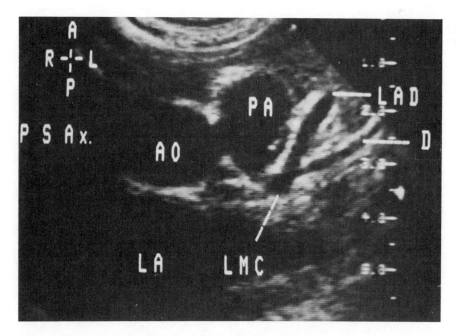

Figure 25. Parasternal short axis of the aortic root. With some cranial angulation, left main coronary artery (LMC) can be seen arising from the posterior part of the pulmonary trunk (PA). The left anterior descending artery (LAD) and the diagonal branch (D) are moderately dilated. Note the large dropout between both great arteries and further dropout at 4 o'clock in the aortic wall at the site of expected origin of LMC.

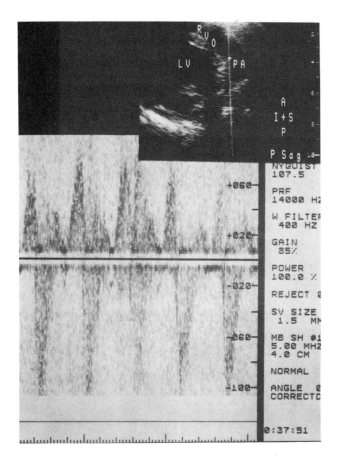

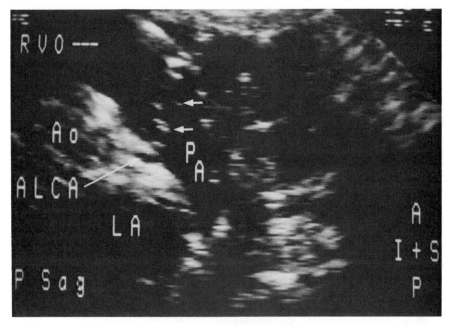

Figure 26. Parasternal parasagittal view, showing the Doppler interrogation at the inferior border of the pulmonary trunk. There is a disturbed flow pattern with diastolic retrograde flow reminiscent of a patent arterial duct but detected only at the site of entry of the anomalous artery on the contralateral side to that site of flow disturbance expected from a duct.

Figure 27. Parasternal parasagittal view. After radial artery injection of 3 ml agitated saline solution retrograde opacification of the aortic root (Ao) is notified, and subsequently contrast bubbles (small arrows) enter the pulmonary trunk (PA) from the anomalous left coronary (ALCA). Note that right ventricular outflow tract (RVO) is free of contrast.

times possible to define the appropriate connection of the anomalous artery with the pulmonary trunk in this plane (Fig. 25).

There are several other echocardiographic features that should lead one to suspect the diagnosis of anomalous left coronary artery. It is only when these points are considered that the diagnosis might be made prospectively with a high degree of accuracy. Any child with poor left ventricular function consistent with the diagnosis of congestive cardiomyopathy should be suspected of having an anomalous left coronary artery until the latter diagnosis can be excluded. It is particularly noteworthy that many of our patients were referred with the diagnosis of cardiomyopathy and had normal-appearing coronary arteries in the parasternal short-axis view. Appropriate imaging using the ductal cut must therefore be used to determine whether the left coronary artery arises from the pulmonary trunk or from the aorta. Special attention should be paid to those children with poor left ventricular myocardial function in whom the right coronary artery is large. When reviewing our patients with anomalous origin of the left coronary artery from the pulmonary trunk, we noted, as did others (Caldwell et al., 1983; Fisher et al., 1981), that the right coronary artery was always prominent and more easily identified than the left. This is probably related to the right coronary artery carrying all the cardiac blood flow.

Other reports have described the use of pulsed Doppler ultrasound in the definition of turbulent flow in the pulmonary trunk, relating this to the aortopulmonary runoff from the anomalously arising left coronary artery (King et al., 1985). It is notable when using pulsed Doppler and flow mapping that the area of turbulence is in a different position from that which is normally described for patency of the arterial duct (Fig. 26). In the latter setting, the turbulent flow hugs the superior wall of the pulmonary trunk in the so-called ductal cut. With anomalous origin of the left coronary artery from the pulmonary trunk, the turbulence is

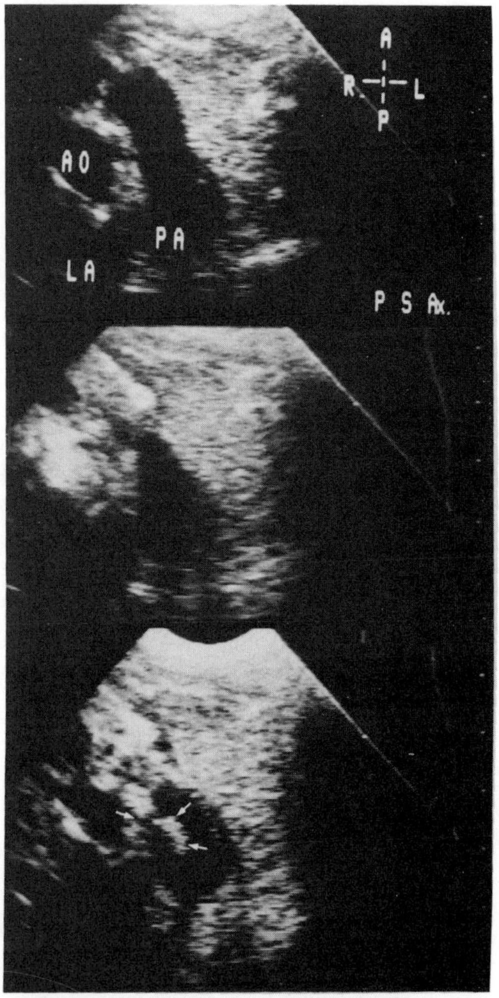

Figure 28. Parasternal short axis. *Top:* Aorta (AO) and pulmonary trunk (PA) can be seen. The dense reflection in the lower left area of the aortic root represents the catheter tip. *Middle:* Contrast injection (3 ml agitated saline solution) opacifies the aortic root. *Bottom:* Later and after the aortic root has cleared the microbubbles enter PA from the site of abnormal originating left coronary artery (small arrows). (Reprinted from Martin et al., 1986, with permission.)

related to the posterior pulmonary sinus adjacent to the ventriculoinfundibular fold. The degree of flow disturbance can be quite minimal and must be carefully sought. In our smaller patients, in whom there had not been a fall in the pulmonary artery pressure

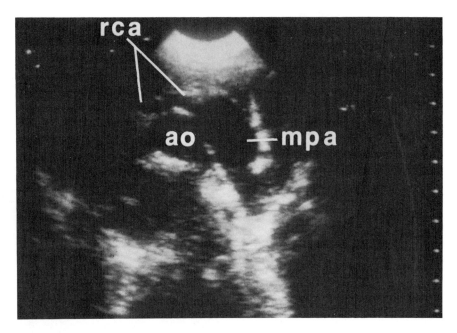

Figure 29. Parasternal short axis. Right coronary artery (RCA) arises from pulmonary trunk (MPA), whereas left coronary origin is visible at its usual site at the aortic root (Ao). (Published with permission of Dr. S.P. Sanders, M.D., Children's Hospital, Boston, MA.)

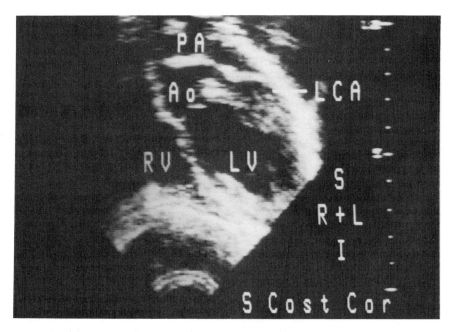

Figure 30. Subcostal coronal view in a patient with a coronary-cameral fistula between the left coronary artery (LCA) and the left ventricle (LV). The LCA is tortuous and dilated.

or in whom the degree of runoff is small, this finding was negative.

It may also be important to establish the diagnosis using contrast echocardiography via the radial artery (Martin et al., 1986). Radial arterial injection of a bolus of 3 ml of agitated aerated saline will demonstrate filling of the pulmonary trunk after the aortic root (Fig. 27). It is important to exclude two alternative routes of contrast arising in the pulmonary artery when using radial artery contrast. First, it must be shown that there is no arteriovenous anastomosis which might produce antegrade appearance of contrast across the pulmonary trunk. In this latter instance, contrast will first be detected in the right ventricle. Second, it must be demonstrated that there are

no other aortopulmonary communications such as patency of the arterial duct. We consider contrast echocardiography a valuable diagnostic aid and worthy of consideration in any child in whom anomalous origin of the coronary artery from the pulmonary trunk is considered.

Establishing the diagnosis by coronary angiography, especially when the collateral flow and pulmonary runoff is small, may be time-consuming and require administration of considerable amounts of angiographic contrast material. Because of this, we have used aortic root saline contrast echocardiography in several patients with coronary artery anomalies, including the four patients with anomalous left coronary artery, to establish the diagnosis rapidly (Fig. 28). No

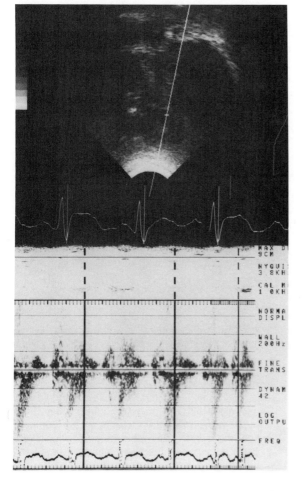

Figure 31. Apical four-chamber view. The cursor of the duplex Doppler is placed at the apical aspect of the ventricular septum within a dilated vascular structure (*top*). There is predominantly diastolic flow pattern, typical of left coronary artery flow (*bottom*). (Reprinted from Cooper et al., 1985, with permission.)

matter how small the shunt, once the blood containing microbubbles passes from the aortic circulation to the left coronary artery, it will enter the pulmonary trunk. Even though a small degree of runoff is present, the amount of saline contrast noted in the coronary arteries can be quite brilliant. This injection technique is achieved with 1 to 3 ml of agitated saline solution injected rapidly by hand into the aortic root. It proved positive in all four of our patients. It is safe and may help identify those patients who do not have an anomalous coronary artery but whose myocardial dysfunction is related to cardiomyopathy and in whom contrast angiography with high volume may prove deleterious to ventricular function.

Despite the ability of ultrasound to define the anomaly, we have been able to recognize prospectively only one of our four patients seen during the last year. The rarity of the lesion suggests that others may have similar lack of success. Saline contrast and Doppler ultrasound techniques should be used routinely when the lesion is suspected. Using all these modalities of ultrasound, and bearing in mind our caveats, we believe it will be possible to make this diagnosis prospectively in the large majority of infants and children with this lesion.

Anomalous origin of the right coronary artery from the pulmonary trunk is a rare condition with minimal symptoms. The lesion has been successfully identified echocardiographically (Worsham et al., 1985). While we have not encountered this abnormality, the descriptions in the literature suggest that adequate recognition is achieved from the parasternal short-axis view (Fig. 29).

Coronary Arteriovenous Fistula

Fistulous communication between one or another coronary artery and the cardiac chambers or the pulmonary arteries is rare but can be demonstrated echocardio-

graphically (Agatston et al., 1984; Reeder et al., 1980; Satomi et al., 1983). We have encountered two such communications involving the left coronary system (Cooper et al., 1985). In each, the left coronary artery was large and tortuous (Fig. 30). In the first case, the coronary-cameral communication was detected by Doppler ultrasound (Fig. 31). Turbulent flow within the left and right ventricles suggested that there was communication between those chambers. The left anterior descending coronary artery was dilated and aneurysmal in one patient. Con-

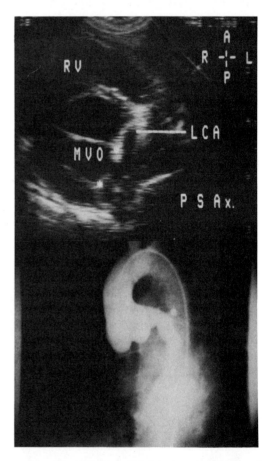

Figure 32. *Top:* Parasternal short-axis view of the left ventricle showing the dilated left circumflex coronary artery (LCA) and its communication (asterisks) with the left ventricle at the site of the mitral valve orifice (MVO). *Bottom:* For comparison, the frontal plane from the aortic root angiogram in this patient is seen, showing the dilated circumflex artery and its connexion to the left ventricle.

trast saline echocardiography in the aortic root was used at cardiac catheterization showing in one case the communications with both the left and right ventricles (Cooper et al., 1985). It was a notable finding because simultaneous left-sided and right-sided communications are rare and because the angiogram suggested only a right-sided communication. Echocardiographic saline contrast demonstrated its connection to both left and right ventricles. An abnormal flow in the coronary artery was demonstrated using the Doppler techniques. This patient was not submitted to surgery and the communication appears to be diminishing in size. A second patient showed a large communication between the circumflex artery and the left ventricle which could be easily seen echocardiographically in the parasternal short-axis and subcostal parasagittal views (Fig. 32). Although we have not encountered any fistula from the right coronary arterial system, we expect that under these circumstances, they would be large. The coronary sinus has been reported to be large when the fistula is arteriovenous (Agatston et al., 1984).

Coronary Artery Abnormalities in Congenital Heart Disease

Tetralogy of Fallot

Abnormalities in the coronary arteries that course across the right ventricular outflow tract may complicate the repair of this defect. We had recognized this abnormality

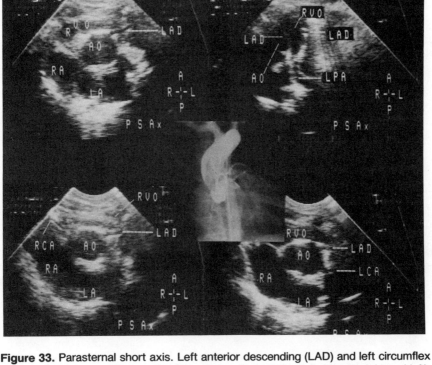

Figure 33. Parasternal short axis. Left anterior descending (LAD) and left circumflex artery (LCA) arise at different sites from the aortic root (*top left, bottom right and left*); LAD crosses the right ventricular outflow tract (RVO, *top right, left, bottom right, left*). Right coronary artery (RCA) is small and arises regularly (*bottom left*). Left coronary artery also arises normally (*bottom right*). *Center:* Aortic angiogram in the same patient. LPA = left pulmonary artery.

prospectively in two patients in whom the diagnosis was subsequently confirmed at angiography and at surgery (Fig. 33). The left anterior descending artery could be traced across the right ventricular outflow tract and could be shown to have a separate origin from the right coronary sinus of the aorta. The coronary artery itself was large. Recognition of this abnormality by echocardiography may prove valuable in helping to select patients for surgery.

Complete Transposition

Recognition of the normal origin and course of the coronary arteries in complete transposition by cross-sectional echocardi-

ography is now possible (Fig. 34). This feature will be of great value in those patients being considered for an arterial switch procedure. While the primary position of the arteries may be identified, we have not had sufficient experience to comment further on the place of echocardiography prior to the switch procedure.

Conclusion

The proximal portions of the normal major coronary arteries can be imaged. Aneurysms are readily recognized and diagnosed by echocardiography such that this technique may be sufficient for the success-

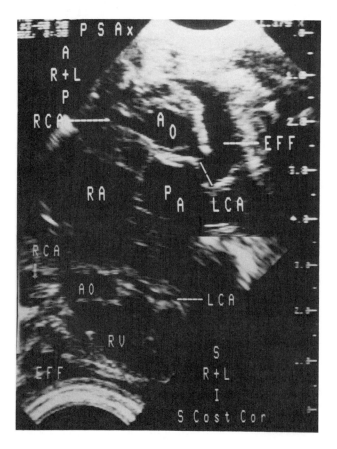

Figure 34. *Top:* Parasternal short-axis view. The aorta (Ao) is anterior and to the right of the pulmonary trunk (PA) and gives rise to both coronaries at 5 and 9 o'clock, respectively. The right coronary artery (RCA) is moderately enlarged. There is a pericardial effusion (EFF) following a intraatrial baffle repair of complete transposition. *Bottom:* Subcostal coronal view in the same patient. Left anterior descending coronary artery (LCA) is seen on the surface of the right ventricle as well as the origin of the right coronary artery (RCA).

ful management of patients with Kawasaki's disease. Anomalous origin of the left and right coronary arteries from the pulmonary trunk can be recognized by echocardiography, although accuracy is poor and the role of the technique remains uncertain. Enlarged coronary arteries due to fistulous communications can be recognized and the site of the fistula identified. Further experience is likely to make echocardiography a valuable additional tool in the hands of the pediatric cardiologist wishing to define the course and origin of the coronary arteries.

References

Agatston AS, Chapman E, Hildner FJ, Samet P. Diagnosis of a right coronary artery-right atrial fistula using two-dimensional and Doppler echocardiography. *Am J Cardiol* 1984;54:238–239.

Caldwell RL, Hurwitz RA, Girod DA, et al. Two-dimensional echocardiographic differentiation of anomalous left coronary artery from congestive cardiomyopathy. *Am Heart J* 1983;106:710–716.

Capannari TE, Daniels SR, Meyer RA, et al. Sensitivity, specificity and predictive value of two-dimensional echocardiography in detecting coronary artery aneurysms in patients with Kawasaki Disease. *J Am Coll Cardiol* 1986;7:355–360.

Chung KJ, Brandt L, Fulton DR, Kreidberg MB. Cardiac and coronary arterial involvement in infants and children from New England with mucocutaneous lymph node syndrome (Kawasaki disease). *Am J Cardiol* 1982;50:136–142.

Cooper MJ, Bernstein D, Silverman NH. Recognition of left coronary artery fistula to the left and right ventricles by contrast echocardiography. *J Am Coll Cardiol* 1985;6:923–926.

Feigenbaum H. *Echocardiography.* 4th ed, Philadelphia: Lea & Febiger, 1986;496–504.

Fisher EA, Sepehri B, Lendrum B, et al. Two-dimensional echocardiographic visualization of the left coronary artery in anomalous origin of the left coronary artery from the pulmonary artery. *Circulation* 1981;63:698–704.

Friedman DM, Rutkowski M. Coronary artery fistula: A pulsed Doppler/two-dimensional echocardiographic study. *Am J Cardiol* 1985; 55:1652–1655.

Gidding SS, Shulman ST, Ilbawi M, et al. Muco-cutaneous lymph node syndrome (Kawasaki disease): Delayed aortic and mitral insufficiency secondary to active valvulitis. *J Am Coll Cardiol* 1986;7:894–897.

Hiraishi S, Yashiro K, Kusano S. Noninvasive visualization of coronary arterial aneurysms in infants and young children with mucocutaneous lymph node syndrome with two dimensional echocardiography. *Am J Cardiol* 1979;43:1225–1233.

King DH, Danford DA, Huhta JC, Gutgesell HP. Noninvasive detection of anomalous origin of the left main coronary artery from the pulmonary trunk by pulsed Doppler echocardiography. *Am J Cardiol* 1985;55:608–609.

Martin GR, Cooper MJ, Silverman NH, Soifer SJ. Contrast echocardiography in the diagnosis of anomalous left coronary artery arising from the pulmonary artery. *Pediatr Cardiol* 1986;6:203–205.

Meyer RA. Kawasaki Syndrome: Coronary artery disease in the young. *Echocardiography* 1984; 1:75–86.

Nakano H, Nojima K, Saito A, Ueda K. High incidence of aortic regurgitation following Kawasaki Disease. *J Pediatr* 1985;107:59–63.

Newburger JW, Takahashi M, Burns JC, et al. The treatment of Kawasaki syndrome with intravenous gamma globuline. *N Engl J Med* 1986;315:341–347.

Pickoff AS, Wolff GS, Bennet VL, et al. Pulsed Doppler echocardiographic detection of coronary artery to right ventricle fistula. *Pediatr Cardiol* 1982;2:145–149.

Reeder GS, Tajik AJ, Smith HC. Visualization of coronary artery fistula by two-dimensional echocardiography. *Mayo Clin Proc* 1980;55:185–189.

Robinson PJ, Sullivan ID, Kumpeng V, et al. Anomalous origin of the left coronary artery from the pulmonary trunk: Potential for false negative diagnosis with cross-sectional echocardiography. *Br Heart J* 1984;52:272–277.

Satomi G, Nakamura K, Narai S, Takao A. Systematic visualization of coronary arteries by two-dimensional echocardiography in children and infants: evaluation in Kawasaki's Disease and coronary arteriovenous fistulas. *Am Heart J* 1984;107:497–505.

Silverman NH, Snider R. *Two-dimensional Echocardiography in Congenital Heart Disease:* Norwalk, Appleton-Century-Crofts, 1982:21–29.

Weyman AE, Feigenbaum H, Dillon JC, et al. Noninvasive visualization of the left main coronary artery by cross-sectional echocardiography. *Circulation* 1976;54:169–174.

Worsham C, Sanders SP, Burger BM, et al. Origin of the right coronary artery from the pulmonary trunk: Diagnosis by two-dimensional echocardiography. *Am J Cardiol* 1985;55:232–233.

Yoshida H, Maeda T, Funabashi T, et al. Subcostal two-dimensional echocardiographic imaging of peripheral right coronary artery in Kawasaki disease. *Circulation* 1982;65:956–961.

Yoshikawa J, Yanagihara K, Owaki T, et al.

Cross-sectional echocardiographic diagnosis of coronary artery aneurysms in patients with the mucocutaneous lymph node syndrome. *Circulation* 1979;59:133–139.

Yoshikawa J, Katao H, Yanagihara K, et al. Noninvasive visualization of the dilated main coronary arteries in coronary artery fistulas by crosssectional echocardiography. *Circulation* 1982;65:600–603.

Origin of the Left Coronary Artery from the Pulmonary Trunk: Clinical Spectrum and Operative Management

Ralph D. Siewers

Anomalous origin of the left coronary from the pulmonary trunk is the most common hemodynamically significant anomaly of the coronary arteries. First reported by Brooks in 1886, the clinical and hemodynamic sequels were described by Bland et al. (1933) and the condition is frequently known eponymously for these latter authors. It is a rare anomaly, estimated to occur in 1 out of 300,000 births, and made up approximately 0.5% of congenital heart disorders seen in Toronto (Keith, 1959). By 1975, 250 cases had been reported (Askenazi and Nadas, 1975). Numerous more recent reports have documented various forms of operative intervention, expanding the numbers of cases available for review. It is now clear that, although in this condition the left coronary artery most often arises from the left posterior sinus of the pulmonary trunk, rarely, both coronaries may arise from the pulmonary trunk (Heifetz et al., 1986), the right coronary alone may arise from the pulmonary trunk (Lerberg et al., 1979), the left coronary artery may arise from the right pulmonary artery (Doty et al., 1976), or a portion of the left coronary arterial system (left anterior descending coronary artery) may arise alone from the pulmonary trunk (Tamer et al., 1984). Other varieties are embryologically possible. Although a small proportion of infants with this anomaly survive infancy, presenting with cardiomegaly and ventricular dysfunction during childhood or even adult life, it is estimated that 90% will die from myocardial ischemia during the first year of life (Perry and Scott, 1970).

From: Anderson, RH, Neches, WH, Park, SC, Zuberbuhler, JR, eds: *Perspectives in Pediatric Cardiology*: Mount Kisco, New York, Futura Publishing Co., © 1988.

Pathophysiology and Clinical Presentation

When the left coronary artery arises from the pulmonary circulation, the myocardium it supplies is perfused with blood at low oxygen tension. As pulmonary resistance drops, the perfusion is at a lower pressure. The low perfusion pressure in turn stimulates the development of collateral branches from the area of myocardium supplied by the right coronary artery, thus augmenting flow in the left coronary arterial system. The benefit of this collateralization is offset by retrograde flow from the left coronary artery to the low-pressure pulmonary trunk, thus creating a left-to-right shunt. Symptoms of congestive heart failure and myocardial ischemia occur during the first four months of life in the majority of infants (Wesselhoeft et al., 1968). Chest radiographs show cardiac enlargement and electrocardiograms demonstrate anterolateral ischemia or infarction. Most patients with symptoms during the first four months of life will die in infancy. The rest present later with mitral regurgitation, angina, a continuous murmur, and sudden death. Although infants with large collateral blood flow to the left coronary artery, demonstrated by an oxygen "step-up" in the pulmonary trunk, will usually survive infancy, those with less abundant collateral flow are at a much higher risk of an early death (Perry and Scott, 1970). Surgical intervention to correct the retrograde left coronary artery blood flow and, ideally, to provide antegrade oxygenated blood flow to the left coronary arterial system will therefore be required in most infants with this anomaly (Neches et al., 1974).

Surgical Intervention

Numerous attempts have been made to improve blood flow to the left coronary artery such that there are now several currently recommended methods for establishment of antegrade flow. Potts used an aortopulmonary fistula for this purpose in 1949, and this was followed in 1955 by banding or constriction of the pulmonary trunk (Kittle et al., 1955). The induction of pericardial adhesions by poudrage or pericardiectomy was also proposed in 1955 (Paul and Robbins, 1957). Direct ligation of the left coronary artery at its origin was frequently used during the 1960s and later following early success in 1960 (Augstsson et al., 1962; Hallman et al., 1966; Nadas et al., 1964). Mustard (1962) then attempted to provide direct antegrade flow in infants by anastomosing the left carotid artery to the left coronary artery but his first two attempts were unsuccessful. Meyer et al. (1968) then successfully used this concept by using the left subclavian artery. Saphenous vein grafts from the aorta to the anomalous left coronary artery with proximal ligation of the artery had been successfully used by Cooley et al. (1966). The use of this technique, however, is limited by the size of the conduit material relative to the coronary artery, being of practical use only in older children and adults.

Attempts at direct transplantation of the anomalously arising left coronary artery from the pulmonary trunk to the aorta were antedated by such treatment used for an anomalously arising right coronary artery from the pulmonary trunk. Burroughs et al. (1962) were the first to use the concept of removal of the anomalously arising coronary artery (the right in his case) together with a surrounding button of pulmonary arterial wall. They implanted this button directly into the aortic root but their patient died of postoperative complications. In 1972, an 11-year-old child with fatigue, frequent upper respiratory infections, and a continuous murmur was admitted to Children's Hospital of Pittsburgh. This child was found on catheterization to have an anomalous right coronary artery arising from the pulmonary trunk. The case, reported by Lerberg and his colleagues (1979), was successfully corrected in June 1972 by direct implantation of the anomalously arising coronary artery into the aorta. Later during 1972, Tingelstad et al. reported a similar repair in a 12-year-old child which had been done in 1971. On the basis of this experience, in August 1973, the group at Children's Hospital of Pittsburgh successfully used the technique of direct implantation of an anomalously arising left coronary artery in a $5\frac{1}{2}$-year-old boy (Neches et al., 1974). Shortly following that case (January 1974), a seven-month-old child with a similar anatomy had repair by interposition of a short segment of right subclavian artery between the aorta and a button of pulmonary trunk continuous with the anomalous left coronary artery. This experience established the feasibility of anatomical correction of the symptomatic infant with anomalous origin of the left coronary artery from the pulmonary trunk. Laborde and his associates (1981) used almost identical techniques, using free segments of the left subclavian artery, saphenous vein homografts, or direct anastomosis in 14 successful operations from a series of 20 between 1970 and 1979. Concern remained over the frequent inability to attach the left coronary artery directly to the aorta in infants, along with uncertainty about the long-term durability of vascular free grafts for bridging the gap between the aorta and detached coronary artery. Takeuchi et al. (1979), therefore, conceptualized an ingenious procedure whereby a tunnel was created across the back wall of the pulmonary trunk which connected an aortopulmonary side-to-side anastomosis to the orifice of the anomalous left coronary artery. This technique has proved with experience to be both relatively simple and highly successful, as demonstrated by Midgley and his colleagues (1984) and in our series here reported.

Patients and Methods

Thirteen patients with a left coronary artery arising anomalously from the pulmo-

nary trunk have been operated upon at Children's Hospital of Pittsburgh between August 1973 and September 1985 (Table 1). Their ages ranged from $1\frac{1}{2}$ months to $5\frac{1}{2}$ years (23.5 months mean, 15 months median). All had electrocardiographic patterns of left ventricular ischemia or infarction. Cardiomegaly was present on chest radiographs in 11 of the 13 with ratios ranging from 0.52 to 0.73 (0.62 mean). Preoperative catheterizations were performed in all patients and documented elevated preangiographic left ventricular end-diastolic pressures in 10 of the 13 (ranging from 9 to 28 mmHg with a mean of 17 mmHg). The end-diastolic pressure was not measured in one 18-month-old child with an ejection fraction of less than 20%. In both $5\frac{1}{2}$-year-old children, the pressure was 5 mmHg and both had measured angiographic left ventricular ejection fractions of 50%. One of these children had severe mitral regurgitation and did not survive the repair. The measured left ventricular ejection fractions in the other 11 patients were 40% in one, 30% in one, and less than 20% in the remaining nine.

The eight patients operated upon prior to 1983 had either direct implantation of the anomalous left coronary artery into the aorta (four) with one death (in the child with severe mitral insufficiency), or implantation by means of an interposed graft (left subclavian arterial segment in one; PTFE tube segment in three) with two deaths. The deaths were thought to be unrelated to the type of repair achieved. The five operations done since 1983 have followed the concept of Takeuchi et al. (1979). Three had the intrapulmonary flap constructed of glutaraldehyde-preserved bovine pericardium while, in the last two, a flap of anterior pulmonary arterial wall was used for the intrapulmonary tunnel as described by Takeuchi et al. The only death in these five patients occurred in an 18-month-old child with no demonstrable right-to-left coronary collateral supply and a diminutive left coronary arterial system. This patient was operated upon in 1983.

Table 1

Anomalous Origin of Left Coronary Artery from Pulmonary Artery, Children's Hospital of Pittsburgh, 1973–1985

Case no.	Age at operation (mo.)	Operative procedure	Operative result	CT ratio Preop	CT ratio Postop	LVEDP Preop	LVEDP Postop	LV ejection fraction Preop	LV ejection fraction Postop[2]	Mitral insufficiency[3] Preop	Mitral insufficiency[3] Postop
1	66	Direct	Survived	0.55	0.50	5	5	0.65	0.65	0	0
2	7	Graft	Survived	0.73	0.50	20	6	<0.20	0.60	2+	0
3	40	Direct	Survived	0.55	0.50	9	8	0.30	0.60	2+	1+
4	64	Direct	Death	0.60	—	5	—	0.50	—	4+	—
5	15	Graft	Death	0.66	—	16	—	<0.20	—	0	—
6	7	Graft	Survived	0.61	0.48	23	17	<0.20	0.56	1+	0
7	3.5	Graft	Death	0.52	—	28	—	<0.20	—	0	—
8	5	Direct	Survived	0.65	0.50	19	20[1]	<0.20	0.56	0	0
9	18	IP baffle	Death	0.67	—	16	—	<0.20	—	1+	—
10	18	IP baffle	Survived	0.65	0.59	—	18	<0.20	0.60	0	0
11	1.5	IP baffle	Survived	0.62	0.50	20	14	<0.20	0.58	3+	0
12	4.5	IP baffle	Survived	0.52	0.50	12	10	0.40	0.58	0	0
13	2	IP baffle	Survived	0.68	0.60	13	12	<0.20	0.42	2+	1+

Direct = direct implantation of left coronary into aorta; Graft = interposition of subclavian artery[1] or PTFE[3] between the aorta and removed left coronary; IP Baffle = Takeuchi type procedure; CT ratio = cardiothoracic ratio on chest x-ray.
[1] Measured one month postoperatively.
[2] Calculated from the most recent MUGA scan or echo study.
[3] Angiographic grade.

Postoperative catheterizations have been done in all nine survivors, one month to six years following repair. All reconstructions were found to be patent. The left ventricular end-diastolic pressure was reduced in eight of nine cases, even in the studies performed one to six months postrepair. The one infant operated upon at five months of age with a preoperative end-diastolic pressure of 19 continued to show this abnormal level at a postrepair study two months later. Four years after repair, evaluation of this child using a multigated acquisition scan yielded an ejection fraction of 56%. There have been no late deaths among the early survivors and each child has undergone echocardiographic evaluation of the segmental shortening fraction of the left ventricular wall, demonstrating improvement or normal values in all cases. Estimates of left ventricular ejection fraction late after repair have shown striking improvement with values above 56% in all but the most recent case, whose multigated acquisition scan at seven months postrepair revealed an ejection fraction of 42%. The value, nonetheless, was less than 20% before the operation.

Mitral valve regurgitation was present as judged angiographically in 6 of the 13 patients prior to repair. One of these six children ($5\frac{1}{2}$ years old) had severe regurgitation and did not survive. Her death was thought to be due to mitral insufficiency in the early postoperative period. This child, in retrospect, should have had mitral valve replacement. Three of the survivors with mitral regurgitation before the repair have lost all trace of mitral insufficiency. In two others, the degree of regurgitation has been reduced by a full grade. Postrepair cardiac ratios measured by chest radiograph at the last follow-up visit were less than 0.50 in seven of the nine survivors. One infant seen seven months after the repair continues to show a cardiothoracic ratio of 0.60. Another child seen two years later had a cardiothoracic ratio of 0.59. Both had ratios of over 0.65 prior to the repair.

Conclusions

Anomalous origin of the left coronary artery is a rare, but important, cause of ventricular dysfunction, cardiopulmonary decompensation, and death. Infants with this anomaly require intervention early in life, often during the first 12 to 18 months. Experience has shown that the establishment of antegrade systemic arterial blood flow to the left coronary system will yield the greatest improvement in cardiac function and provide the best chance for long-term return to normal myocardial performance. Cardiomegaly, mitral valve dysfunction, impaired left ventricular ejection fraction, and poor left ventricular wall shortening fractions all predictably improve toward normal following correction by the establishment of antegrade blood flow in the left coronary artery in these infants and small children.

The anomalous origin of the left coronary is usually located in the base of the pulmonary trunk, situated posteriorly and to the left. The left coronary artery, however, may arise from branches of the pulmonary trunk or may partially arise anomalously as a part of the left coronary system (left anterior descending coronary artery or circumflex coronary artery). The entire coronary supply rarely will arise from the pulmonary trunk, requiring urgent early intervention as pulmonary vascular resistance diminishes during the neonatal period.

Surgical intervention designed to establish antegrade systemic blood flow to the left coronary system is recommended for any infant or child found to have an anomalous origin of the left coronary artery from the pulmonary trunk or pulmonary branch arteries. In symptomatic infants with this anomaly the operation should be done as soon as the diagnosis is established. Rarely, older children are found to have well-preserved left ventricular function and the diagnosis is made during evaluation of an obscure murmur or mild degree of cardiomegaly. Surgical intervention in these older children is less urgent, but is recommended electively to avoid the late sequels resulting from changes in the coronary system due to progressive enlargement of collateral vessels from the right to the left coronary system and "left-to-right" shunting through retrograde blood flow in the left coronary system into the pulmonary artery circulation.

Operative correction by the procedure described by Takeuchi et al. (1979) has resulted in excellent early survival and good long-term results in our series reported here and in other centers (Burton et al., 1985; Laborde et al., 1981; Midgley et al., 1984). The operation is especially useful when the left coronary artery orifice is located posteriorly and to the left in the base of the pulmonary trunk. Careful attention to enlargement of the anterior portion of the pulmonary trunk will avoid supravalvular pulmonary stenosis, although mild degrees of pulmonary artery narrowing with turbulent flow following this correction are often detectable. When the orifice of the left coronary artery is found to be posterior in the base of the pulmonary trunk and is in close proximity to the ascending aorta, removal of the left coronary artery with a button of pulmonary artery and direct implantation into the aorta does not require extensive coronary mobilization and is an excellent alternative. We and others have found this approach to be acceptable and to provide excellent long-term results (Laborde et al., 1981; Neches et al., 1974). It avoids possible distortion of the pulmonary trunk and pulmonary valve. In the unusual cases when the anomalous left coronary artery arises from the right or left pulmonary artery, use of the right or left subclavian artery by end-to-end attachment to the removed anomalous left coronary artery as described by Meyer et al. (1968) and Doty et al. (1976) will provide adequate blood flow into the left coronary artery system. In rare situations in older children or adults with this anomaly, conventional methods of coronary revascularization combined with closure of the left coronary artery-pulmonary artery communication may be satisfactory (Cooley et al., 1966). Simple ligation of the anomalous left coronary artery to correct retrograde left coronary artery to pulmonary artery blood flow is associated with an unacceptably high operative mortality and less satisfactory long-term results. It is no longer recommended.

References

Augstsson MH, Gasul BM, Fell EH, et al. Anomalous origin of left coronary artery from pulmonary artery: Diagnosis and treatment of infantile and adult types. *JAMA* 1962;180:15–21.

Askenazi J, Nadas AS. Anomalous left coronary artery originating from the pulmonary artery: Report of 15 cases. *Circulation* 1975;51:976–987.

Bland EF, White PD, Garland J. Congenital anomalies of coronary arteries: Report of an unusual case associated with cardiac hypertrophy. *Am Heart J* 1933;8:787–801.

Brooks HSJ. Two cases of an abnormal coronary artery arising from the pulmonary artery. *J Anat Physiol* 1886;20:26–29.

Burroughs JT, Schmutzer KJ, Linder F, Neuhaus G. Anomalous origin of the right coronary artery with aortico-pulmonary window and ventricular septal defect. Report of a case with complete operative correction. *J Cardiovasc Surg* 1962;3:142–148.

Burton RW, Jones RA, Long AR, Castaneda AR. Anomalous origin of the left coronary artery from pulmonary artery: Ligation versus establishment of a two coronary system. *J Thorac Cardiovasc Surg* 1987;93:103.

Cooley DA, Hallman GL, Bloodwell RD. Definitive surgical treatment of anomalous origin of left coronary artery from pulmonary artery: Indications and results. *J Thorac Cardiovasc Surg* 1966;52:798–808.

Doty DB, Chandramouli B, Schicken RE, et al. Anomalous origin of the left coronary artery from the right pulmonary artery. *J Thorac Cardiovasc Surg* 1976;71:787–791.

Hallman GL, Cooley DA, Singer DB. Congenital anomalies of the coronary arteries: Anatomy, pathology and surgical treatment. *Surgery* 1966;59:133–144.

Heifetz SA, Rabinovitz M, Mueller KH, Virmani R. Total anomalous origin of the coronary arteries from the pulmonary artery. *Pediatr Cardiol* 1986;7:11–18.

Keith JD. The anomalous origin of the left coronary artery from the pulmonary artery. *Br Heart J* 1959;21:149–161.

Kittle CF, Diehl AM, Heilbrunn A. Anomalous left coronary arising from the pulmonary artery —Report of a case and surgical consideration. *J Pediatr* 1955;47:198–206.

Laborde F, Marchand M, Leca F, Jarreau MM, et al. Surgical treatment of anomalous origin of the left coronary artery in infancy and childhood. *J Thorac Cardiovasc Surg* 1981;82:423–428.

Lerberg DB, Ogden JA, Zuberbuhler JR, Bahnson HT. Anomalous origin of the right coronary artery from the pulmonary artery. *Ann Thorac Surg* 1979;27:87–94.

Meyer BW, Stefanik G, Stiles QR, et al. A method for definitive surgical treatment of anomalous origin of left coronary artery. *J Thorac Cardiovasc Surg* 1968;56:104–107.

Midgley FM, Watson DC, Scott LP, et al. Repair of anomalous origin of left coronary artery in the infant and small child. *J Am Coll Cardiol* 1984;4:1231–1234.

Mustard WH. Anomalies of the coronary artery. In Benson CD, Mustard WH, Ravitch MM (Eds): *Pediatric Surgery*, vol 1. Chicago: Year Book Medical, 1962:433.

Nadas AS, Gamboa R, Hugenholz PG. Anomalous left coronary originating from the pulmonary artery: Report of 2 surgically treated cases with a proposal of hemodynamic and therapeutic classification. *Circulation* 1964;29:167–175.

Neches WH, Mathews RA, Park SC, et al. Anomalous origin of the left coronary artery from the pulmonary artery: A method of repair. *Circulation* 1974;50:582–587.

Paul RN, Robbins SG. Surgical treatment proposed for either endocardial fibroelastosis or anomalous left coronary artery. *Pediatrics* 1955;16:147–163.

Perry LW, Scott LP. Anomalous left coronary artery from the pulmonary artery. *Circulation* 1970;41:1043–1052.

Takeuchi S, Imamura H, Katsumoto K, et al. New surgical method for repair of anomalous left coronary artery from pulmonary artery. *J Thorac Cardiovasc Surg* 1979;78:7–11.

Tamer DF, Mallon SM, Garcia OL, Wolff GS. Anomalous origin of the left anterior descending coronary artery from the pulmonary artery. *Am Heart J* 1984;108:341–345.

Tingelstad JB, Lower RR, Eldredge WJ. Anomalous origin of the right coronary artery arising from the main pulmonary artery. *Am J Cardiol* 1972;30:670–673.

Wesselhoeft H, Fawcett JS, Johnson AL. Anomalous origin of the left coronary artery from the pulmonary trunk: Its clinical spectrum, pathology and pathophysiology based on a review of 140 cases with seven further cases. *Circulation* 1968;38:403–425.

7.4

Kawasaki Syndrome

William H. Neches

In 1967, Dr. Tomisaku Kawasaki reported an unusual illness that he had seen in 50 patients and named this disorder the mucocutaneous lymph node syndrome (Kawasaki, 1967). Since that time, a virtual epidemic of this disorder has occurred in Japan, over 30,000 cases having been reported within the last two decades. In 1974 the first report of this disease appeared in the English language literature (Kawasaki, 1974). Since then, what has now become known as Kawasaki disease (or Kawasaki syndrome) has been reported to occur in all parts of the world and in all racial groups.

The principle features of this disorder are outlined in Table 1. The six major findings include fever of over five days' duration, bilateral conjunctivitis, and involvement of the mucous membranes of the oral cavity (Fig. 1). These patients also have a polymorphous rash which is truncal in distribution and without vesicles or crusts. Involvement of the extremities consists of erythema of the palms and soles accompanied by indurative edema. Subsequently, desquamation of the fingertips and toes occurs toward the end of the second week of the illness (Fig. 2). Most patients have signifi-

cant cervical lymphadenopathy. Indeed, some of our early patients were referred for evaluation after having undergone a surgical incision and drainage of what was thought to be suppurative cervical lymphadenitis. Other striking findings in most of these patients, especially the infants under one year of age, are that they are extremely irritable, often lethargic, and they generally appear moderately to severely ill.

A number of organ systems are affected (Table 2). Involvement of the cardiovascular system has occurred in 18% of our patients and will be considered in detail shortly. The gastrointestinal and musculoskeletal systems are each involved in about a third of our patients. One-fourth of our patients have involvement of the genitourinary system, usually with proteinuria and a sterile pyuria secondary to a nonspecific urethritis. Aseptic meningenitis occurred in 13% of patients in our early experience, although the current incidence is not specifically known since we no longer commonly perform lumbar punctures in these patients.

The laboratory findings are nonspecific and are summarized in Table 3. All patients have a leukocytosis with a "shift to the left"

From: Anderson, RH, Neches, WH, Park, SC, Zuberbuhler, JR, eds: *Perspectives in Pediatric Cardiology*: Mount Kisco, New York, Futura Publishing Co., © 1988.

Table 1

Principal Diagnostic Features of Kawasaki Syndrome, Children's Hospital of Pittsburgh (n = 144)

	Incidence (%)
1. Fever over 5 days' duration	100
2. Bilateral conjunctivitis	85
3. Oral cavity	
a. dry, fissured lips	100
b. pharyngitis	100
c. strawberry tongue	95
4. Polymorphous rash	95
a. truncal	
b. no vesicles or crusts	
5. Extremities	
a. erythema, palms and soles	95
b. indurative edema	87
c. desquamation of fingertips	95
6. Cervical lymphadenopathy	85

Most are irritable, often lethargic and generally appear moderately to severely ill.

and white counts ranging from 15,000 to 25,000 cells per mm³ or more. Thrombocytosis is a striking feature, with platelet counts ranging from 500,000 to well over 1 million. The erythrocyte sedimentation rate is elevated in most patients. Seventy percent have sedimentation rates over 50 mm/hr and, in some cases, sedimentation rates are as high as 150 mm/hr. Tests for the C-reactive protein are positive in over 70% of patients and there is also elevation of the alpha-2 globulin, immunoglobulin-E, transaminase and lactic acid dehydrogenase. Although all these laboratory data indicate the presence of a significant inflammatory process with widespread systemic involvement, none of these findings is diagnostic for Kawasaki syndrome.

The typical clinical course is illustrated in Figure 3. The acute phase, which lasts for approximately 14 days, is characterized by the onset of fever. Very shortly thereafter there is involvement of the mucous membranes and the appearance of cervical lymphadenopathy. These latter two findings usually begin to subside a few days before the fever defervesces. Erythema of the palms and soles is usually present by the third or fourth day and is followed quickly

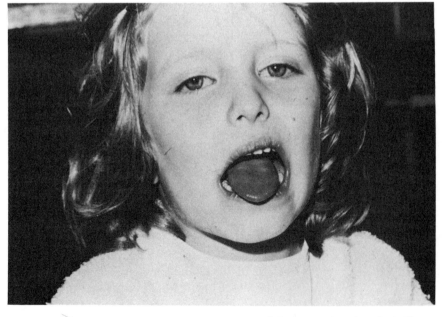

Figure 1. Involvement of the mucous membranes of the eye and oral cavity in Kawasaki syndrome.

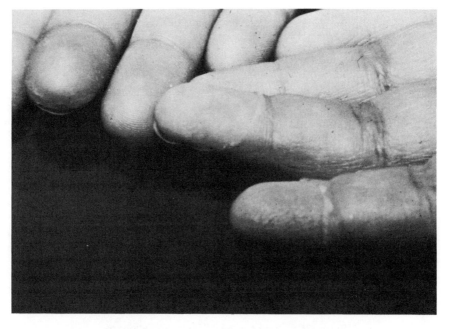

Figure 2. Desquamation of the fingertips in Kawasaki syndrome.

by edema of the hands and feet as well as a polymorphous exanthem. All of these findings usually subside between 10 and 14 days of the onset of illness and are followed by desquamation of the fingertips and toes which usually then lasts for about a week or so.

The experience with mucocutaneous lymph node syndrome at the Children's Hospital of Pittsburgh over the last decade is outlined in Table 4. We saw 144 children with this diagnosis from October 1976 through May 1986. They ranged in age from 3 months to 13 years with a mean age of 2.9 years. Eighty-seven of the patients (63%) were under 2 years of age at the time of the onset of their illness while 32 patients (22%) were less than 1 year of age. There has been some seasonal variation in incidence with

Table 2
Organ Systems Involved in Kawasaki Syndrome, Children's Hospital of Pittsburgh (n = 144)

	Incidence (%)
1. Cardiac	18
2. Gastrointestinal	
a. vomiting, diarrhea	31
b. jaundice	15
c. gall bladder hydrops	10
3. Arthralgia or arthritis	31
4. Genitourinary	26
a. proteinuria, sterile pyuria	
b. urethritis	
5. Aseptic meningitis	13

Table 3
Laboratory Data in Kawasaki Syndrome

1. Leukocytosis with "shift to left"
2. Thrombocytosis
3. ▲ ESR (70% over 50 mm/hr)
4. Positive CRP
5. ▲ Alph-2-globulin
6. ▲ IgE
7. ▲ Transaminases, LDH

CRP = C-reactive protein; ESR = erythrocyte sedimentation rate; IgE = immunoglobulin E; LDH = lactic acid dehydrogenase.

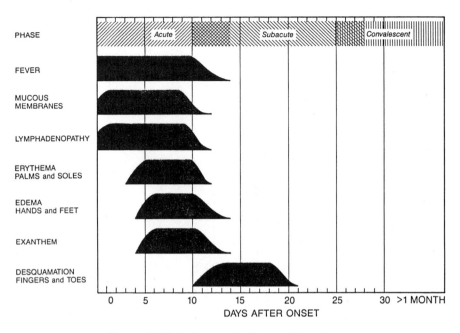

Figure 3. Clinical course in Kawasaki syndrome.

more patients being seen in the first four months of the year than at other times. The disease is usually sporadic, although we have seen a clustering of cases with a total of 3 "mini-epidemics" during this 10-year period.

Table 4

Mucocutaneous Lymph Node Syndrome (Kawasaki Syndrome), Children's Hospital of Pittsburgh, October 1976–May 1986

Year	Number of patients	Age (years)			
		<1	1–2	3–4	5 or more
1976	1	—	—	1	—
1977	1	—	—	—	1
1978	17	6	5	4	2
1979	10	1	5	4	—
1980	8	2	2	3	1
1981	10	2	3	3	2
1982	10	3	2	1	4
1983	20	4	6	6	4
1984	14	2	6	4	2
1985	33	7	17	5	4
1986	20	5	9	2	4
Total	144	32	55	33	24

Age range: 3 months–13 years (mean = 2.9 years)

Cardiac Involvement

Involvement of the cardiovascular system is the most serious feature of Kawasaki syndrome and is the only one with permanent sequelae. The clinical features which suggest cardiovascular involvement are summarized in Table 5. Electrocardiographic changes are infrequent in our experience and usually minimal. The changes that have been reported in the literature are transient and nonspecific, usually occurring during the first two weeks of illness. They include decreased QRS amplitude, prolonged PR and/or QT interval, and minor alterations in the ST segment. A number of other clinical findings indicate, in our experience, a high risk of cardiac involvement. These include fever of greater than 14 days' duration or recurrence of fever after it had subsided. Recurrence of the rash or of the desquamation of the fingertips and toes

Table 5
Cardiac Involvement in Kawasaki Syndrome

A. Suggestive
  1. Electrocardiographic changes
    a. Usually nonspecific
    b. First 2 weeks, then normal
    c. Decreased R wave, prolonged PR and/or QT interval
  2. Fever > 14 days
  3. Recurrent fever
  4. Recurrent rash
  5. Recurrent desquamation
  6. Elevated cardiac enzymes
  7. Elevated acute phase reactants > 1 month
    a. White blood cell count
    b. Erythrocyte sedimentation rate
    c. C-reactive protein
B. Definite
  1. Apical systolic murmur
  2. Cardiomegaly
  3. Pericarditis, effusion
  4. Congestive heart failure
  5. Significant abnormalities on electrocardiogram
    a. Arrhythmia
    b. Ischemia
    c. Infarction
  6. Cardiogenic shock

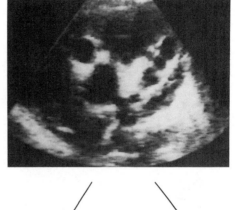
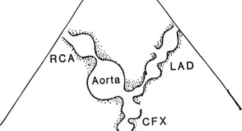

Figure 4. Echocardiogram in Kawasaki syndrome demonstrating aneurysms of the coronary arteries.

after initial resolution are also suggestive signs. Elevation of cardiac enzymes at any time, or elevated acute-phase reactants (such as white blood cell count, erythrocyte sedimentation rate, or C-reactive protein) for more than one month are also useful indicators of possible cardiac involvement.

Although the true incidence of involvement of the cardiovascular system in patients with Kawasaki syndrome is unknown, it is currently believed to occur in approximately 20% of patients. The most common cardiac problem is the development of aneurysms of the coronary arteries. All three major coronary arteries may be involved (Fig. 4). When coronary arterial aneurysms are present, they are usually found in the proximal course of one of the major coronary arteries. Thus, cross-sectional echocardiography is an extremely valuable screening tool for coronary arterial involvement since the proximal portions of the coronary arteries are the areas most readily visualized with this technique. Quantification of the size, number, and location of coronary arterial aneurysms, however, is not possible with echocardiography, and angiography remains the "gold standard" by which other techniques should be judged.

Aneurysms of the right and left anterior descending arteries, as well as dilation of the circumflex artery, are seen in the aortogram in Figure 5. Involvement of the coronary arteries in this patient consisted of long areas of large, fusiform dilations rather than the rounded, beaded aneurysms demonstrated in Figure 6. An important angiographic finding, which is not demonstrated by viewing a single frame from the angiogram, is the extraordinarily sluggish flow through the coronary arteries. When an aortogram is performed, the coronary arteries normally fill during the first diastolic cycle. As soon as the injection ceases, the contrast material is

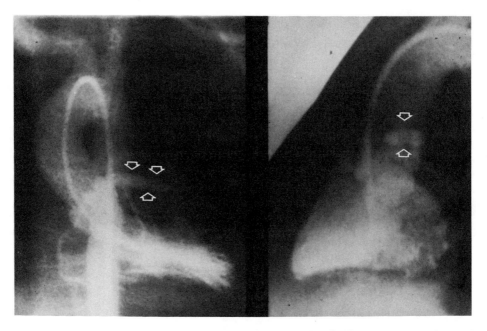

Figure 5. Angiography in Kawasaki syndrome demonstrating fusiform aneurysms (arrows) of the coronary arteries. (Left = AP view; Right = lateral view.)

rapidly cleared from the ascending aorta and the coronary arteries remain visualized for only three or four more cardiac cycles. In contrast, when the coronary arteries are in-volved in Kawasaki syndrome, even when there is only mild dilation, clearing of the coronary arteries is markedly delayed. Con-trast material commonly remains in the cor-

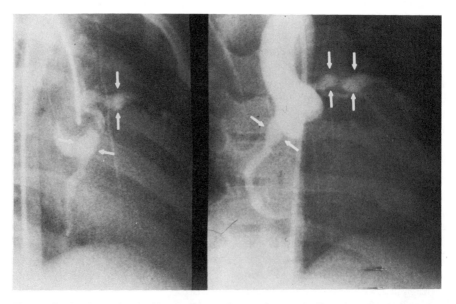

Figure 6. Angiography in Kawasaki syndrome demonstrating saccular aneurysms (arrows) of the coronary arteries. (Left = RAO view; Right = AP view.)

onary arteries for as many as 12 to 15 cardiac cycles thereafter. The presence of dilation and aneurysms of the coronary arteries, extremely sluggish flow, and the marked thrombocytosis would seem to combine to make those patients with all three features at considerable risk for development of thrombosis.

Although the Kawasaki syndrome was described almost two decades ago, the long-term outlook remains largely unknown for patients who develop aneurysms of the coronary arteries after having this disease. The natural history of these lesions has been studied in a number of centers and is best illustrated by the data of Kato et al. (1982). They performed serial angiographic evaluations in a group of 43 patients with coronary arterial aneurysms and found that, in about 50% of cases, the aneurysms disappeared during the first year after the onset of the illness. The aneurysms improved in some of the remaining patients but all patients continued to have coronary arterial abnormalities one year after the onset of the disease. In our series, a number of factors seem to be related to the resolution of the coronary arterial lesions. Aneurysms that occurred during the early stage of the illness in infants and were small and fusiform rather than saccular, were more likely to resolve. In contrast, lesions appearing during later stages of the disease in older children that were large in size and saccular, tended to persist. These findings are similar to those of others, although a recent study (Nakano et al., 1985) reported that the progress of the coronary arterial disease depended upon only the size and distribution of aneurysms at initial angiography. It is interesting that occasional reports of "congenital coronary arterial aneurysms" have long appeared in the literature (Wilson et al., 1975). Although these coronary arterial abnormalities resemble the lesions of Kawasaki syndrome anatomically, the clinical descriptions do not.

Mortality from Kawasaki syndrome has been reported to occur in 1 to 2% of the cases. More recently the mortality in Japan has been 1% or less. This decrease may be related to the increased number of less severe cases that are being reported. Mortality is more common in younger children and 70% of fatal cases have been reported in infants less than one year of age. All deaths have been related to cardiovascular involvement. Indeed, 90% of fatal cases occurred suddenly in patients who were not felt to be seriously ill. Death is most common during the convalescent phase, occurring some three to seven weeks after the onset of the illness, although some deaths have occurred many years later (Nakanishi et al., 1985). One of our patients, a six-year-old girl who had an episode of Kawasaki syndrome at four years of age, awoke one morning, complained of abdominal pain, and died. This was before the availability of cross-sectional echocardiography, and cardiac involvement had not been suspected. At postmortem examination, thrombosis was found within a solitary aneurysm of the midportion of the anterior descending coronary artery. Postmortem examination in other patients with Kawasaki syndrome who have died within the first few months after the onset of the illness has usually revealed a necrotizing coronary arteritis with aneurysm formation. In almost all cases, there has been thrombosis of the aneurysms with subsequent myocardial infarction. Although rupture of a coronary arterial aneurysm has been suggested as a possible complication, this is extremely rare.

The incidence of cardiovascular involvement in the series of patients seen at Children's Hospital of Pittsburgh is outlined in Table 6. In the period from October 1976 through May 1986, 26 of the 144 patients with Kawasaki syndrome were found to have cardiac involvement (18%). In all cases this was confirmed by angiography. The incidence of cardiac involvement was greatest in the youngest age group, 10 of 32 patients (31%) developing aneurysms. The incidence was lowest (9%) in patients between 1 and 3 years of age. Note, however, that these

Table 6
Cardiac Involvement in Mucocutaneous Lymph Node Syndrome (Kawasaki Syndrome), Children's Hospital of Pittsburgh, October 1976–May 1986

Age (yrs)	Number of patients	CAD	Number of deaths (% CAD)	Current status	
				Persistent	Resolved
<1	32	10 (31%)	3 (30%)	4	3
1–2	55	5 (9%)	1 (20%)	0	4
3–4	33	8 (24%)	1 (14%)	5	2*
5 or more	24	3 (13%)	0	2	1*
Total	144	26 (18%)	5 (19%)	11	10

CAD = coronary arterial disease.
* = 1 patient lost to follow-up.

numbers are relatively small. Death has occurred in 5 patients. This represents 3% of our total series and 19% of the patients with cardiac involvement. The highest incidence of mortality occurred in infants under one year of age, and 3 of 10 (30%) with cardiac involvement died. The incidence of mortality in the other groups decreased with increasing age. Although these numbers are too small for meaningful statistical analysis, it at least appears that there is a tendency for the cardiac involvement to be more severe in infancy. Our experience with long-term follow-up suggests that, in infants who do survive, there is a greater chance of resolution of the coronary artery aneurysms than in older patients. Although aneurysms have been observed to persist in a few infants in this series, most have had their illness within the last year. On the basis of our past experience, we anticipate that these aneurysms may resolve. In contrast, the incidence of mortality in older children is extremely low but the aneurysms may persist for as long as eight years.

Our experience with a seven-month-old infant, one of the first patients whom we had seen with Kawasaki syndrome, graphically demonstrates the potential severity and extent of cardiac involvement. This infant had a febrile illness with all the characteristic features of Kawasaki syndrome. In

contrast to the usual patient with this disease, however, irritability and fever persisted for approximately 3.5 weeks. This was before the days of cross-sectional echocardiography and was early in our experience so cardiac involvement was not suspected. A few days after apparent recovery, the child had a cardiac arrest while being prepared for discharge. Cardiac catheterization was performed a few hours after resuscitation and aortography demonstrated extremely large saccular aneurysms of the major coronary arteries (Fig. 7). Arteriography also demonstrated involvement of peripheral arteries (Fig. 8). The child subsequently died and postmortem examination revealed massive coronary arterial aneurysms (Fig. 9). These coronary arteries were larger in diameter than the patient's ascending aorta and contained false channels that were thrombosed.

The relationship between Kawasaki syndrome and the pathological entity of infantile periarteritis nodosa is worthy of mention. We reviewed the five specimens from infants with this latter diagnosis who died at our institution between 1950 and 1970. The gross and microscopic findings are identical to those of Kawasaki syndrome. Although the clinical features were similar, infantile periarteritis nodosa only occurred in infants and often had a more

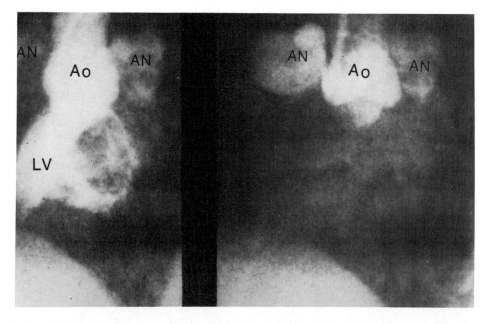

Figure 7. Angiography in Kawasaki syndrome demonstrating massive aneurysms of the coronary arteries. (Left = left ventricular angiogram in the LAO view; Right = aortogram in LAO view; AN = aneurysms; AO = aorta; LV = left ventricle.)

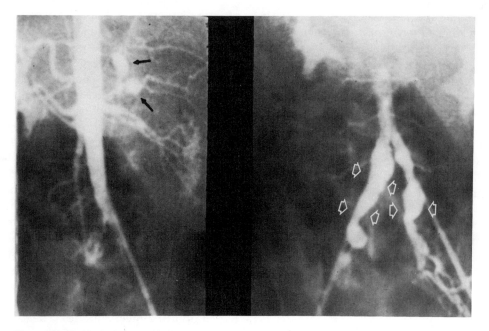

Figure 8. Abdominal aortogram in the same patient as in Fig. 7 demonstrating involvement of abdominal vessels (arrows).

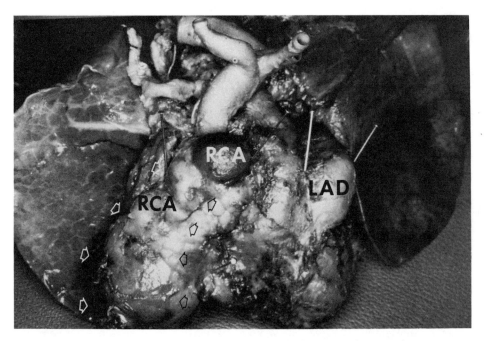

Figure 9. Pathological specimen in Kawasaki syndrome demonstrating massive aneurysms of the coronary arteries. (LAD = left anterior descending coronary artery. Note aneurysms between pins and between arrows.)

prolonged course which included renal involvement and peripheral vascular insufficiency. In addition, despite careful review of the records of these patients and of the literature, I have been unable to find any mention of desquamation of the fingertips and toes. This phenomenon, which is so characteristic of Kawasaki syndrome, is such a striking feature that it is difficult to imagine that it would not have been reported. Thus, although the pathological features are identical and the clinical features of these two diagnoses are similar, they differ enough to obscure the issue as to whether they represent two separate entities or are just a different means of clinical expression of the same disorder.

Management

Acute Phase

There is no standard management of patients with Kawasaki syndrome since no specific therapy is available for this disorder of unknown etiology. With this in mind, I will describe our approach at the Children's Hospital of Pittsburgh. Aspirin (acetylsalicylic acid) is given in a dosage of at least 100 mg/kg/day during the acute phase. Many patients with this disorder seem to have a defect in absorption and/or exhibit excess excretion of this drug. It is thus often necessary to administer 150 mg/kg/day or more in order to achieve a salicylate level of between 15 and 20 mg%. A word of caution! If this higher dosage is used, then one must remember to decrease the dosage of salicylate as soon as the acute phase of the illness begins to subside. The abnormality of salicylate metabolism disappears rapidly during this phase. If the dosage is not decreased, then salicylate intoxication will rapidly ensue. High-dose salicylate therapy is continued until the fever subsides. The salicylate dosage is then reduced to 5 mg/kg/day for approximately two months.

Unfortunately, the etiology of this disorder is still unknown and thus far, preventive measures and specific therapy are not available. Kawasaki syndrome is, nonetheless, an inflammatory process. It seems logical therefore that agents modifying an inflammatory response might also modify the course of this disease. Prednisone and/or other corticosteroids are among the most potent antiinflammatory agents. Steroids, however, have acquired a reputation as being harmful in patients with Kawasaki syndrome and most state that their use is contraindicated. One such study (Kato et al., 1979) is quoted in almost all of the English language literature. This study was not only poorly controlled but the authors also chose to disregard the small group of patients who received both aspirin and prednisone and had a zero incidence of coronary artery aneurysms. Although the conclusions of this study may be correct, a more carefully controlled investigation of the use of this potent antiinflammatory agent in the management of Kawasaki syndrome should be undertaken.

The use of intravenous gammaglobulin has recently been recommended for the treatment of patients with Kawasaki syndrome during the first 10 days of the illness. In a cooperative study from a number of centers in the United States (Newberger et al., 1986), intravenous gammaglobulin in a dose of 400 mg/kg/day was given for 5 days to patients who were between the 3rd and 10th day after the onset of their illness. These investigators reported prompt remission of symptoms and a significantly lower incidence of coronary artery "abnormalities" in those who received intravenous gammaglobulin as compared to a similar group of patients who received aspirin therapy alone. It would seem at first glance that this study conclusively proved the effectiveness of gammaglobulin and that, furthermore, this drug should now be used as the treatment of choice in all patients with Kawasaki disease. There are, however, serious deficiencies in the data that have been presented. Certain points should be clarified or investigated further before this treatment regimen becomes universally accepted. Pa-

tients in this study were described as having "coronary artery involvement" solely on the basis of echocardiography. There was no attempt to classify the patients with these abnormalities into those who had simply dilation of one or more coronary arteries and those who had true aneurysms. Interobserver variation in the assessment of dilation of these coronary arteries occurred in almost one-fifth of the patients with cardiac involvement in this series. Simply having a third observer as a "tie-breaker" is not adequate. If it should transpire that there are more patients with simple dilation than aneurysms in one or the other of the treatment groups, then the data could be skewed. No comment was made about whether the incidence of coronary arterial involvement was any different if gammaglobulin was administered on the 3rd or 4th day of illness as compared to the 9th or 10th day. In addition, since no patient who had passed the 10th day of illness had received treatment, no conclusion can be made regarding the effectiveness of administration of intravenous gammaglobulin after this point in time. Intravenous gammaglobulin may prove to be an important advance in therapy for patients with Kawasaki syndrome. But it is costly and may involve some risks in its administration. I would, therefore, add my own word of caution to those of others (Feigin, 1986) about the universal application of this form of treatment until other carefully controlled investigations have conclusively documented its efficacy.

Demonstration of Cardiac Involvement

At Children's Hospital of Pittsburgh, cardiac catheterization is recommended for all patients with Kawasaki syndrome who are suspected of having cardiac involvement. Echocardiography is also an excellent screening tool (See Chap. 7.2) and is extremely useful in the follow-up of patients with coronary arterial lesions. Cross-sec-

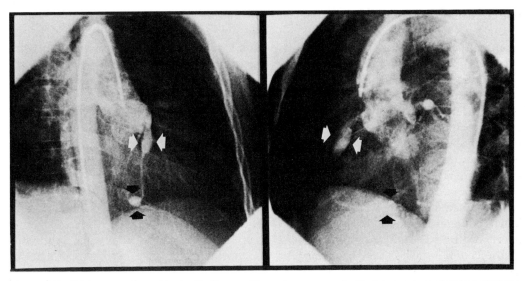

Figure 10. Angiogram of a patient with Kawasaki syndrome reported to have a normal right coronary artery by echocardiogram. There is some dilation of the proximal right coronary artery and a saccular aneurysm distally. (Left = RAO view; Right = LAO view of aortograms.)

tional echocardiography with special attention to the coronary arteries is performed during the acute phase and again at four to six weeks after the onset of the illness in all patients. False-positive echocardiograms can occur (coronary artery dilation as suggested by echocardiography with normal coronary arteries angiographically) in addition to false-negative echocardiographic studies. Recently, a patient with right and left coronary artery aneurysms documented two years before was reported echocardiographically to have a normal right coronary artery and persistence of an aneurysm in the left coronary artery. Angiography (Fig. 10) demonstrated dilation of the right coronary artery and revealed a saccular aneurysm in the distal portion of this vessel which had not been visualized by echocardiography. Although this patient had coronary artery involvement on the basis of an abnormal left coronary artery, the involvement of the right coronary artery was missed echocardiographically. Because of these concerns, we continue to advocate cardiac catheterization and angiocardiography for the evaluation and follow-up of patients suspected of

coronary arterial involvement (Table 7). It is rarely necessary to perform selective coronary arteriography at the time of the initial study in patients with this disorder since

Table 7
Kawasaki Syndrome Management, Cardiac Catheterization

—Document extent of coronary arterial involvement
—Quantify: type, size, number, and location of aneurysms
—Indications
  A. Patients with cardiac findings
     1. Persistent electrocardiographic changes
     2. Gallop, mitral regurgitation
     3. Cardiomegaly
     4. Pericardial effusion
     5. Congestive heart failure
  B. Patients without cardiac findings
     1. Fever > 14 days
     2. Acute-phase reactants elevated over 1 month
     3. Recurrence of fever, rash, or desquamation

aortography with a good volume of contrast media (1 ml/kg over 2 sec) is usually adequate to visualize the entire coronary arterial system. However, selective coronary arteriography is usually performed on subsequent studies. Angiography is the only way to document the extent of coronary artery involvement adequately and to quantify the type, size, number, and location of coronary arterial aneurysms. We perform this procedure in all patients with cardiac findings or in those patients without cardiac findings who are in the group previously defined as being at high risk for having cardiac involvement (those with fever of greater than 14 days' duration; prolonged elevation of acute-phase reactants over one month after the onset of illness; or those patients with recurrence of fever, rash, or desquamation).

If patients with Kawasaki syndrome are found to have coronary arterial involvement, we continue salicylate therapy at a dose of 5 mg/kg/day and add dipyridamole at a dose of 2 mg/kg/day. Drug therapy is continued until patients are demonstrated angiographically no longer to have coronary arterial abnormalities. Echocardiographic follow-up is performed every three to six months. It is particularly important to visualize those areas that had previously been found to be abnormal in order to document the progression or regression of the abnormalities. Repeat cardiac catheterization is recommended approximately one year following the previous procedure. If the patient has had negative echocardiograms, then this procedure will document that the coronary arteries are now definitely normal. On the other hand, if the patient still has abnormal echocardiographic findings, repeat angiography will confirm this involvement and document its extent as well as any changes that have occurred since the first study. Further routine follow-up is then by echocardiography. Repeat angiography is not recommended until the patient is found to be completely free of echocardiographic abnormalities.

Summary

Kawasaki syndrome is an increasingly recognized disorder whose etiology, natural history, and relationship to other disorders remains unknown. It is self-limited in most cases. When death does occur, it is always on the basis of cardiovascular involvement and is usually sudden and unexpected. Even patients with documented coronary arterial abnormalities who have died have rarely had cardiac symptoms more than 24 hours or so in advance of their demise. Coronary arterial involvement occurred in 18% of patients in our series, an incidence similar to that reported from other centers. The significance of coronary arterial involvement remains unclear since a mortality of only 1% is reported in the literature and was only 3% in our series. Although the majority of our patients with coronary artery involvement have persistent lesions, none has had symptoms. The long-term outlook for these patients is unknown. Treatment of the disease is still controversial. Salicylates are used by most centers in the treatment of the acute disease but questions remain about the use of corticosteroids, anticoagulants, and intravenous gammaglobulin in the management of patients with this very puzzling disorder.

References

Feigin RD, Barron KS. Treatment of Kawasaki syndrome. *N Engl J Med* 1986;315:388–390.

Kato H, Koike S, Yokoyama T. Kawasaki disease: Effect of treatment on coronary artery involvement. *Pediatrics* 1979;63:175–179.

Kato H, Ichinose E, Yoshioka F, et al. Fate of coronary aneurysms in Kawasaki disease: Serial coronary angiography and long-term follow-up study. *Am J Cardiol* 1982;49:1758–1766.

Kawasaki T: Acute febrile mucocutaneous lymph node syndrome: Clinical observations of 50 cases. *Jpn J Allerg* (Japanese) 1967;16:178–222.

Kawasaki T, Kosaki F, Okawa S, et al. A new infantile acute febrile mucocutaneous lymph node syndrome (MLNS) prevailing in Japan. *Pediatrics* 1974;54:271–276.

Nakanishi T, Takao A, Nakazawa M, et al. Mucocutaneous lymph node syndrome: Clinical hemodynamic and angiographic features of coronary obstructive disease. *Am J Cardiol* 1985;55:662–668.

Nakano H, Ueda K, Saito A, Nojima K. Repeated quantitative angiograms in coronary arterial aneurysm in Kawasaki Disease. *Am J Cardiol* 1985;56:846–851.

Newburger JW, Takahashi M, Burns JC, et al. The treatment of Kawasaki syndrome with intravenous gamma globulin. *N Engl J Med* 1986;315:341–347.

Wilson CS, Weaver WF, Zeman ED, Forker AD. Bilateral nonfistulous congenital coronary arterial aneurysms. *Am J Cardiol* 1975;35:319–323.

VIII

Miscellaneous Topics

8.1

The Cardiac Pathologist in the 1990s

Anton E. Becker

Pathologists traditionally teach the basic principles of disease, both at a fundamental level and in applied medicine. It is on this basis that the pathologist provides a hospital service, including quality control in medical health care and basic and applied researches in an attempt to improve the understanding of disease processes. It is the continuous feedback between pathology, research, and clinician that marks the standard of pathology today and should guarantee its future.

In this respect it is important that organ pathology should never be detached from the broad base where basic principles of diseases are taught and researched. An abundance of examples can be provided where organ pathologists, working in isolation, lose contact with achievements in basic general pathology and, hence, are unable to cope with specific problems that arise in their particular field. It is for this reason that the cardiac pathologist should work in close harmony with the general pathologist and other "organ pathologists," today as well as in the future.

Quality Control

One of the important tools available in medicine to control the quality of medical health care is the autopsy. It is regrettable, therefore, that the current worldwide trend is to underestimate its importance. A steady decline in the autopsy rate testifies to this fact (Roberts, 1978; Williams and Peery, 1978). It is probably related, at least in part, to the fact that new diagnostic devices have been developed, which according to a new generation of doctors make unnecessary such time-consuming and basically unpleasant procedures as an autopsy (Robinson, 1983). Despite advanced technology, however, today's autopsy still provides information that is new to the clinician (Britton, 1974; de Vries et al., 1986; Laissue et al., 1986; Pounder et al., 1983). Such information, if known during the clinical episode, might have changed the medical regimen.

Within this context, cardiac pathology plays an important role. In my experience,

From: Anderson, RH, Neches, WH, Park, SC, Zuberbuhler, JR, eds: *Perspectives in Pediatric Cardiology*: Mount Kisco, New York, Futura Publishing Co., © 1988.

heart and vessel diseases are among the most common conditions encountered and, to the extent demonstrated, are often unexpected. Furthermore, particularly in the field of heart diseases, the study of tissues and cells during life is limited. Feedback from autopsies is therefore mandatory. Much knowledge can be gained from the proper study of the heart at autopsy together with an adequate correlation between morphology and clinical data. Such a correlation is essential to make the findings meaningful.

Considering quality control in the 1990s, and taking the autopsy as the optimal tool for such control, we can only hope that the medical profession will realize that the autopsy is necessary. The pathologist, on the other hand, should realize that his approach to the autopsy should stretch beyond the "classic path." Much can be gained by applying new techniques, particularly immunopathology and electron microscopy.

Diagnosis

The dominant role of tissue and cell diagnosis as it applies to many fields of clinical medicine is less obvious in diseases of the heart and vessels. Improvements in the field of endomyocardial and lung biopsies, nonetheless, provide the pathologist with unique material to exercise diagnostic skills. Thus far, endomyocardial biopsies are particularly indicated in cardiac transplantation patients and in patients with idiopathic dilated congestive cardiomyopathy. In the latter category, the biopsy is mainly intended to rule out disease that may be amenable to treatment, such as myocarditis. The overall effect of endomyocardial biopsies for the diagnosis of dilated congestive cardiomyopathies, however, appears to be extremely limited. Light and electron microscopic studies and morphometric analysis thus far have not yielded spectacular results

(Baandrup and Olsen, 1981; Fowles and Mason, 1984; Rose and Beck, 1985; Yonesaka and Becker, 1986). Indeed, the criteria for diagnosis of dilated congestive cardiomyopathy from endomyocardial biopsies are still uncertain. Research devoted to understand the disease remains unfruitful. It is in this particular arena that the application of new techniques available to the pathologist should be expanded. Immunopathological methods, in particular immuno-histocytochemistry at the ultrastructural level, may have promise for the near future. Similarly, methods of studying the functional capacity of the myocardial cells, harvested through endomyocardial biopsies, may open new gateways to a better understanding of the disease.

Within this context, the possible role of endomyocardial biopsies in congenital heart disease may be considered. Thus far, endomyocardial biopsies in pediatric patients have been limited mainly to patients with dilated congestive cardiomyopathy (Schmaltz et al., 1982). In such instances the early stages of development of endocardial fibroelastosis can be detected. This is important not only from the scientific viewpoint in understanding the cellular mechanisms involved in endocardial thickening, but also since it may indicate the turning point from a reversible to an irreversible disease process. Endomyocardial biopsies may also contribute to the evaluation of myocardial fibrosis by enabling quantification. A preliminary study of biopsies taken from heart specimens performed in our laboratories showed that this was indeed the case (Fig. 1). Whether or not this may become a useful clinical tool in the management of patients with congenital heart disease remains to be seen. Not all pediatric cardiologists and pediatricians will be enthusiastic about taking a biopsy in a severely ill baby. Nevertheless, one may anticipate that in the near future the availability of tissue, investigated with sophisticated pathological techniques, could provide information that plays a role in the decision-making

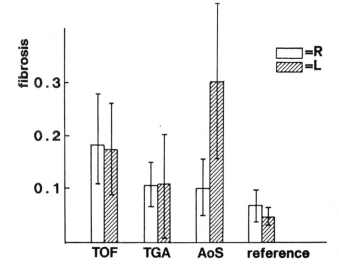

Figure 1. The degree of myocardial fibrosis is judged from postmortem endomyocardial biopsies. The differences between right and left ventricular myocardial fibrosis in heart specimens with aortic stenosis (AoS) is highly significant ($p < 0.001$). TOF = tetralogy of Fallot; TGA = complete transposition; reference = hearts without cardiovascular pathology.

processes such as the optimal timing for surgery.

Along the same lines, the role of lung biopsies may be considered a subject of debatable clinical significance. From a purely diagnostic point of view, not all pediatric cardiologists will accept that there is a place for lung biopsies. It is our experience, however, that (particularly in patients whose calculated pulmonary vascular resistance is borderline) lung biopsy may be a valuable additional tool in the process of deciding whether or not to correct the underlying cardiac defect (Marcelletti et al., 1979). It is important to note that the hemodynamic data on which the clinician has to base the calculations of pulmonary vascular resistance are often far from precise (Johnson and Haworth, 1984; McGregor and Sniderman, 1985; Murgo and Westerhof, 1984; Nihill et al., 1976).

The role of lung biopsies has thus far been evaluated mainly in the setting of a left-to-right shunt, regardless of the detailed anatomy of the underlying cardiac malformation, which leads potentially to plexogenic pulmonary arteriopathy. Lung biopsies, however, may also play a role in evaluating the pulmonary vascular structural condition in patients considered candidates for a Fontan procedure. Here the

problems encountered are of a totally different nature, since diminished pulmonary flow is the hallmark of the disease. In a number of these patients there is concomitant pulmonary venous hypertension. To what extent the structural changes that accompany this hemodynamic feature may ultimately lead to a change in the reservoir function of the pulmonary venous bed remains unknown (Fig. 2). If they do, one may anticipate that structural changes at the venous end of the pulmonary circulation are important and may become a limiting factor for the execution of the Fontan procedure.

Research

Research in pathology is the cornerstone for further achievements in understanding disease processes and, hence, their diagnosis and treatment. At this stage it is important to state that the classic approach is by no means outdated. One may expect that the detailed description of cardiac abnormalities will retain its importance for a long time to come. One of the main reasons for this is that cardiac pathology has the serious drawback that little tissue is available for study during the life span of the

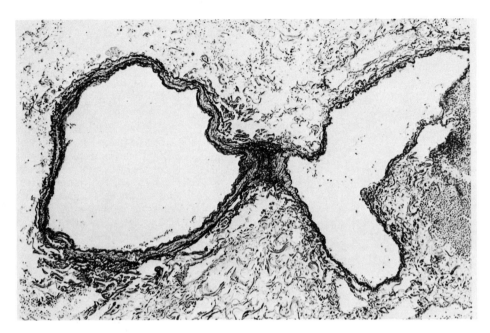

Figure 2. Arterialization of pulmonary veins, as an expression of longstanding pulmonary venous hypertension. The significance of this structural adaptation for pulmonary venous compliance remains to be settled. Elastic tissue stain.

patient. This applies to both congenital and acquired heart disease. A meticulous description of "well-known" malformations still may reveal new facts of clinical relevance that are beneficial to the patient. The importance of the "classic" approach can be illustrated by numerous examples of which the following, taken from the arena of congenital heart disease, can be exemplary.

The Classic Approach

Complete transposition is a well-defined congenital heart malformation. Much knowledge has been gained regarding right ventricular outflow tract characteristics, the connections and relations of the great arteries, and origin and course of the main coronary arteries. All of these features are considered of paramount importance in view of current surgical techniques such as the arterial switch procedure. It is surprising, there-

fore, that little is known regarding the process of myocardial remodeling, during either the intrauterine or the postnatal periods. Apart from myocyte adaptation, the microvasculature must develop in proportion to the myocardial muscle mass. Preliminary studies in our laboratory have shown that the development of the intramyocardial resistance arterioles (those with an external diameter between 30 and 100 μm) lags behind that of the mature myocardium in the normal heart (Kurosawa et al., 1986). This is a peculiar finding that raises questions both with respect to fundamental aspects, such as myocardial growth and adaptation, and with regard to immediate clinical aspects, such as impact on management.

A second example is the well-known underdevelopment of segments of the aorta. It is widely acknowledged presently that diminished flow during the development of an artery will affect its growth. Basically, structural units will be present but further growth into the fully mature state with an adequate luminal diameter is hampered be-

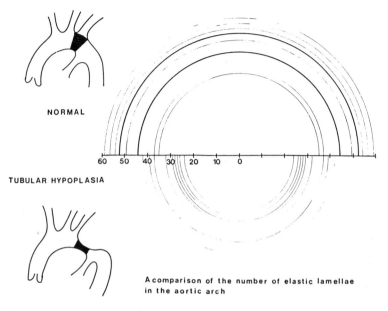

NORMAL

TUBULAR HYPOPLASIA

A comparison of the number of elastic lamellae
in the aortic arch

Figure 3. A comparison of the number of elastic units in the aortic arch of the normal and tubular hypoplasia shows a statistically significant difference ($p < 0.01$).

cause of lack of flow as the initiating event (Berry, 1973). A preliminary study of the number of elastic lamellae in the aorta, comparing tubular hypoplasia of the aortic arch with the hypoplastic ascending aorta in cases of aortic atresia, has revealed that significant differences exist. In the hypoplastic segment of the aortic arch, the number of elastic lamellae was markedly lower than that encountered in a normal arch at the site of origin of the left subclavian artery (Fig. 3). In the ascending aorta of hearts with aortic atresia, on the other hand, the number of elastic lamellae was almost equal to that in the normal (Fig. 4). Thus, the question is raised whether this is a genetically transmitted difference or whether the findings can still be considered in the light of the flow concept, taking into account that the hemodynamic impact may vary and that in this respect the stage of preexistent development could play a role.

The conduction tissue of the heart has been extensively studied and fundamental concepts regarding its position and course have been worked out (Becker and Ander-

son, 1983). Nevertheless, it has been shown recently that new and valuable additional information can be gathered from the ongoing study of heart specimens with congenital malformations (Kurosawa and Becker, 1984). Recently, the study of a heart with congenitally corrected transposition and a straddling right-sided mitral valve revealed that the atrioventricular node and bundle were in a posterior location, rather anteriorly as anticipated. The main conduction axis extended anteriorly as a dead-end tract and disappeared in the fibrous tissue of the cardiac skeleton supporting the pulmonary valve (Kurosawa and Becker, unpublished observations). Here is an exception to the "rule," which necessitates modulation of concepts regarding the position of the atrioventricular node and bundle in hearts with congenitally corrected transposition.

Surgical repair of hearts with an atrioventricular septal defect is now performed worldwide. The anatomy of this particular heart malformation has been described extensively and left ventricular outflow tract narrowing is a well-known intrinsic prob-

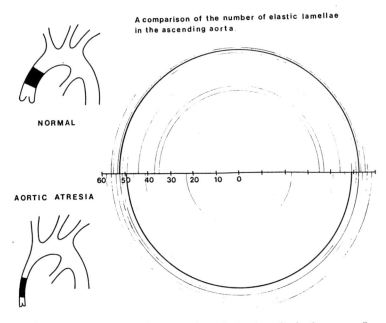

Figure 4. A comparison of the number of elastic units in the ascending aorta of the normal and aortic atresia shows no statistically significant difference.

lem (Ebels et al., 1986; Piccoli et al., 1982). A recent study in our laboratory with respect to the mode of attachment of the valve leaflets has revealed that the presence of a fibrous shelf together with thick and often fused tendinous cords contributed markedly to the stenosis. On that basis, a modification of the existent surgical techniques has been suggested in which part or all of the valve attachments in cases with the so-called Rastelli type A are detached from the crest of the septum. This procedure leads to relief of the left ventricular outflow tract obstruction by mobilizing the superior leaflet (Fig. 5). This study may thus contribute to a further improvement of the current surgical techniques and will, one hopes, diminish the potential risk of early and late postoperative complications due to left ventricular outflow tract obstruction.

It is clear that the "classic" descriptive approach to the pathology of heart disease can still provide new facts and may lead to modulation of existing concepts.

The New Approach

The 1990s, however, will definitely bring further progress in cardiac research through the application of modern sophisticated techniques, such as immuno-histo-cytochemistry, electron microscopy, tissue cell culture, in situ hybridization techniques, and the application of technology relative to DNA and RNA production. Some of the pathways already trodden may exemplify this point.

It has been known for a considerable time that coronary arteries, very early in life, show changes of the intima characterized by a proliferation of vascular smooth-muscle cells. This process has been related to atherosclerosis as it occurs in older patients although the precise interaction between cellular intimal proliferation in infants and children and the atherosclerotic process in adults remains uncertain. The question arises to what extent preexistent cell differentiation plays a role in the process of pro-

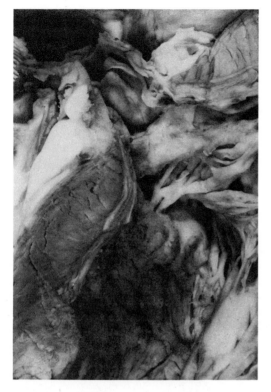

Figure 5. Left-sided view of a heart with an atrioventricular septal defect and intrinsic left ventricular outflow tract stenosis. Part of the stenosis relates to immobilization of the superior leaflet. Detachment during surgical repair may relieve the stenosis.

liferation and outgrowing of the cellular components. Recent immunohistochemical techniques have made it possible to demonstrate proteins of the cytoskeleton, such as vimentin and desmin. Preliminary studies reveal that, early in life, the inner layer of cells in the media do not stain for desmin, as would be anticipated because of their smooth-muscle cell nature, but rather for vimentin (Fig. 6). Similarly, the proliferating cells within the intima stain for vimentin and not for desmin. This raises questions regarding the adjustment of the cell to circumstances that have apparently switched the cell from one designed for contraction to a cell coded to produce intercellular matrix.

Endomyocardial biopsies and heart tissue available through transplantation programs may be studied with modern techniques with particular emphasis on functional morphology. For instance, it has been shown previously that myocardial tissue specimens taken at open heart surgery provide information regarding the contractile capacity of the cell and thus have predictive value in a given patient for the postoperative result (Canković-Darracott, 1982). The same technique is presently applied to donor hearts. It has indeed provided valuable information regarding donor heart function after transplantation. It is along these lines that one may anticipate disclosing similar functional characteristics of myocytes, but in the posttransplantation heart, the samples will be obtained through endomyocardial biopsies. Such techniques could be particularly important in the subset of patients with dilated congestive cardiomyopathy. It may well be that the study of the functional pathomorphology will provide a better insight in the mid- and long-term prognosis than those presently available with morphometric techniques. Moreover, the available tissue can be used for different studies, including in-situ hybridization. For instance, the hypothesis that dilated congestive cardiomyopathy may be due to cellular derangement caused by a viral myocarditis could be tested using DNA probes. This could lead to a breakthrough in the basic understanding of some of the cardiomyopathies. Similar techniques are used already in the study of endothelial cells and their interaction with smooth-muscle cells in relation to the genesis of atherosclerosis.

Immuno-histo-cytochemical techniques, furthermore, are applied to the study of myosin isozymes, both in developing hearts and in mature hearts undergoing adaptation. Studies in developing chicken hearts have already demonstrated that there are different types of isozymes that change during development (de Jong et al., 1986).

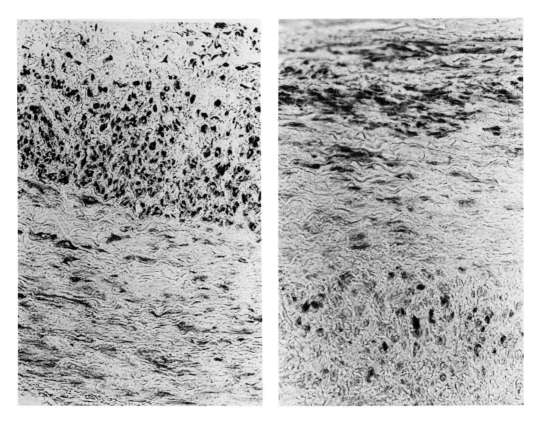

Figure 6. Coronary artery with intimal proliferation. *A:* Desmin stain revealing positivity concentrated mainly in the outer medial layers. *B:* Vimentin stain showing positivity throughout the media and also in the proliferating intimal cells.

The same group of investigators have recently demonstrated that fetal myosin no longer detectable in the adult heart reappears in old rats. Likewise, the question can be raised whether when it comes to the myosin component, all forms of myocardial hypertrophy are alike. Since pressure-load hypertrophy and volume-load hypertrophy are different, and since the functional consequences of both compensatory mechanisms are not exactly the same, it is interesting to see which types of myosin isozymes are active under these circumstances. It is not beyond reality to expect that further study of this intriguing field may lead to a much better insight in cardiac adaptation and its sequels.

Teaching

Finally, the pathologist must retain his or her principal role in teaching, at both undergraduate and postgraduate levels. This is vital, since today's complex technology tends to distract the trainee from the basics of pathology. It is astounding that cardiologists can be "fully trained" without ever having touched a heart. Indeed, in some instances, they may not have a proper conception of the heart's intricate anatomy. Echocardiography, which depends so heavily on a good understanding of cardiac anatomy and pathology, then becomes a matter of pattern recognition rather than true understanding.

The impact of ongoing research on the teaching of cardiac disease is obvious and necessary in order not to lose touch with the current trends in clinical medicine.

Conclusions

Pathologists in general, and for that reason cardiac pathologists in particular, have an important role to fulfill at present and in the decades ahead. They have the tools at their fingertips, but optimal usage of sophisticated techniques will at the same time necessitate a good understanding and feedback with the clinical cardiologist. It is essential that the cardiac pathologist speak the language of the cardiologist. Otherwise, he or she will become isolated within the "ivory tower" laboratory and ultimately will produce results that are either useless or destined never to be used.

References

Baandrup U, Olsen EGJ. Critical analysis of endomyocardial biopsy from patients suspected of having cardiomyopathy. I. Morphologic and morphometric aspects. *Br Heart J* 1981;45:475–486.

Becker AE, Anderson RH. *Cardiac Pathology. An Integrated Text and Colour Atlas.* London-New York: Gower Medical Publishing, 1983.

Berry CL. Growth development and healing of large arteries. *Ann Coll Surg* 1973;53:246–257.

Britton M. Diagnostic errors discovered at autopsy. *Acta Med Scand* 1974;196:203–210.

Canković-Darracott S. Methods for assessing preservation techniques—Invasive methods (enzymatic, cytochemical). In Engelman RM, Levitsky S (Eds): *A Textbook of Clinical Cardioplegia.* Mount Kisco, NY: Futura, 1982:43–61.

de Jong F, Geerts WJC, de Groot IJM, et al.

Changing isomyosin expression pattern in tubular stages of chicken heart development: A 3D immunohistochemical analysis, Submitted for publication, 1986.

de Vries M, Zwertbroek W, Becker AE. De obductie: Zin of onzin. *Nederlands Tijd Genees* 1986;130:1273–1276.

Ebels T, Ho SY, Anderson RH, et al. The surgical anatomy of the left ventricular outflow tract in atrioventricular septal defect. *Ann Thorac Surg* 1986;41:483–488.

Fowles RE, Mason JW. Role of cardiac biopsy in the diagnosis and management of cardiac disease. *Prog Cardiovasc Dis* 1984;27:153–172.

Greenwald SG, Johnson RJ, Haworth SG. Pulmonary vascular imput impedance in the newborn and infant pig. *Cardiovasc Res* 1984;18:44–50.

Kurosawa H, Becker AE. Modification of the precise relationship of the atrioventricular conduction bundle to the margins of the ventricular septal defects by the trabecula septomarginalis. *J Thorac Cardiovasc Surg* 1984;87:605–615.

Kurosawa S, Kurosawa H, Becker AE. The coronary arterioles in newborns, infants and children. A morphometric study of normal hearts and hearts with aortic atresia and complete transposition. *Int J Cardiol* 1986;10:43–56.

Laissue JA, Altermatt HJ, Zürcher B, et al. Bedeutung der Autopsie. Fortlaufende internistische Wertung von Autopsie-ergebnissen. *Schweiz Med Woch* 1986;116:130–134.

Marcelletti C, Wagenvoort CA, Losekoot TG, et al. Palliative Mustard or Rastelli operation in complete transposition of the great arteries. Option decided by lung biopsy. *J Thorac Cardiovasc Surg* 1979;77:677–681.

McGregor M, Sniderman A. On pulmonary vascular resistance: The need for more precise definition. *Am J Cardiol* 1985;55:217–221.

Murgo JP, Westerhof N. Input impedance of the pulmonary arterial system in normal man. Effects of respiration and comparison to systemic impedance. *Circ Res* 1984;54:666–673.

Nihill MR, McNamara DG, Vick RK. The effects of increased blood viscosity on pulmonary vascular resistance. *Am Heart J* 1976;92:65–75.

Piccoli GP, Ho SY, Wilkinson JL, et al. Left-sided obstructive lesions in atrioventricular septal defects. An anatomic study. *J Thorac Cardiovasc Surg* 1982;83:453–460.

Pounder DJ, Horowitz M, Rowland R, Reid DP. The value of the autopsy in medical audit—A combined clinical and pathological assessment of 100 cases. *Austr NZ J Med* 1983;13:478–482.

Roberts WC. The autopsy: Its decline and a suggestion for its revival. *N Engl J Med* 1978; 288:332–338.

Rose AG, Beck W. Dilated (congestive) cardiomyopathy: A syndrome of severe cardiac function with remarkable few morphological features of myocardial damage. *Histopathology* 1985; 9:367–379.

Robinson MJ. The autopsy 1983: Can it be revived? *Human Pathol* 1983;14:566–568.

Schmaltz AA, Apitz J, Hort W. Endomyocardial biopsy in infants and children: technique; indications and results. *Eur J Pediatr* 1982;138:211–215.

Williams MJ, Peery TM. The autopsy, a beginning, not an end. *Am J Clin Pathol* 1978;69:215–216.

Yonesaka S, Becker AE. Dilated cardiomyopathy. Diagnostic accuracy of endomyocardial biopsies. Submitted for publication, 1986.

8.2

Cardiopulmonary Transplantation

Bartley P. Griffith

Cardiopulmonary transplantation has shown promise as a potential treatment for end-stage heart and lung disease and has given hope to potential recipients where none previously existed. In reality, however, the procedure remains experimental. Since 1980 there have been more than 200 procedures performed worldwide, and the regional availability has expanded, but survival averages only 50%. It is likely that short-term survival will improve based on the lessons learned about selection of candidates and donors, the operative procedure, and organ preservation. Since deaths related to infection predominate, the susceptibility of the pulmonary allograft to pneumonia must be studied. Finally, a better understanding of early and late pulmonary rejection is required before a therapeutic result can be anticipated. The four-year experience in Pittsburgh, which includes 46 cases, generally reflects the current status of cardiopulmonary transplantation (Griffith et al., 1987).

Patient Population

All potential recipients have end-stage pulmonary vascular or parenchymal diseases, and most have associated severe secondary failure of the right ventricle. Children and infants likely to benefit include those with congenital heart disease with pulmonary vascular disease, those with primary pulmonary hypertension, and patients with parenchymal and airway disease (Penkoske et al., 1984). Candidates have required supplemental oxygen, and all but the most determined have led a profoundly disabled home or hospital-bound existence. Patients with previous thoracic surgeries should be avoided. None of the three patients with previous sternotomies, who were operated upon in Pittsburgh, survived, and all of those with thoracotomies had extensive bleeding and required reoperation. Other exclusionary criteria include severe cachexia, congestive hepatic dysfunction,

From: Anderson, RH, Neches, WH, Park, SC, Zuberbuhler, JR, eds: *Perspectives in Pediatric Cardiology*: Mount Kisco, New York, Futura Publishing Co., © 1988.

ventilator dependence, and established pulmonary infection. While the upper age limit has been around 50 years, a minimum age has not been established, and there is concern about the potential of the tracheal anastomosis to grow. Our youngest patient was nine years old, but younger children have been treated elsewhere.

In Pittsburgh, specific diseases treated include primary pulmonary hypertension (22 cases), Eisenmenger's syndrome (15), emphysema (3), multiple pulmonary emboli (1), cystic fibrosis (1), eosinophilic granuloma (1), sarcoidosis (1), fibrosing alveolitis (1), and idiopathic fibrosis (1).

Operative Procedure

A hemostatic removal of the recipient's diseased heart and lungs poses the greatest technical challenge of the operative procedure. Extreme care must be exercised to avoid postoperative hemorrhage from bronchial and mediastinal collateral circulation. Although it is possible to remove the organs in one block, dissection is facilitated when the ventricles are removed first, followed by common hilar ligation and amputation of the lungs. The unexpected occurrence of dense pleural adhesions is now an indication to abort the procedure. The carina is approached directly from between the superior caval vein and the ascending aorta, the airway is divided just above the carina, and the left and right bronchi can be removed to the previous suture line along their adventitial planes.

En bloc implantation of the heart and lungs of the donor is by sequential supracarinal to tracheal, right atrial, and aortic anastomoses. Because dehiscence of the continuous Polypropylene anastomosis has occurred in three patients, the suture line is interrupted in four places and is wrapped by a tongue of omentum.

Procurement of Donor's Organs

The ideal cardiopulmonary donor must pass the criteria for cardiac donation (Hardesty and Griffith, 1987), and in addition, must have a clear chest radiograph, an arterial oxygen tension of more than 300 mmHg with an inspired oxygen fraction of 1.0, and produce a clean sputum. This strict selection severely limits the number of potential donors, but we have learned that more liberal acceptance of donors is ill-advised and that the most important determinant of early survival has been the quality of the transplanted lungs. Seldom does a donor qualify who has been ventilated more than 24 hours. The recipient and donor are matched by blood group, weight, and thoracic circumference. The use of a blood group O donor in a blood group A recipient resulted in hemolysis which caused acute tubular necrosis and temporary dependence on dialysis.

Initially, the inability to preserve the lung reliably for more than one hour required that all donors be local or transported as "heart-beating" cadavers to the transplant institution. Because this did not meet the demand for organs, we experimented with the use of autoperfusion of the heart and lungs for preservation during distant procurement. This was first used clinically in August 1984, and our clinical experience now includes 22 cases (Hardesty and Griffith, 1987). While we are confident that autoperfusion of the heart-lung block has provided well-preserved organs, we recently favor a simple flush of the organs with a solution of modified Euro-collins and prostaglandin E_1. This method is based upon the experimental work performed at Stanford (Haverich et al., 1985; Starkey et al., 1986) and Cambridge (Wallwork J, personal communication, 1987), and has been used in our last eight patients with excellent results and ex vivo times beyond four hours. Finally, hypothermia induced by cardiopulmonary bypass has successfully cooled the donor's heart and lungs for local and distant procurement (Hardesty and Griffith, 1987; Yacoub M, personal communication, 1987).

Immunosuppression

All patients receive 500 mg of methylprednisolone following release of the aortic cross-clamp. Postoperatively, cyclosporine is begun when the patient is hemodynamically stable, and the doses are adjusted to a blood level of 700 ng/ml (RIA, whole blood, Sandoz). To maximize the potential for healing of the tracheal anastomosis, steroids are withheld during the first two postoperative weeks. During this period the patients receive a three- to five-day course of rabbit antithymocyte globulin, and azathioprine is given at a dose of 2 mg/kg/day during the first two postoperative weeks. After two weeks, prednisone is instituted at maintenance doses of 10–20 mg/day, and patients receive maintenance therapy with the regime of triple drugs. Rejection has generally been controlled with intravenous pulses of methylprednisolone.

Surveillance for Rejection and Infection

The endomyocardial biopsy is useful only in that sometimes it confirmed the clinical impression of pulmonary rejection (Griffith et al., 1985; McGregor et al., 1985). Significant myocyte necrosis is rarely found in the absence of an abnormal chest roentgenogram. Rejection of the lung, however, is found to occur frequently without significant abnormalities detected on the endomyocardial biopsy. The most common abnormality associated with pulmonary rejection has been the gradual onset over 24 to 36 hours of a radiographic homogeneous or nonhomogeneous opacification of the

parenchyma. Rapid clearing following intravenous methylprednisolone has been the rule. During mild phases of this process, clinical manifestations of cough and shortness of breath are mild. With more severe abnormalities, patients become markedly short of breath and experience significant reductions in their arterial oxygen saturation. Rejection of the allograft is common between 7 and 14 days postoperatively and has occurred in more than one-half of our survivors (Griffith et al., 1987).

Bronchoalveolar lavage is a rich source of immunocompetent cells and is performed at least once during the first month after transplantation, at two- to three-month intervals thereafter, and whenever an episode of infection or rejection is suspected. The analysis of the cells recovered by lavage provides useful information regarding infection, rejection, and the allogenic response. The results of HLA phenotyping of lymphocytes and macrophages obtained by lavage have revealed that, during the first six weeks, transplanted cells of the donor are incompletely replaced by those of the recipient, suggesting a cause for the common occurrence of early rejection (Paradis et al., 1985; Zeevi et al., 1985). While clear distinction between the cellular profiles obtained during episodes of rejection and infection has not been possible to date, the absence of an organism in the lavage fluid has strengthened the clinical decision to treat for rejection.

Lymphocytes exhibited significant spontaneous proliferation and Interleuken-2 response. Lymphocytes were far more likely than peripheral blood lymphocytes to express high levels of cell-mediated lympholysis during episodes of rejection.

Results

Survival

Twenty-seven of 46 patients have been discharged from the hospital following cardiopulmonary transplantation, and 22 continue to survive between one and 49 months postoperatively. One patient is approaching the fifth anniversary of his procedure. Their functional status generally has been in class I of New York Heart Association's Classification and has been influenced more by preoperative disability than by cardiopulmonary limitation. The survivors agree on the immensely improved quality of their lives.

Most deaths have occurred within the first two months after operation. Operative deaths have predominated and have been due either to exsanguination from pleuropulmonary adhesions in poorly selected recipients or to cardiopulmonary failure. Infection, usually of thoracic origin, has been responsible for the majority of deaths that occurred between 30 and 70 days. The two early postoperative deaths of noninfectious etiology included one from hemorrhage related to dehiscence of the tracheal suture line and one from an unexplained seizure disorder.

Infection

Cardiopulmonary transplant recipients have had a higher rate of infection in our institution than have cardiac transplant recipients, and nearly all infections have been life-threatening. In the survivors, 67% of the infections involved the lung or thoracic cavity as the primary site, while most of the others were disseminated viral or fungal infections. Fifty percent of the infections were bacterial; 19% viral; 19% protozoal, and 12% fungal. Morbid cytomegalic viral infection is more likely to occur in children and adults not previously exposed and is commonly transmitted at operation through blood products and the donor's organs. A nine-year-old patient tested for primary pulmonary hypertension died with pneumonia due to cytomegalic virus which was initially believed to be rejection. Currently, staining techniques for the virus in fluid obtained at lavage have improved, and incorrect diagnoses will now, hopefully, be rare.

Most of these infections occurred during the first six postoperative months (Dummer et al., 1986). Bacterial pneumonia was the most common infection during the first six postoperative weeks. This type of infection was seen as early as five days after transplantation and had a peak incidence around two weeks. Bacterial pneumonia was less frequent beyond six weeks, but infections with Pneumocystis carinii have been common.

Chronic Allograft Function

Annual coronary arteriography has not demonstrated occlusive coronary arterial disease in any of the long-term survivors, and the cardiac function has been normal. A moderate restrictive defect (decreased forced vital capacity and FEV_1) and a mild impairment of the diffusing capacity has been present at 1.5 months after transplantation. After the first six months following transplantation, only a mild, restrictive defect remains. There was also a significant improvement in the diffusing capacity over the first 12 postoperative months. Function of the airway, which was normal 1.5 months posttransplant, does decline with time, but this change has been generally minimal and not significant.

Two patients have developed chronic inflammation of the airway, and one patient has significant radiographic interstitial infiltrates after a severe pneumocystis infection, and one patient has obliterative bronchiolitis. The obstructive process in the latter improved with the institution of chest physiotherapy and bronchodilators and has remained stable in the last year. Histologic evaluation showed focal submucosal fibrosis of the bronchioles with occasional areas of round-cell inflammation consistent with obliterative bronchiolitis (Burke et al., 1984). Unfortunately, over the last 18 months, the obstructive defect has been increasing slowly, and the patient's FEV_1 is 1.2 liters.

Summary

We continue to pursue a therapeutic procedure, but to do so we must improve our operative mortality through selection of donor and recipients and by decreasing the high incidence of early pneumonia. The latter is related in part to the selection of donors but also to our inadequate understanding of the immunological interaction between the recipient and the donated lung. It is likely that the usual defense mechanisms (including mucociliary clearance and infectious antigen processing) are disordered. The late occurrence of obstructive disease of the airway is likely a result of chronic rejection but might be stimulated by chronic infection and facilitated by the absence of any bronchial collateral circulation. Animal models will be necessary to study this problem in greater detail.

Because it has given hope, the possibility of cardiopulmonary transplantation likely has done more for potential recipients than the number of successful results would indicate. The future of pediatric recipients will depend upon refinements in immunosuppression and answers to the questions raised by the few procedures to date.

References

Burke CM, Theodore J, Dawkins KD, et al. Post-transplant obliterative bronchiolitis and other late lung sequelae in human heart-lung transplantation. *Chest* 1984;86:824–829.

Dummer JS, Montero CG, Griffith BP, et al. Infections in heart-lung transplant recipients. *Transplantation* 1986;41:725–729.

Griffith BP, Hardesty RL, Trento A, et al. Heart-lung transplantation: Lessons learned and future hopes. *Ann Thorac Surg*, 1987;43:6–17.

Griffith BP, Hardesty RL, Trento A, Bahnson HT. Asynchronous rejection of heart and lungs following cardiopulmonary transplantation. *Ann Surg* 1985;40:488–493.

Griffith BP, Durham SJ, Hardesty RL, et al. Acute rejection of the heart-lung allograft and methods of its detection. *Transplant Proc* 1987;19:2527–2530.

Hardesty RL, Griffith BP. Autoperfusion of the heart and lungs for preservation during distant procurement. *J Thorac Cardiovasc Surg* 1987;87:11–18.

Haverich A, Scott WC, Aziz S, Jamieson SW. Influence of perfusate flow and volume on preservation of the lungs for transplantation. *Heart Transplant* 1985;4:129.

McGregor CGA, Baldwin JC, Jamieson SW, et al. Isolated pulmonary rejection after combined heart-lung transplantation. *J Thorac Cardiovasc Surg* 1985;90:623–626.

Paradis IL, Marrari M, Zeevi A, et al. HLA phenotype of lung lavage cells following heart-lung transplantation. *Heart Transplant* 1985;4:422–425.

Penkoske PA, Freedom RM, Rowe RD, Trusler GA. The future of heart and heart-lung transplantation in children. *Heart Transplant* 1984;3:233–238.

Starkey TD, Sakakibara N, Hagberg RC, et al. Successful six-hour cardiopulmonary preservation with simple hypothermic crystalloid flush. *Heart Transplant* 1986;5:291–297.

Zeevi A, Fung JJ, Paradis IL, et al. Lymphocytes of bronchoalveolar lavages from heart-lung transplant recipients. *Heart Transplant* 1985;4:417–421.

INDEX

Index